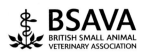

Small Animal
Formulary
8th edition

Editor-in-Chief:

Ian Ramsey BVSc PhD DSAM DipECVIM-CA FHEA MRCVS
School of Veterinary Medicine, University of Glasgow,
Bearsden Road, Bearsden, Glasgow G61 1QH

Published by:
British Small Animal Veterinary Association
Woodrow House, 1 Telford Way, Waterwells Business Park,
Quedgeley, Gloucester GL2 2AB

A Company Limited by Guarantee in England.
Registered Company No. 2837793.
Registered as a Charity.

Copyright © 2014 BSAVA

First edition 1994
Second edition 1997
Third edition 1999
Reprinted with corrections 2000
Fourth edition 2002
Reprinted with corrections 2003
Fifth edition 2005
Reprinted with corrections 2007
Sixth edition 2008
Reprinted with corrections 2009, 2010
Seventh edition 2011
Reprinted with corrections 2012, 2013
Eighth edition 2014
Reprinted with corrections 2015 (twice)

A catalogue record for this book is available from the British Library.

ISBN 978 1 905 319 65 7

The publishers, editors and contributors cannot take responsibility for information
provided on dosages and methods of application of drugs mentioned or referred to
in this publication. Details of this kind must be verified in each case by individual
users from up to date literature published by the manufacturers or suppliers of those
drugs. Veterinary surgeons are reminded that in each case they must follow all
appropriate national legislation and regulations (for example, in the United Kingdom,
the prescribing cascade) from time to time in force.

Printed in India by Imprint Digital
Printed on ECF paper made from sustainable forests.   3320MDC15

Other titles from BSAVA:

Guide to Procedures in Small Animal Practice
Guide to the Use of Veterinary Medicines (available online)
Manual of Canine & Feline Abdominal Imaging
Manual of Canine & Feline Abdominal Surgery
Manual of Canine & Feline Advanced Veterinary Nursing
Manual of Canine & Feline Anaesthesia and Analgesia
Manual of Canine & Feline Behavioural Medicine
Manual of Canine & Feline Cardiorespiratory Medicine
Manual of Canine & Feline Clinical Pathology
Manual of Canine & Feline Dentistry
Manual of Canine & Feline Dermatology
Manual of Canine & Feline Emergency and Critical Care
Manual of Canine & Feline Endocrinology
Manual of Canine & Feline Endoscopy and Endosurgery
Manual of Canine & Feline Gastroenterology
Manual of Canine & Feline Haematology and Transfusion Medicine
Manual of Canine & Feline Head, Neck and Thoracic Surgery
Manual of Canine & Feline Musculoskeletal Disorders
Manual of Canine & Feline Musculoskeletal Imaging
Manual of Canine & Feline Nephrology and Urology
Manual of Canine & Feline Neurology
Manual of Canine & Feline Oncology
Manual of Canine & Feline Ophthalmology
Manual of Canine & Feline Radiography and Radiology
*Manual of Canine & Feline Rehabilitation, Supportive and Palliative
    Care: Case Studies in Patient Management*
Manual of Canine & Feline Reproduction and Neonatology
Manual of Canine & Feline Surgical Principles
Manual of Canine & Feline Thoracic Imaging
Manual of Canine & Feline Ultrasonography
Manual of Canine & Feline Wound Management and Reconstruction
Manual of Exotic Pet and Wildlife Nursing
Manual of Exotic Pets
Manual of Feline Practice
Manual of Ornamental Fish
Manual of Practical Animal Care
Manual of Practical Veterinary Nursing
Manual of Psittacine Birds
Manual of Rabbit Medicine
Manual of Rabbit Surgery, Dentistry and Imaging
Manual of Raptors, Pigeons and Passerine Birds
Manual of Reptiles
Manual of Rodents and Ferrets
Manual of Small Animal Fracture Repair and Management
Manual of Small Animal Practice Management and Development
Manual of Wildlife Casualties

For information on these and all BSAVA publications please visit our
website: www.bsava.com

Contents

Editorial Panel

Daniel S. Mills BVSc PhD CBiol FSBiol FHEA CCAB DipECAWBM(BM) MRCVS
School of Life Sciences, University of Lincoln, Riseholme Park, Lincoln LN2 2LG

Jo Murrell BVSc(Hons) PhD DipECVAA MRCVS
Department of Clinical Veterinary Science, University of Bristol, Langford, Bristol BS40 5DU

Jacques Penderis BVSc MVM PhD CertVR DipECVN MRCVS
School of Veterinary Medicine, University of Glasgow, Bearsden Road, Bearsden, Glasgow G61 1QH

Ian Ramsey BVSC PhD DSAM DipECVIM-CA FHEA MRCVS
School of Veterinary Medicine, University of Glasgow, Bearsden Road, Bearsden, Glasgow G61 1QH

Richard A. Saunders BSc(Hons) BVSc CBiol MSB CertZooMed DZooMed (Mammalian) MRCVS
Veterinary Department, Bristol Zoo Gardens, Clifton, Bristol BS8 3HA

Preface to the eighth edition

Welcome to the 8th edition of the *BSAVA Small Animal Formulary*. Everyone involved in its production hopes you find it a useful resource. There are 12 new drug monographs and there have been many deletions since the last edition as older drugs become unavailable or newer drugs make them obsolete. Most of the remaining monographs have had minor revisions and some have had major changes. The Appendix has been thoroughly revised and some of the information has been moved to the BSAVA website, where it is accessible to BSAVA members.

The labelling of veterinary medicines has also been examined in greater depth than ever before. The law is clear, but not practical, and veterinary surgeons must tread a fine line between compliance and practical solutions. Client Information Leaflets (CILs) are available from the BSAVA for a number of the drugs listed in the Formulary which do not have a marketing authorization for veterinary use in the UK. These leaflets go a long way towards providing practical information in a client-friendly format. However, they are not a substitute for explaining the 'Cascade' system to owners and the details of the particular drugs that have been prescribed.

Drug formularies are progressively evolving works and the latest updates are available on the BSAVA website. The doses provided should always be read in conjunction with the rest of the monograph, which contains important information on the use of the drug. In an ideal world, all the information in this book would be based on peer-reviewed literature. In reality, we rely on the experience of our Editorial Panel to integrate, and often extrapolate from, the variable sources of information.

I would, once again, like to thank the dedication of my colleagues on the Editorial Panel who have examined each monograph for scientific accuracy, relevance and practical application. I am also grateful to the publishing team at Woodrow House for their assistance and patience. I am indebted to the many readers and BSAVA members who have taken time to discuss with me and comment on entries in the Formulary.

Ian Ramsey
January 2014

Foreword

The *BSAVA Small Animal Formulary* continues to be one of the Association's most valued practical resources for veterinary surgeons and is one of our key membership benefits. The availability of the Formulary as an app version for mobile devices has enhanced enormously the rapid accessibility of this fundamental information in a practice setting.

Professor Ian Ramsey and his team are to be congratulated on bringing out this new and updated 8th edition of the Formulary. As with previous editions of the Formulary, a number of new drug monographs have been added, whilst those drugs that are no longer available to the veterinary profession have been removed. The major new addition to this 8th edition of the Formulary is the introduction of examples of immunosuppressive protocols to the Appendix.

In recent years the prescribing of veterinary medicines has continued to have political prominence. In particular, concerns over antimicrobial resistance in human and veterinary medicine have captured attention on a global scale. BSAVA, in collaboration with the Small Animal Medicine Society (SAMSoc), has led the response of small animal practitioners to this debate. The PROTECT poster and accompanying literature (freely available on the BSAVA website) provides practitioners with key facts and strategies to minimize antimicrobial resistance in small animal practice. It is pleasing that the PROTECT concept has been adopted by other UK and international associations in promoting this important message.

Professor Michael J. Day BSc BVMS(Hons) PhD DSc DipECVP FASM
FRCPath FRCVS
BSAVA President 2013–14

Introduction
Notes on the monographs

- **Name**. The rINN generic name is used where this has been agreed. When a choice of names is available the more commonly used in the UK has been provided. The list of trade names is not necessarily comprehensive, and the mention or exclusion of any particular commercial product is not a recommendation or otherwise as to its value. Any omission of a product that is authorized for a particular small animal indication is purely accidental. All monographs were updated in the period July–December 2013. Products that are not authorized for veterinary use by the Veterinary Medicines Directorate are marked with an asterisk. Note that an indication that a product is authorized does not necessarily mean that it is authorized for all species and indications listed in the monograph; users should check individual data sheets. You may also wish to refer to the VMD's Product Information Database (www.vmd.defra.gov.uk/ProductInformationDatabase/).
- **Formulations**. Only medicines and formulations that are available in the UK have been included – many others are available outside the UK and some medicines in different formulations. Common trade names of human medicines are provided. In many cases they are available as generic formulations and may be cheaper. However, be careful of assuming that the bioavailability of one brand is the same as that of another. Avoid switching between brands unnecessarily.
- **Action** and **Use**. Veterinary surgeons using this publication are warned that **many of the drugs and doses listed are not currently authorized** by the Veterinary Medicines Directorate (VMD) or the European Agency for the Evaluation of Medicinal Products (EMEA) (either at all or for a particular species), or manufacturers' recommendations may be limited to particular indications. **The decision, and therefore the responsibility, for prescribing any drug for an animal lies solely with the veterinary surgeon.** Expert assistance should be obtained when necessary. The 'cascade' and its implications are discussed below.
- **Safety and handling.** This section only outlines specific risks and precautions for a particular drug that are in addition to the general advice given below in the 'Health and safety in dispensing' section. A separate Appendix deals with chemotherapeutic drugs.
- **Contraindications and Adverse reactions:** The list of adverse reactions is not intended to be comprehensive and is limited to those effects that may be of clinical significance. The information for both of these sections is taken from published veterinary and human references and not just from product literature.
- **Drug interactions.** A listing of those interactions which may be of clinical significance.
- **Doses.** These are based on those recommended by the manufacturers in their data sheets and package inserts, **or** are

based on those given in published articles or textbooks, **or** are based on clinical experience. These recommendations should be used only as guidelines and should not be considered appropriate for every case. Clinical judgement must take precedence. Where possible, doses have been given for individual species; however, sometimes generalizations are used. 'Small mammals' includes ferrets, lagomorphs and rodents. 'Birds' includes psittacines, raptors, pigeons and others. 'Reptiles' includes chelonians, lizards and snakes. Except where indicated, all doses given for ectothermic animals (reptiles) assume that the animal is kept within its Preferred Optimum Temperature Zone (POTZ). Animals that are maintained at different temperatures may have different rates of metabolism and therefore the dose (and especially the frequency) that is required may require alteration.

Distribution categories

Authorized small animal medicines now fall within the first four categories below and all packaging supplied by drug manufacturers and distributors was changed in 2008. Medical products not authorized for veterinary use retain their former classification (e.g. P, POM). Some nutritional supplements (nutraceuticals) are not considered medicinal products and therefore are not classified. Where a product does not have a marketing authorization it is designated 'general sale'.

AVM-GSL: Authorized veterinary medicine – general sales list (formerly GSL). This may be sold by anyone.

NFA-VPS: Non-food animal medicine – veterinarian, pharmacist, Suitably Qualified Person (SQP) (formerly PML companion animal products and a few P products). These medicines for companion animals must be supplied by a veterinary surgeon, pharmacist or SQP. An SQP has to be registered with the Animal Medicines Training Regulatory Authority (AMTRA). Veterinary nurses can become SQPs but it is not automatic.

POM-VPS: Prescription-only medicine – veterinarian, pharmacist, SQP (formerly PML livestock products, MFSX products and a few P products). These medicines for food-producing animals (including horses) can only be supplied on an oral or written veterinary prescription from a veterinary surgeon, pharmacist or SQP and can only be supplied by one of those groups of people in accordance with the prescription.

POM-V: Prescription-only medicine – veterinarian (formerly POM products and a few P products). These medicines can only be supplied against a veterinary prescription that has been prepared (either orally or in writing) by a veterinary surgeon to animals under their care following a clinical assessment, and can only be supplied by a veterinary surgeon or pharmacist in accordance with the prescription.

Exemptions for Small Pet Animals (ESPA): Schedule 6 of the Veterinary Medicine Regulations 2013 (unofficially known as the Small Animal Exemption Scheme) allows for the use of medicines in certain pet species (aquarium fish, cage birds, ferrets, homing pigeons, rabbits, small rodents and terrarium animals) the active ingredient of which has been declared by the Secretary of State as not requiring veterinary control. These medicines are exempt from the requirement for a marketing authorization and are not therefore required to prove safety, quality or efficacy, but must be manufactured to the same standards as authorized medicines and are subject to pharmacovigilance reporting.

CD: Controlled Drug. A substance controlled by the Misuse of Drugs Act 1971 and Regulations. The CD is followed by (Schedule 1), (Schedule 2), (Schedule 3), (Schedule 4) or (Schedule 5) depending on the Schedule to The Misuse of Drugs Regulations 2001 (as amended) in which the preparation is included. You could be prosecuted for failure to comply with this act. *Prescribers are reminded that there are additional requirements relating to the prescribing of Controlled Drugs. For more information see the* BSAVA Guide to the Use of Veterinary Medicines *at www.bsava.com.*

Schedule 1: Includes LSD, cannabis, lysergide and other drugs that are not used medicinally. Possession and supply are prohibited except in accordance with Home Office Authority.

Schedule 2: Includes etorphine, morphine, papaveretum, pethidine, diamorphine (heroin), cocaine and amphetamine. Record all purchases and each individual supply (within 24 hours). Registers must be kept for 2 calendar years after the last entry. Drugs must be kept under safe custody (locked secure cabinet), except secobarbital. Drugs may not be destroyed except in the presence of a person authorized by the Secretary of State.

Schedule 3: Includes buprenorphine, pentazocine, the barbiturates (e.g. pentobarbital and phenobarbital but not secobarbital – which is Schedule 2) and others. Buprenorphine, diethylpropion and temazepam must be kept under safe custody (locked secure cabinet); it is advisable that all Schedule 3 drugs are locked away. Retention of invoices for 2 years is necessary.

Schedule 4: Includes most of the benzodiazepines (temazepam is now in Schedule 3), and androgenic and anabolic steroids (e.g. clenbuterol). Exempted from control when used in normal veterinary practice.

Schedule 5: Includes preparations (such as several codeine products) which, because of their strength, are exempt from virtually all Controlled Drug requirements other than the retention of invoices for 2 years.

INTRODUCTION

The prescribing cascade

Veterinary medicinal products must be administered in accordance with the prescribing cascade, as set out in the Medicines (Restrictions on the Administration of Veterinary Medicinal Products) Regulations 1994 as amended. These Regulations provide that when no authorized veterinary medicinal product exists for a condition in a particular species, veterinary surgeons exercising their clinical judgement may, in particular to avoid unacceptable suffering, prescribe for one or a small number of animals under their care other suitable medications in accordance with the following sequence:

1   A veterinary medicine authorized for use in another species, or for a different use in the same species ('off-label' use).
2   A medicine authorized in the UK for human use or a veterinary medicine from another country with an import certificate from the Veterinary Medicines Directorate (VMD).
3   A medicine to be made up at the time on a one-off basis by a veterinary surgeon or a properly authorized person.

'Off-label' use of medicines

'Off-label' use is the use of medicines outside the terms of their marketing authorization. It may include medicines authorized outside the UK that are used in accordance with an import certificate issued by the VMD. A veterinary surgeon with detailed knowledge of the medical history and clinical status of a patient, may reasonably prescribe a medicine 'off-label' in accordance with the prescribing cascade. Authorized medicines have been scientifically assessed against statutory criteria of safety, quality and efficacy when used in accordance with the authorized recommendations on the product literature. Use of an unauthorized medicine provides none of these safeguards and may, therefore, pose potential risks that the authorization process seeks to minimize.

Medicines may be used 'off-label' for a variety of reasons including:

*   No authorized product is suitable for the condition or specific subpopulation being treated
*   Need to alter the duration of therapy, dosage, route of administration, etc., to treat the specific condition presented
*   An authorized product has proved ineffective in the circumstances of a particular case (all cases of suspected lack of efficacy of authorized veterinary medicines should be reported to the VMD).

Responsibility for the use of a medicine 'off-label' lies solely with the prescribing veterinary surgeon. He or she should inform the owner of the reason why a medicine is to be used 'off-label' and record this reason in the patient's clinical notes. When electing to use a medicine 'off-label' always:

- Discuss all therapeutic options with the owner
- Use the cascade to determine your choice of medicine
- Obtain signed informed consent if an unauthorized product is to be used, ensuring that all potential problems are explained to the client
- Administer unauthorized medicines against a patient-specific prescription. Do not administer to a group of animals if at all possible.

An 'off-label' medicine must show a comparative clinical advantage to the authorized product in the specific circumstances presented (where applicable). Medicines may be used 'off-label' in the following ways (this is not an exhaustive list):

- Authorized product at an unauthorized dose
- Authorized product for an unauthorized indication
- Authorized product used outwith the authorized age range
- Authorized product administered by an unauthorized route
- Authorized product used to treat an animal in an unauthorized
- physiological state, e.g. pregnancy (i.e. an unauthorized indication)
- Product authorized for use in humans or a different animal species to that being treated.

Adverse effects may or may not be specific for a species, and idiosyncratic reactions are always a possibility. If no adverse effects are listed, consider data from different species. When using novel or unfamiliar drugs, consider pharmaceutical and pharmacological interactions. In some species, and with some diseases, the ability to metabolize/excrete a drug may be impaired/enhanced. Use the lowest dose that might be effective and the safest route of administration. Ensure that you are aware of the clinical signs that may suggest toxicity.

Information on 'off-label' use may be available from a wide variety of sources (see Appendix).

Drug storage and dispensing

For further information on the storage and dispensing of medicines see the *BSAVA Guide to the Use of Veterinary Medicines* available at www.bsava.com. Note the recent change in legislation, which states that veterinary surgeons may only supply a veterinary medicine from practice premises that are registered with the RCVS and that these premises must be inspected. It is recommended that, in general, medications are kept in and dispensed in the manufacturer's original packaging. Medicines can be adversely affected by adverse temperatures, excessive light, humidity and rough handling. Loose tablets or capsules that are repackaged from bulk containers should be dispensed in child-resistant containers and supplied with a package insert (if one exists). Tablets and capsules in foil strips should be sold in their original packaging or in a similar cardboard box for smaller quantities. Preparations for external application should be dispensed in coloured fluted bottles. Oral liquids should be dispensed in plain glass bottles with child-resistant closures.

All medicines should be labelled. The label should include:

- The owner's name and address
- Indentification of the animal
- Date (and, if applicable, the expiry date)
- Product name (and strength)
- Total quantity of the product supplied in the container
- Instructions for dosage
- Practice name and address
- The name of the veterinary surgeon who prescribed the medication (if not an authorized use)
- Any specific pharmacy precautions (including storage, disposal, handling)
- The wording 'Keep out of reach of children' and 'For animal treatment only'
- Any other necessary warnings.

The words 'For external use only' should be included on labels for products for topical use. All labels should be typed. If this information cannot be fitted on a single label then it is permissible to include the information on a separate sheet.

For medicines that are not authorized for veterinary use, and even for some that are, it is useful to add to the label or on a separate sheet the likely adverse effects, drug interactions and the action to be taken in the event of inadvertent mis-dosing or incorrect administration written in plain English. Samples of such Client Information Leaflets (shown as **CIL** in the monographs) for many commonly used, but unauthorized, drugs are available for BSAVA members to download from www.bsava.com.

In order to comply with the current Veterinary Medicines Regulations, records of all products supplied on prescription must be kept for 5 years. When a batch is brought into use in a practice, the batch number and date should be recorded. It is not necessary to record the batch number of each medication used for a given animal.

Health and safety in dispensing

All drugs are potentially poisonous to humans as well as animals. Toxicity may be mild or sever e and includes carcinogenic and teratogenic effects. Warnings are given in the monographs. However, risks to humans dispensing medicines are not always well characterized and idiosyncratic reactions may occur. **It is good practice for everyone to wear protective clothing (including gloves) when directly handling medicines, not to eat or drink (or store food or drink) near medicines**, and to wash their hands frequently when working with medicines. Gloves, masks and safety glasses should be worn if handling potentially toxic liquids, powders or broken tablets. Do not break tablets of antineoplastic cytotoxic drugs and use laminar flow cabinets for the preparation and dispensing of these medications. See Appendix for more information.

Many prescribers and users of medicines are not aware of the carcinogenic potential of the drugs they are handling. Below are lists of medicines included in the *BSAVA Formulary* that are known or potential carcinogens or teratogens. The lists are not all-inclusive: they include only those substances that have been evaluated. Most of the drugs are connected only with certain kinds of cancer. The relative carcinogenicity of the agents varies considerably and some do not cause cancer at all times or under all circumstances. Some may only be carcinogenic or teratogenic if a person is exposed in a certain way (for example, ingesting as opposed to touching the drug). For more detailed information refer to the International Agency for Research on Cancer (IARC) or the National Toxicology Program (NTP) (information is available on their respective websites).

Examples of drugs known or suspected to be human carcinogens (c) or teratogens (t):

- ACE inhibitors (t), e.g. benazepril, enalapril, ramipril
- Androgenic (anabolic) steroids (t, c)
- Antibiotics (c), e.g. metronidazole, chloramphenicol
- Antibiotics (t) e.g. aminoglycosides, doxycycline, trimethoprim, sulphonamides
- Antifungals (c), e.g. fluconazole, itraconazole, flucytosine
- Antineoplastic drugs (c, t) – all
- Antithyroid drugs (t), e.g. carbimazole/methimazole
- Beta-blockers (t)
- Dantron (c)
- Deferoxamine (t)
- Diltiazem (t)
- Finasteride (t)
- Immunosuppressives (c), e.g. azathioprine, ciclosporin
- Lithium (t)
- Methotrexate (t)
- Misoprostol (t)
- NSAIDs (t)
- Penicillamine (t)
- Phenoxybenzamine (c)
- Progesterone (c) and some oestrogens (c)
- Vitamin A (t)

Note that most carcinogens are also likely to be teratogens.

Acepromazine (ACP)
(ACP) POM-V

Formulations: Injectable: 2 mg/ml solution. Oral: 10 mg, 25 mg tablets.

Action: Phenothiazine with depressant effect on the CNS, thereby causing sedation and a reduction in spontaneous activity.

Use: Sedation or pre-anaesthetic medication in dogs, cats, small mammals and other exotic species. ACP raises the threshold for cardiac arrhythmias and has antiemetic properties. Sedation is unreliable when ACP is used alone; combining ACP with an opioid drug improves sedation (neuroleptanalgesia) and the opioid provides analgesia. The depth of sedation is dose-dependent up to a plateau (0.1 mg/kg). Increasing the dose above 0.1 mg/kg does little to improve the predictability of achieving adequate sedation but increases the risk of incurring adverse effects, the severity of adverse effects and the duration of action of any effects (desirable or adverse) that arise. The lower end of the dose range should be used for giant-breed dogs to allow for the effects of metabolic body size. Onset of sedation is 20–30 min after i.m. administration; clinical doses cause sedation for up to 6 hours. The oral dose of ACP tablets required to produce sedation varies between individual animals and high doses can lead to very prolonged sedation. Also used for the management of thromboembolism in cats because of its peripheral vasodilatory action. The use of ACP in the management of sound phobias in dogs, such as firework or thunder phobia, is not recommended by behaviourists.

Safety and handling: Normal precautions should be observed.

Contraindications: Hypotension due to shock, trauma or cardiovascular disease. Avoid in animals <3 months and animals with liver disease. In Boxers spontaneous fainting and syncope can occur due to sinoatrial block caused by excessive vagal tone; use low doses or avoid. Lowers the seizure threshold in susceptible strains of gerbil.

Adverse reactions: Rarely, healthy animals may develop profound hypotension following administration of phenothiazines. Supportive therapy to maintain body temperature and fluid balance is indicated until the animal is fully recovered. Can lead to seizures in gerbils.

Drug interactions: Other CNS depressant agents (e.g. barbiturates, propofol, alfaxalone, volatile anaesthetics) will cause additive CNS depression if used with ACP. Doses of other anaesthetic drugs should be reduced when ACP has been used for premedication. Quinidine given with phenothiazines may cause additional cardiac depression. Increased levels of both drugs may result if propranolol is administered with phenothiazines. As phenothiazines block alpha-adrenergic receptors, concomitant use with adrenaline may lead to unopposed beta activity, thereby causing vasodilation and tachycardia. Antidiarrhoeal mixtures (e.g. kaolin/pectin, bismuth salicylate) and antacids may cause reduced GI absorption of oral phenothiazines.

A B C D E F G H I J K L M N O P Q R S T U V W X Y Z

2 BSAVA Small Animal Formulary 8th edition

DOSES

When used for sedation is generally given as part of a combination. See Appendix for sedation protocols in all species.

Dogs (not Boxers), Cats: 0.01–0.02 mg/kg slowly i.v.; 0.01–0.05 mg/kg i.m., s.c.; 1–3 mg/kg p.o. Boxers: 0.005–0.01 mg/kg i.m. or avoid (when given alone).

Small mammals: Ferrets: 0.2–0.5 mg/kg i.m., s.c., p.o.; Rabbits: 0.1–1.0 mg/kg i.m., s.c.; Guinea pigs: 2.5–5 mg/kg i.m., s.c., p.o.; Hamsters: 5 mg/kg i.m., s.c., p.o.; Gerbils: 3 mg/kg i.m., s.c., p.o.; Rats: 2.5 mg/kg i.m., s.c., p.o.; Mice: 1–5 mg/kg i.m., s.c., p.o.

Birds: Not recommended.

Reptiles: 0.1–0.5 mg/kg i.m.

Acetaminophen see Paracetamol

Acetazolamide

(Diamox*, Diamox SR*) **POM**

Formulations: Injectable: 500 mg vial (powder for reconstitution). Oral: 250 mg tablets, capsules.

Action: Systemic carbonic anhydrase inhibitor.

Use: Treatment of acute and chronic glaucoma in dogs, though topical carbonic anhydrase inhibitors and prostaglandin analogues are preferred. Concurrent use of a topical and a systemic carbonic anhydrase inhibitor is not beneficial as there is no additional decrease in intraocular pressure compared with the sole use of either route. Used as treatment for the management of episodic falling in the Cavalier King Charles Spaniel experiencing a high frequency of collapse episodes which are refractory to other treatments (clonazepam and diazepam). If there is no favourable response after two weeks on q12h dose then the drug should be stopped.

Safety and handling: Normal precautions should be observed.

Contraindications: Avoid in anorexic dogs, those with hepatic or renal dysfunction and those with sulphonamide hypersensitivity. Cats are particularly susceptible to the adverse effects of systemic carbonic anhydrase inhibitors; avoid in this species.

Adverse reactions: Weakness, GI disturbances (anorexia, vomiting, diarrhoea), panting, metabolic acidosis, diuresis, electrolyte disturbances in particular potassium depletion.

Drug interactions: Acetazolamide alkalinizes urine; thus, excretion rate of weak bases may be decreased but weak acid excretion increased. Concomitant use of corticosteroids may exacerbate potassium depletion, causing hypokalaemia.

DOSES

Dogs: Glaucoma: 5–10 mg/kg i.v. single dose, 4–8 mg/kg p.o. q8–12h.
CKCS episodic falling syndrome: 31.5 mg/dog p.o. q24h for 2 weeks,
if no response then try same dose at q12h.
Cats: Do not use.
Small mammals, Birds, Reptiles: No information available.

Acetylcysteine
(Ilube*, Parvolex*) **POM**

Formulations: Injectable: 200 mg/ml solution. Topical: 5%
ophthalmic solution in combination with 0.35% hypromellose
ophthalmic drops in 10 ml bottle.

Action: Decreases the viscosity of bronchial secretions, maintains
glutathione levels in the liver and has some anticollagenase activity.

Use: Reduces the extent of liver injury in cases of paracetamol
poisoning and can also be used as a mucolytic in respiratory disease.
Oral solution should be diluted to a 5% solution and given via a
stomach tube as it tastes unpleasant. Acetylcysteine may be useful in
the treatment of keratoconjunctivitis sicca (KCS) (dry eye), or in
'melting' corneal ulcers although there is limited *in vivo* work to
confirm this. In the eye it may be used in conjunction with
hypromellose. In rabbits direct application into the ear has been
reported as beneficial in cases of secretory otitis media, reducing
inflammation and preventing long-term fibrotic changes.

Safety and handling: Normal precautions should be observed.

Contraindications: No information available.

Adverse reactions: Acetylcysteine has caused hypersensitivity and
bronchospasm when used in the pulmonary tree. When given orally
for paracetamol poisoning it may cause GI effects (nausea, vomiting)
and, rarely, urticaria.

Drug interactions: In cases of paracetamol poisoning the
concurrent administration of activated charcoal is controversial as it
may also reduce acetylcysteine absorption.

DOSES

Dogs, Cats:
- Mucolytic: Either nebulize 50 mg as a 2% (dilute with saline)
  solution over 30–60 min or instil directly into the trachea 1–2 ml
  of a 20% solution.
- Paracetamol poisoning: After inducing emesis give 140–280 mg/
  kg diluted in 12–25 ml/kg of 5% dextrose i.v. by slow infusion over
  6 hours, followed by further slow infusions of 70 mg/kg (similarly
  diluted) every 6 hours for at least 7 doses, depending on dose of
  paracetamol consumed (seek advice from a poisons information
  service). The intravenous solution can be administered orally but
  should be diluted to improve palability and lessen pungent aroma.

- KCS: 1 drop of the ophthalmic solution topically to the eye q6–8h. Rarely used now for this indication.
- Melting corneal ulcers: 1 drop of the ophthalmic solution q1–4h in the affected eye for 24–48 hours. Topical autologous serum is more effective for the treatment of a melting corneal ulcer and is preferred.

Small mammals: Ferrets, Rabbits, Rodents: Mucolytic: nebulize 50 mg as a 2% (dilute with saline) solution over 30–60 min; Otic lavage: 1–2 ml of a 20% solution.
Birds: Mucolytic: as for rabbits (2–5 drops in 15 ml saline for nebulization).
Reptiles: Mucolytic: 2% solution (dilute with saline) nebulized for 15 min.

Acetylsalicyclic acid see Aspirin

Aciclovir
(Aciclovir, Zovirax*) **POM**

Formulations: Ophthalmic: 3% ointment in 4.5 g tubes. Oral: 200 mg, 800 mg tablets; 200 mg/5 ml and 400 mg/5 ml suspension. Injectable: 250 mg, 500 mg vials for reconstitution. Skin: 5% ointment in 10 g, 25 g tubes.

Action: Inhibits viral replication (viral DNA polymerase); depends on viral thymidine kinase for phosphorylation.

Use: Management of ocular feline herpesvirus-1 (FHV-1) infections. *In vitro* studies show that aciclovir is ineffective against FHV-1 but suggest that the combination of aciclovir and recombinant human interferon may be effective; *in vivo* efficacy of the combination is not known. The clinical efficacy of aciclovir on its own is questionable but frequent application (5 times daily) may achieve corneal concentrations. Aciclovir is virostatic and is unable to eradicate latent viral infection. In refractory and severe cases of FHV-1 ulceration, combined therapy including topical antiviral medication, oral interferon and lysine, can be used. Also used to treat herpesvirus infections of other species (e.g. Pacheco's disease in psittacid birds).

Safety and handling: Normal precautions should be observed.

Contraindications: No information available.

Adverse reactions: Ocular irritation may occur and the frequency of application should be reduced if this develops. Treatment should not be continued for >3 weeks. May cause vomiting in birds.

Drug interactions: No information available.

DOSES
Dogs: Not applicable.

Cats: Apply a small amount to affected eye q4–6h for a maximum of 3 weeks (5 times daily more effective than three times daily).
Small mammals: No information available.
Birds: Raptors: 330 mg/kg p.o. q12h for 7–14 days; Psittacids: 80 mg/kg p.o., i.v., i.m. q8h or 240 mg/kg in food in aviaries.
Reptiles: 80 mg/kg p.o. q8–24h; topically to oral lesions q8–24h. There is a suggestion that q8h dosing is more successful than q24h dosing.

ACP see **Acepromazine**
ACTH see **Tetracosactide**
Actinomycin-D see **Dactinomycin**
Activated charcoal see **Charcoal**
ADH see **vasopressin**

Adrenaline (Epinephrine)
(Adrenaline*, Epinephrine*) **POM**

Formulations: Injectable: Range of concentrations for injection: 0.1–10 mg/ml, equivalent to 1:10,000 to 1:100.

Action: Adrenaline exerts its effects via alpha-1, -2 and beta-1 and -2 adrenoreceptors.

Use: Cardiac resuscitation, status asthmaticus and to offset the effects of histamine release in severe anaphylactoid reactions. The ophthalmic preparation is used in open angle glaucoma. The effects of adrenaline vary according to dose. Infusions of low doses mainly result in beta-adrenergic effects (increases in cardiac output, myocardial oxygen consumption, and a reduced threshold for arrhythmias with peripheral vasodilation and a fall in diastolic blood pressure). At high doses alpha-1 effects predominate, causing a rise in systemic vascular resistance, diverting blood to the central organs; however, this may improve cardiac output and blood flow. Adrenaline is not a substitute for fluid replacement therapy. Respiratory effects include bronchodilation and an increase in pulmonary vascular resistance. Renal blood flow is moderately decreased. The duration of action of adrenaline is short (2–5 min). Beware of using in animals with diabetes mellitus (monitor blood glucose concentration), hypertension or hyperthyroidism. Use with caution in hypovolaemic animals. Overdosage can be fatal so check dose, particularly in small patients. Intracardiac injection is not recommended.

Safety and handling: Do not confuse adrenaline vials of different concentrations. Adrenaline is sensitive to light and air: do not use if it is pink, brown or contains a precipitate. It is unstable in 5% dextrose.

Contraindications: The use of human adrenaline pen injections is not recommended for the treatment of suspected anaphylaxis. The doses in such pens are usually too small to be effective in most normal animals and by the time the dog has collapsed would be unlikely to have any effect on outcome. If such pen injections are administered by owners, then, in common with medical practice, patients must be carefully monitored for at least 6 hours.

Adverse reactions: Increases myocardial oxygen demand and produces arrhythmias including ventricular fibrillation. These may be ameliorated by administering oxygen and slowing the heart rate with beta-2 antagonists. Other adverse effects include tachycardia, arrhythmias, dry mouth and cold extremities. Repeated injections can cause necrosis at the injection site.

Drug interactions: Toxicity may occur if used with other sympathomimetic amines because of additive effects. The effects of adrenaline may be potentiated by antihistamines and thyroxine. Propranolol may block the beta effects of adrenaline, thus facilitating an increase in blood pressure. Alpha blocking agents or diuretics may negate or diminish the pressor effects. When adrenaline is used with drugs that sensitize the myocardium (e.g. halothane, high doses of digoxin) monitor for signs of arrhythmias. Hypertension may result if adrenaline is used with oxytocic agents.

DOSES
Dogs: 20 µg (micrograms)/kg of a 1:1000 solution (1000 µg/ml) diluted to 5–10 ml in normal saline and given i.v. or intraosseously. Can be given intratracheally for resuscitation of intubated animals, but higher doses may be required. A long catheter should be used to ensure the drug is delivered into the bronchi beyond the end of the endotracheal tube. For dogs <10 kg use a 1:10,000 solution. Use lower doses for the management of bronchoconstriction. The i.v. route is preferred if hypotension accompanies an anaphylactoid reaction. In cardiac resuscitation, repeated and/or higher doses (up to 100 µg/kg) may be required at intervals of 2–5 min.
Cats: 20 µg (micrograms)/kg of a 1:10,000 solution (100 µg/ml) i.v., intraosseous, intratracheal. In cardiac resuscitation, repeated and/or higher doses (up to 100 µg/kg) may be required at intervals of 2–5 min.
Small mammals: Ferrets: 20 µg (micrograms)/kg s.c., i.m., i.v., intratracheal; Rabbits: cardiac resuscitation: 100 µg (micrograms)/kg i.v., repeated and/or higher doses (up to 200 µg/kg) may be required at intervals of 2–5 min; Guinea pigs: 3 µg (micrograms)/kg i.v.; Other rodents: 10 µg (micrograms)/kg i.v. as required.
Birds: 0.1–1.0 mg/kg i.v., intraosseous, intracardiac, intratracheal.
Reptiles: 0.5 mg/kg i.v., intraosseous, 1 mg/kg intratracheally diluted in 1 ml/100 g body weight.

Aglepristone
(Alizin) **POM-V**

Formulations: Injectable: 30 mg/ml solution.

Action: Progesterone receptor blockage leads to reduced progesterone support for pregnancy.

Use: Termination of pregnancy in bitches up to 45 days and in queens up to 35 days after mating. In bitches confirmed as pregnant, a partial abortion may occur in up to 5%; owners should be warned. A clinical examination (uterine palpation) is always recommended 10 days after treatment and at least 30 days after mating in order to confirm termination. After induced abortion an early return to oestrus is frequently observed (the oestrus-to-oestrus interval may be shortened by 1–3 months). Can also be used for the treatment of pyometra in dogs, although recurrence is fairly common. Bitches will usually be able to carry subsequent pregnancies successfully. May also be used to induce parturition and to treat progesterone-induced acromegaly in dogs. In cats can be used to treat progesterone-induced fibroadenomatous mammary hyperplasia.

Safety and handling: Use with care. Accidental injection may be a hazard to women who are pregnant or intending to become pregnant.

Contraindications: Consider avoiding in dogs with diagnosed or suspected hypoadrenocorticism or diabetes mellitus.

Adverse reactions: Transient pain at the injection site; any local inflammation produced resolves uneventfully. In bitches/queens treated beyond the 20th day of gestation, abortion may be accompanied by the physiological signs of parturition, i.e. fetal expulsion, anorexia, mammary congestion.

Drug interactions: Aglepristone binds to glucocorticoid receptors and may therefore interfere with the actions of glucocorticoids; however, the clinical significance of this is unclear.

DOSES
Dogs: Maximum of 5 ml injected at any one site.
- Pregnancy termination: 10 mg/kg s.c. q24h for two doses.
- Acromegaly: 10 mg/kg s.c. q24h for two doses and then q7d for 3 more doses.
- Pyometra: 10 mg/kg s.c. on days 1, 2 and 7. Additional doses may be given on days 14 and 21 if there is an inadequate response.

Cats: Maximum of 5 ml injected at any one site.
- Pregnancy termination: 15 mg/kg s.c. q24h for two doses.
- Fibroadenomatous hyperplasia: 20 mg/kg s.c. q7d (also consider atenolol if cat is tachycardic with heart rate >200 bpm).
- Pyometra: 15 mg/kg s.c. on days 1, 2 and 7. Additional doses may be given on days 14 and 21 if there is an inadequate response.

Small mammals: Rabbits: pregnancy termination: 10 mg/kg on days 6 and 7 post implantation; Guinea pigs: pyometra/metritis: 10 mg/kg on days 1, 2 and 8.
Birds, Reptiles: No information available.

Aledronate see Clodronate

A

Alfaxalone
(Alfaxan) **POM-V**

B
C
D
E
F
G
H
I
J
K
L
M

Formulations: Injectable: 10 mg/ml solution; the alfaxalone is solubilized in a cyclodextrin.

Action: Anaesthesia induced by the CNS depressant effect of the alfaxalone.

Use: Induction agent used before inhalational anaesthesia, or as a sole anaesthetic agent for examination or surgical procedures. As with all i.v. anaesthetic drugs, premedication will reduce the dose required for induction and maintenance of anaesthesia. The drug should be given slowly and to effect in order to prevent inadvertent overdose. The dose recommended by the manufacturer for induction of anaesthesia can usually be reduced in all animals. Analgesia is insufficient for surgery: other analgesic drugs such as opioids should be incorporated into the anaesthetic protocol. Alfaxalone is shorter acting and causes less excitement during recovery than the alfaxalone/alfadalone combination previously available. The cyclodextrin carrier does not cause histamine release in dogs (cf. the cremaphor EL of the combination). Alfaxalone can be given i.m. or s.c. to provide sedation in cats and dogs although it is not licensed for these routes. Do not use in combination with other i.v. anaesthetic agents. Although not licensed for animals <12 weeks of age, safety in dogs between 6 and 12 weeks old has been demonstrated using a similar dose for induction of anaesthesia as adult dogs.

N
O

Safety and handling: Does not contain an antimicrobial preservative; thus it is recommended that the remainder of an opened bottle is discarded after single use.

P

Contraindications: No information available.

Q
R
S

Adverse reactions: A slight increase in heart rate can occur immediately after i.v. injection as a compensatory response to maintain blood pressure in the face of mild hypotension. This effect can be minimized by slow i.v. injection. As with all anaesthetic drugs, respiratory depression can occur with overdoses.

T

Drug interactions: No information available.

DOSES
See Appendix for sedation protocols in all species.
Dogs:

U
V
W
X
Y
Z

- Induction of anaesthesia: 3 mg/kg i.v. in unpremedicated dogs; 2 mg/kg i.v. in premedicated dogs, although commonly lower doses can be used.
- Maintenance: 6–9 mg/kg/h is recommended as a continuous rate infusion or top-up boluses of 1–1.5 mg/kg q10min.

Cats:
- Induction of anaesthesia: 2–5 mg/kg i.v.; the lower end of the dose range is often adequate.
- Maintenance: 7–10 mg/kg/h is recommended as a continuous rate infusion or top-up boluses of 1–1.5 mg/kg q10min.

Small mammals: Unpremedicated: Ferrets: 9–12 mg (0.5–0.75 ml)/kg i.v., i.m.; Rabbits: 1–3 mg/kg i.v. or 3 mg/kg i.m.; Guinea pigs: 40 mg/kg i.m. or i.p.; Other rodents: 20 mg/kg i.m. or 120 mg/kg i.p.; Rabbits: 5 mg/kg i.m. following premedication with medetomidine at 0.25 mg/kg s.c.
Birds: For large birds and those with a dive response: 2–4 mg/kg i.v. to effect.
Reptiles: 2–4 mg/kg i.v. or intraosseously for induction; Chelonians: has been used at 10–20 mg/kg intracoelomically; Green iguanas: 10 mg/kg i.m. (light sedation) up to 30 mg/kg i.m. for surgical anaesthesia.

Alfentanil
(Rapifen*) **POM CD SCHEDULE 2**

Formulations: Injectable: 0.5 mg/ml solution, available in 2 ml or 10 ml vials; 5 mg/ml solution.

Action: Pure mu agonist of the phenylpiperidine series.

Use: Very potent opioid analgesic (10–20 times more potent than morphine) used to provide intraoperative analgesia during anaesthesia in dogs and cats. Use of such potent opioids during anaesthesia contributes to a balanced anaesthesia technique but they must be administered accurately. It has a rapid onset (15–30 seconds) and short duration of action. It is best given using continuous rate infusions. The drug is not suited to provision of analgesia in the postoperative period.

Safety and handling: Normal precautions should be observed.

Contraindications: No information available.

Adverse reactions: A reduction in heart rate is likely whenever alfentanil is given; atropine can be administered to counter bradycardia if necessary. Respiratory depression leading to cessation of spontaneous respiration is likely following administration. Do not use unless facilities for positive pressure ventilation are available (either manual or automatic). Rapid i.v. injection can cause a severe bradycardia, even asystole. In rabbits seizures have been noted with the use of alfentanil as part of a midazolam, medetomidine and alfentanil combination.

Drug interactions: Alfentanil reduces the dose requirements of concurrently administered anaesthetics, including inhaled anaesthetics, by at least 50%. In humans it is currently recommended to avoid giving alfentanil to patients receiving monoamine oxidase inhibitors due to the risk of serotonin toxicity.

DOSES
Dogs: 0.001–0.005 mg/kg i.v. as a single bolus or 0.001–0.0025 mg/kg/min continuous rate infusion.

Cats: 0.001 mg/kg i.v. as a single bolus or 0.001 mg/kg/min continuous rate infusion.

Small mammals: Rabbits: 0.03–0.07 mg/kg i.v.; Rodents: no information available.

Birds, Reptiles: No information available.

Allopurinol   `CIL`
(Zyloric*) **POM**

Formulations: Oral: 100 mg, 300 mg tablets.

Action: Xanthine oxidase inhibition decreases formation of uric acid by blocking the conversion of hypoxanthine to xanthine, and of xanthine to uric acid.

Use: In dogs, the treatment and prevention of recurrent uric acid uroliths and hyperuricosuric calcium oxalate urolithiasis and, in combination with meglumine antimonite or miltefosine, to treat leishmaniosis. Use with caution in patients with impaired renal function. May predispose to xanthine urolithiasis especially if used for several months and not fed a purine restricted diet. In birds, the dosage should be reduced as plasma uric acid levels decrease.

Safety and handling: Normal precautions should be observed.

Contraindications: No information available.

Adverse reactions: In humans, allopurinol may enhance the effects of azathioprine and theophylline.

Drug interactions: No information available.

DOSES
Dogs:
- Uric acid urolithiasis: 10 mg/kg p.o. q8h for 1 month, then 10–15 mg/kg p.o. q12h.
- Leishmaniosis: 10 mg/kg p.o. q12h for 6–12 months with meglumine antimonate for 1–2 months, or miltefosine for 1 month (note that this does not result in complete parasitological cure).

Cats, Small mammals: No information available.

Birds: 10–30 mg/kg p.o. q12h (all species); Pigeons: 830 mg/l drinking water; Psittacids: 10 mg/30 ml drinking water.

Reptiles: 10–20 mg/kg p.o. q24h (most species); Chelonians: 50 mg/kg p.o. q24h for 30 days then q72h.

Alphaxalone see Alfaxalone

Alprazolam

(Alprazolam*, Xanax*) **POM**

Formulations: Oral: 0.25 mg, 0.5 mg, 1 mg, 2 mg tablets.

Action: Increases GABA activity within the CNS, resulting in anxiolysis and a range of cognitive effects including the inhibition of memory.

Use: Treatment of anxiety and fear-related disorders in dogs and cats, especially where there are signs of panic. Best if used approximately 30 minutes before a fear-inducing event. Its short half-life and rapid onset of action make it useful for the management of acute episodes, with treatment given as needed within the dosing limits described. In addition, its anterograde and retrograde amnesic properties, especially on subjective memory, mean it can be used before, during or immediately following an aversive experience to minimize the emotional impact of such exposure. This may be necessary during a long-term behavioural therapy programme to avoid relapses due to exposure to an intense fear-inducing stimulus during treatment. In experimental circumstances, single higher range doses (>0.25 mg/kg) have been found to block memory significantly and may be useful in companion animals, but may result in temporary sedation. Alprazolam may be used as an adjunct to clomipramine for the management of phobic responses. It can also be used for the management of urine spraying in cats but a high relapse rate upon withdrawal should be expected.

Safety and handling: Normal precautions should be observed.

Contraindications: Hypersensitivity to benzodiazepines, glaucoma, significant liver or kidney disease, though appears to be less hepatotoxic than diazepam or clorazepate. Not recommended in pregnant or lactating animals.

Adverse reactions: Drowsiness and mild transient incoordination may develop. A general concern with benzodiazepines concerns disinhibition and the subsequent emergence of aggression.

Drug interactions: Caution is advised if used in association with antifungals such as itraconazole, which inhibit its metabolism.

DOSES

Dogs: 0.01–0.1 mg/kg p.o. as needed up to 4 times a day.
Cats: 0.125–0.25 mg/kg p.o. as needed up to twice a day.
Small mammals, Birds, Reptiles: No information available.

A

Aluminium antacids (Aluminium hydroxide)

(Alucap*. With alginate: Acidex*, Gastrocote*, Gaviscon Advance*, Peptac*. With magnesium salt: Asilone*, Maalox*, Mucogel*) **P, GSL**

Formulations: Oral: Aluminium hydroxide is available as a dried gel. Other products are composite preparations containing a variety of other compounds including magnesium oxide, hydroxide or trisilicate, potassium bicarbonate, sodium carbonate and bicarbonate, alginates and dimeticone. Aluminium hydroxide content varies.

Action: Neutralizes gastric hydrochloric acid. May also bind bile acids and pepsin and stimulate local prostaglandin (PGE-1) production. Also binds inorganic phosphate (PO_4^{3-}) in the GI tract, making it unavailable for absorption.

Use: Management of gastritis and gastric ulceration. In renal failure, to lower serum phosphate levels in cats and dogs with hyperphosphataemia. Frequent administration is necessary to prevent rebound acid secretion. Phosphate-binding agents are usually only used if low-phosphate diets are unsuccessful. Monitor serum phosphate levels at 10–14 day intervals and adjust dosage accordingly if trying to normalize serum concentrations. Thoroughly mix the drug with food to disperse it throughout the GI tract and to increase its palatability.

Safety and handling: Long-term use (many years) of oral aluminium products in humans has been associated with aluminium toxicity and possible neurotoxicity. This is unlikely to be a problem in veterinary medicine.

Contraindications: No information available.

Adverse reactions: Constipation may occur. This is an effect of the aluminium compound and is counteracted by inclusion of a magnesium salt.

Drug interactions: Do not administer digoxin, tetracycline or fluoroquinolone products orally within 2 hours of aluminium salts as their absorption may be impaired.

DOSES

Dogs, Cats: Initially 10–30 mg/kg p.o. q6–8h (tablets) or 0.5–1.0 ml/kg (2–30 ml) p.o. q6–8h (gel) with or immediately after meals. Dosages are empirical; none have been properly defined in dogs or cats.
Small mammals: Rabbits: 30–60 mg/kg p.o. q8–12h; Rodents: 20–40 mg/animal p.o prn.
Birds: No information available.
Reptiles: 100 mg/kg p.o. q24h.

Aluminium hydroxide see **Aluminium antacids**

Amantadine
(Lysovir*, Symmetrel*) **POM**

Formulations: Oral: 100 mg capsule; 10 mg/ml syrup.

Action: Provides analgesia through NMDA antagonist action which may potentiate the effects of other analgesics.

Use: Adjunctive analgesic in animals that are unresponsive to opioids, or that require chronic pain relief in a home environment (e.g. osteoarthritis or cancer pain). In dogs with osteoarthritis that were refractory to an NSAID physical activity was improved, suggesting that amantadine might be a useful adjunct in the clinical management of canine osteoarthritic pain.

Safety and handling: Normal precautions should be observed.

Contraindications: No information available.

Adverse reactions: In humans minor GI and CNS effects have been reported, although these have not been reported in animals.

Drug interactions: No information available.

DOSES
Dogs: 3.0–5.0 mg/kg q24h.
Cats: 1.0–4.0 mg/kg q24h; start at the lowest dose and increase slowly. This dose recommendation is anecdotal and is not based on evidence from clinical research.
Small mammals: Ferrets: 3–5 mg/kg (anecdotal).
Birds, Reptiles: No information available.

Amethocaine see **Tetracaine**

Amikacin
(Amikacin*, Amikin*) **POM**

Formulations: Injectable: 50 mg/ml, 250 mg/ml solutions.

Action: Aminoglycosides inhibit bacterial protein synthesis. They are bactericidal and their mechanism of killing is concentration-dependent, leading to a marked post-antibiotic effect, allowing prolonged dosing intervals (which may reduce toxicity).

Use: Active against many Gram-negative bacteria, *Staphlococcus aureus* and *Nocardia* spp., including some that may be resistant to gentamicin. Streptococci and anaerobes are usually resistant. Its use is only indicated after sensitivity testing has been performed and the organism shown to be resistant to other aminoglycosides such as gentamicin. Activity at low oxygen sites may be limited. Movement across biological membranes may also be limited, hence systemic levels require parenteral administration, and access to sites such as the CNS and ocular fluids is very limited. Monitoring serum amikacin levels should be considered to ensure therapeutic levels and minimize toxicity, particularly in neonates, geriatric patients and those with reduced renal function. Monitoring renal function is also advisable during treatment of any animal. Intravenous doses should be given slowly, generally over 30–60 min. Concurrent fluid therapy is advised.

Safety and handling: Normal precautions should be observed.

Contraindications: If possible avoid use in animals with reduced renal function.

Adverse reactions: Nephrotoxic and ototoxic. Oral doses can cause fatal enterotoxaemia in rabbits. Use with caution in birds, as it is toxic.

Drug interactions: Synergism may occur *in vivo* when aminoglycosides are combined with beta-lactam antimicrobials. Avoid the concurrent use of other nephrotoxic, ototoxic or neurotoxic agents (e.g. amphotericin B, furosemide). Aminoglycosides may be inactivated *in vitro* by beta-lactam antibiotics (e.g. penicillins, cephalosporins) or heparin; do not give these drugs in the same syringe. Can potentiate neuromuscular blockade so avoid use in combination with neuromuscular blocking agents.

DOSES
See Appendix for guidelines on responsible antibacterial use.
Dogs: 15–30 mg/kg i.v, i.m., s.c. q24h.
Cats: 10–15 mg/kg i.v, i.m., s.c. q24h.
Dogs, Cats: For both dogs and cats, higher doses are recommended by some authors for managing sepsis, although there is an increased risk of adverse effects with such high doses.
Small mammals: Ferrets: 8–16 mg/kg i.v., i.m., s.c. q8–24h; Rabbits: 2–10 mg/kg i.v., i.m., s.c. q8–12h; Rodents: 5–15 mg/kg i.v., i.m., s.c. q8–12h. Concurrent fluid therapy advised, especially if hydration status poor or uncertain.
Birds: 10–20 mg/kg i.m., s.c., i.v. q8–12h.
Reptiles: 5 mg/kg i.m. once, then 2.5 mg/kg i.m. q72h at 25°C. Concurrent fluid therapy is advised due to nephrotoxicity.

Amiloride
(Amiloride Hydrochloride*) **POM**

Formulations: Oral: 5 mg tablets; 1 mg/ml solution. Also present in compound preparations with hydrochlorothiazide (Moduret, Moduretic) and furosemide (Frumil, Lasoride).

Action: Potassium-sparing diuretic which inhibits sodium absorption in the distal tubule and collecting duct. This leads to a failure of the normal renal concentration gradient. It is a weak diuretic when used alone, so is almost always used in combination with a thiazide or furosemide.

Use: Oedema or ascites due to liver or heart failure. Often added to more potent diuretics such as furosemide in cases of refractory heart failure. Doses have not been widely reported in the veterinary literature.

Safety and handling: Normal precautions should be observed.

Contraindications: No information available.

Adverse reactions: Hypotension, hyperkalaemia, acidosis and hyponatraemia may develop.

Drug interactions: Avoid the concomitant administration of potassium.

DOSES
Dogs, Cats: 0.1 mg/kg p.o. q12h is used in humans and has been suggested for dogs and cats.
Small mammals, Birds, Reptiles: No information available.

Amino acid solutions
(Duphalyte, Aminoplasmal*, Aminoven*, Clinimix*, Glamin*, Hyperamine*, Intrafusin*, Kabiven*, Kabiven Peripheral*, Nutriflex*) **POM, POM-V**

Formulations: Injectable: synthetic crystalline L-amino acid solutions for i.v. use only. Numerous human products are available, varying in concentrations of amino acids. Most products also contain electrolytes. Some products contain varying concentrations of glucose.

Action: Support protein anabolism, arrest protein and muscle wasting, and maintain intermediary metabolism.

Use: Amino acid solutions supply essential and non-essential amino acids for protein production. They are used parenterally in patients requiring nutritional support but unable to receive enteral support. The authorized veterinary preparation (Duphalyte) contains insufficient amino acids to meet basal requirements for protein production and is intended as an aid for i.v. fluid support. None of the human formulations contains taurine, which is essential for cats and in specific conditions in dogs. All products are hyperosmolar. The use of concentrated amino acid solutions for parenteral nutrition support should not be undertaken without specific training and requires central venous access and intensive care monitoring. Parenteral nutrition may also be able to meet the patient's requirements for fluids, essential electrolytes (sodium, potassium, magnesium) and phosphate. Additionally if treatment is prolonged, vitamins and trace elements may need to be given. Intravenous lines for parenteral nutrition should be dedicated for that use alone and not used for other medications. As many of the available amino acids solutions contain potassium, the maximal acceptable rates of infusion will depend on the potassium content of the amino acid preparation.

Safety and handling: Normal precautions should be observed.

Contraindications: Dehydration, hepatic encephalopathy, severe azotaemia, shock, congestive heart failure and electrolyte imbalances.

Adverse reactions: The main complications of parenteral nutrition are metabolic, including hyperglycaemia, hyperlipidaemia, hypercapnia, acid-base disturbances and electrolyte disturbances. Other complications include catheter-associated thrombophlebitis, bacterial colonization of the catheter and resulting bacteraemia and septicaemia. Potentially life-threatening electrolyte imbalances including hypophosphataemia may also be seen (also referred to as refeeding syndrome). As with other hyperosmolar solutions, severe tissue damage could occur if extravasated, though this has not been reported.

Drug interactions: Consult specific product data sheet(s).

DOSES
Dogs: 4–6 g protein/100 kcal (418 kJ) energy requirements.
Cats: 6–8 g protein/100 kcal (418 kJ) energy requirements.
Dogs, Cats: Up to 10 ml/kg (Duphalyte).
Small mammals: Rabbits, Rodents: Anecdotally, these products have been used either alone or diluted with lactated Ringer's solution at a 1:5 ratio and given at a total volume of approximately 100 ml/kg/day.
Birds, Reptiles: No information available.

Aminophylline
(Aminophylline*) **POM**

Formulations: Injectable: 25 mg/ml solution. Oral: 100 mg tablet. For modified-release preparations see Theophylline (100 mg of aminophylline is equivalent to 79 mg of theophylline).

Action: Aminophylline is a stable mixture of theophylline (q.v.) and ethylenediamine. Causes inhibition of phosphodiesterase, alteration of intracellular calcium, release of catecholamine, and antagonism of adenosine and prostaglandin, leading to bronchodilation and other effects.

Use: Spasmolytic agent and has a mild diuretic action. It is used in the treatment of small airway disease. Beneficial effects include bronchodilation, enhanced mucociliary clearance stimulation of the respiratory centre, increased sensitivity to P_aCO_2, increased diaphragmatic contractility, stabilization of mast cells and a mild inotropic effect. Aminophylline has a low therapeutic index and should be dosed on a lean body weight basis. Administer with caution in patients with severe cardiac disease, gastric ulcers, hyperthyroidism, renal or hepatic disease, severe hypoxia or severe hypertension. Therapeutic plasma aminophylline values are 5–20 μg/ml.

Safety and handling: Do not mix aminophylline in a syringe with other drugs.

Contraindications: Patients with known history of arrhythmias or seizures.

Adverse reactions: Vomiting, diarrhoea, polydipsia, polyuria, reduced appetite, tachycardia, arrhythmias, nausea, twitching, restlessness, agitation, excitement and convulsions. Hyperaesthesia is seen in cats. Most adverse effects are related to the serum level and may be symptomatic of toxic serum concentrations. The severity of these effects may be decreased by the use of modified-release preparations. They are more likely to be seen with more frequent administration. Aminophylline causes intense local pain when given i.m. and is very rarely used or recommended via this route.

Drug interactions: Agents that may increase the serum levels of aminophylline include cimetidine, diltiazem, erythromycin, fluoroquinolones and allopurinol. Phenobarbital may decrease the serum concentration of aminophylline. Aminophylline may decrease the effects of pancuronium. Aminophylline and beta-adrenergic blockers (e.g. propranolol) may antagonize each other's effects. Aminophylline administration with halothane may cause an increased incidence of cardiac dysrhythmias and with ketamine an increased incidence of seizures.

DOSES
Dogs: 10 mg/kg p.o., i.v. q8h or slowly i.v. (diluted) for emergency bronchodilation.
Cats: 5 mg/kg p.o. q12h or 2–5 mg/kg slowly i.v. (diluted) for emergency bronchodilation.
Small mammals: Ferrets: 4.4–6.6 mg/kg p.o., i.m. q12h; Rabbits: 2.0 mg/kg i.v.; Guinea pigs: 50 mg/kg p.o.
Birds: 4–5 mg/kg i.m., i.v. q6–12h.
Reptiles: 2–4 mg/kg i.m. once.

Amiodarone `CIL`
(Amiodarone*, Cordarone*) **POM**

Formulations: Oral: 100 mg, 200 mg tablets. Injectable: 50 mg/ml for dilution and use as an infusion.

Action: Antiarrhythmic agent with primarily class 3 actions, but also potent class 1 and ancillary class 2 and 4 actions. Prolongs action potential duration and therefore effective refractory period in all cardiac tissues, including bypass tracts (class 3 action), inhibits sodium channels (class 1 action), blocks alpha- and beta-adrenergic receptors (class 2 action), slows the sinus rate, prolongs sinus node recovery time, and inhibits AV nodal conduction.

Use: Used to treat ventricular arrhythmias and supraventricular arrhythmias in dogs. It may be useful in ventricular pre-excitation syndromes because it can prolong AV nodal and bypass tract effective refractory periods. It has been successfully used for rate control or conversion to sinus rhythm in some dogs with atrial fibrillation. Use as an i.v. infusion in dogs with recent onset atrial fibrillation has been reported, with a variable efficacy for restoring sinus rhythm but high frequency of severe adverse effects. It has slow and variable GI absorption, a slow onset of action and a long elimination half-life (up to 3.2 days after repeated dosing). Because numerous side effects have been documented in humans and dogs, its use is advised for patients in which other antiarrhythmic agents have not been effective or are not tolerated. Owing to the risks of thyroid dysfunction and hepatotoxicity, it is advisable to evaluate hepatic enzyme activities and thyroid function prior to starting therapy and at 1–3 monthly intervals during maintenance therapy.

Safety and handling: Normal precautions should be observed.

Contraindications: Avoid in dogs with sinus bradycardia, AV block or thyroid dysfunction.

Adverse reactions: Amiodarone can cause bradycardia, AV block and prolongation of the QT interval. It is a negative inotrope and can cause hypotension. Systemic side effects described in dogs include anorexia, GI disturbances, hepatotoxicity, keratopathy and positive Coombs' test. Pulmonary fibrosis and thyroid dysfunction have also been reported in humans. In dogs T4 level decreases with amiodarone administration, but clinically apparent hypothyroidism is less common. Adverse effects associated with i.v. administration include pain at injection site, hypotension, hypersalivation and hypersensitivity reactions, which may be a reaction to the carrier solvent.

Drug interactions: Amiodarone may significantly increase serum levels and/or pharmacological effects of anticoagulants, beta-blockers, calcium-channel blockers, ciclosporin, digoxin, lidocaine, methotrexate, quinidine and theophylline. Cimetidine may increase serum levels of amiodarone.

DOSES
Dogs: Oral: 10–15 mg/kg p.o. q12h for 7 days, then 5–7.5 mg/kg p.o. q12h for 14 days; thereafter 5–7.5 mg/kg p.o. q24h. Intravenous: not well defined. Doses of 0.03–0.05 mg/kg/min have been administered as an infusion for cardioversion of atrial fibrillation. Bolus administration of 2.5–5 mg/kg given very slowly i.v. has been used in ventricular tachycardia.
Cats, Small mammals, Birds, Reptiles: No information available.

Amitraz
(Aludex, Promeris Duo) **POM-V**

Formulations: Topical: 5% w/v concentrated liquid; spot-on 150 mg/ml amitraz combined with metaflumizone in pipettes of various sizes.

Action: Increases neuronal activity through its action on octopamine receptors of mites.

Use: To treat generalized mite infestation, specifically canine demodicosis and sarcoptic acariasis. Dip to be left on coat. Clipping long hair coats will improve penetration. Monthly application of the spot-on product for demodicosis is not uniformly effective. Concurrent bacterial skin infections should be treated appropriately. Treatment and prevention of fleas and ticks, and treatment of lice and demodicosis in dogs. Use with care in small dogs. Used for generalized demodicosis in ferrets and hamsters and for acariasis in rodents.

Safety and handling: Do not store diluted product.

Contraindications: Do not use in dogs <3 months (<8 weeks for spot-on product), in Chihuahuas, cats or diabetic animals.

Adverse reactions: Sedation and bradycardia; can be reversed with an alpha-2 antagonist, e.g. atipamezole. Can cause irritation of the skin.

Drug interactions: No information available.

DOSES
Dogs:
- Generalized demodicosis: 0.05% solution (1 ml Aludex concentrated liquid in 100 ml water) q5–7d until two negative skin scrapings/hair plucks are achieved 2 weeks apart.
- Sarcoptic acariasis: 0.025% solution (1 ml Aludex concentrated liquid in 200 ml water) weekly for 2–6 weeks.
- Prophylactic: spot-on product: 20 mg/kg each amitraz and metaflumizone monthly.

Cats: Do not use.

Small mammals: Ferrets, Guinea Pigs: 0.3% solution (1 ml Aludex concentrated liquid in 17 ml water) applied topically to skin q14d for 3–6 treatments; Hamsters, Rats, Mice: 1.4 ml/l topically applied with a cotton bud q7d; Gerbils: 0.007% solution (1.4 ml Aludex concentrated liquid in 1000 ml water) applied with a cotton bud q14d for 3–6 treatments.

Birds, Reptiles: No information available.

Amitriptyline
(Amitriptyline*) **POM**   **CIL**

Formulations: Oral: 10 mg, 25 mg, 50 mg tablets; 5 mg/ml, 10 mg/ml solutions.

Action: Blocks noradrenaline and serotonin re-uptake in the brain, resulting in antidepressive activity.

Use: Management of chronic anxiety problems, including 'compulsive disorders', separation anxiety in dogs and 'compulsive disorders', psychogenic alopecia, hypervocalization and idiopathic cystitis in cats. The atypical tricyclic antidepressant clomipramine exists as an authorized preparation for use in dogs and is claimed to have better anticompulsive properties. Amitriptyline is bitter and can be very distasteful to cats. Some caution and careful monitoring is warranted in patients with cardiac or renal disease. Used for a minimum of 30 days for feather plucking in birds.

Safety and handling: Normal precautions should be observed.

Contraindications: Hypersensitivity to tricyclic antidepressants, glaucoma, history of seizures or urinary retention, severe liver disease.

Adverse reactions: Sedation, dry mouth, vomiting, excitability, arrhythmias, hypotension, syncope, increased appetite, weight gain and, less commonly, seizures and bone marrow disorders have been reported in humans. The bitter taste can cause ptyalism in cats.

Drug interactions: Should not be used with monoamine oxidase inhibitors or drugs metabolized by cytochrome P450 2D6, e.g. chlorphenamine, cimetidine. If changing medication from one of these compounds, a minimal washout period of 2 weeks is recommended (the washout period may be longer if the drug has been used for a prolonged period of time).

DOSES
Dogs: 1–2 mg/kg p.o. q12–24h.
Cats: 0.5–1 mg/kg p.o. q24h.
Small mammals: Rats: 5–20 mg/kg.
Birds: 1–2 mg/kg p.o. q12–24h; can be increased to 5 mg/kg if needed.
Reptiles: No information available.

Amlodipine

(Amlodipine*, Istin*) **POM**

Formulations: Oral: 5 mg, 10 mg tablets.

Action: Dihydropyridine calcium-channel blocker, with predominant action as a peripheral arteriolar vasculature, causing vasodilation and reducing afterload. Has mild negative inotropic and chronotropic effects, which are negligible at low doses.

Use: Treatment of systemic hypertension in cats and appears to be safe even when there is concurrent renal failure. Has been used in dogs for treatment of systemic hypertension and in normotensive dogs as adjunctive therapy for refractory heart failure due to mitral regurgitation. It is a very effective antihypertensive agent in cats and is frequently used in this species. It has also been shown to decrease proteinuria in cats with systemic hypertension. It is a less effective antihypertensive in dogs. Amlodipine is metabolized in the liver and dosage should be reduced when there is hepatic dysfunction.

Safety and handling: Normal precautions should be observed.

Contraindications: Avoid in cardiogenic shock and pregnancy.

Adverse reactions: Lethargy, hypotension or inappetence are rare side effects.

Drug interactions: Little is known in animals. Hepatic metabolism may be impaired by drugs such as cimetidine. Hypotension is a risk if combined with other antihypertensives, e.g. ACE inhibitors, diuretics, beta-blockers.

DOSES

Dogs: Initial dose 0.05–0.1 mg/kg p.o. q12–24h. The dose may be titrated upwards weekly as required, up to 0.4 mg/kg, monitoring blood pressure regularly.

Cats: 0.625–1.25 mg/cat p.o. q24h. The dose may be increased slowly or the frequency increased to q12h if necessary. Blood pressure monitoring is essential.

Small mammals, Birds, Reptiles: No information available.

Amoxicillin (Amoxycillin)

(Amoxinsol, Amoxycare, Amoxypen, Bimoxyl, Clamoxyl, Duphamox, Vetremox) **POM-V**

Formulations: Injectable: 150 mg/ml suspension. Oral: 40 mg, 200 mg, 250 mg tablets; suspension which when reconstituted provides 50 mg/ml.

Action: Binds to penicillin-binding proteins involved in bacterial cell wall synthesis, thereby decreasing cell wall strength and rigidity, affecting cell division, growth and septum formation. These antimicrobials act in a time-dependent bactericidal fashion.

Use: Active against certain Gram-positive and Gram-negative aerobic organisms and many obligate anaerobes but not against those that produce penicillinases (beta-lactamases), e.g. *Escherichia coli*, *Staphylococcus aureus*. The more difficult Gram-negative organisms (*Pseudomonas*, *Klebsiella*) are usually resistant. Amoxicillin is excreted well in bile and urine. Oral amoxicillin may be given with or without food. Since amoxicillin works in a time-dependent fashion, it is important to maintain levels above the MIC for a high percentage of the time. In practical terms this means that dosing interval is critical and missing doses can seriously compromise efficacy. In ferrets it is used in combination with bismuth subsalicylate, ranitidine or omeprazole and metronidazole ('triple therapy') for treatment of *Helicobacter mustelae* infection. The predominant bacterial infections in reptiles are Gram-negative and many are resistant to penicillins.

Safety and handling: Refrigerate oral suspension after reconstitution; discard if solution becomes dark or after 7 days.

Contraindications: Avoid oral antibiotics in critically ill patients, as absorption from the GI tract may be unreliable. Do not administer penicillins to hamsters, guinea pigs, gerbils or chinchillas. Do not administer oral penicillins to rabbits.

Adverse reactions: Nausea, diarrhoea and skin rashes are the commonest adverse effects.

Drug interactions: Avoid concurrent use with bacteriostatic antibiotics (e.g. tetracycline, erythromycin, chloramphenicol). Do not mix in the same syringe as aminoglycosides. A synergistic effect is seen when beta-lactam and aminoglycoside antimicrobials are used concurrently.

DOSES
See Appendix for guidelines on responsible antibacterial use.
Dogs, Cats: Parenteral: 7 mg/kg i.m. q24h; 15 mg/kg i.m. q48h for depot preparations. Oral: 10 mg/kg p.o. q8–12h. (Doses of 16–33 mg/kg i.v. q8h are used in humans to treat serious infections.) Dose chosen will depend on site of infection, causal organism and severity of the disease.
Small mammals: Ferrets: 10–30 mg/kg s.c., p.o. q12h; Rabbits: 7 mg/kg s.c. q24h; Rats, Mice: 100–150 mg/kg i.m., s.c. q12h.
Birds: 150–175 mg/kg i.m., s.c. q8–12h (q24h for long-acting preparations); Parrots, Raptors: 150–175 mg/kg p.o. q12h; Pigeons: 1–1.5 g/l drinking water (Vetremox pigeon) q24h for 3–5 days or 100–200 mg/kg p.o. q6–8h; Waterfowl: 1 g/l drinking water (Amoxinsol soluble powder) alternate days for 3–5 days, 300–500 mg/kg soft food for 3–5 days; Passerines 1.5g/l drinking water (Vetremox pigeon).
Reptiles: 5–10 mg/kg i.m., p.o. q12–24h (most species); Chelonians: 5–50 mg/kg i.m., p.o. q12h.

Amoxicillin/Clavulanate see Co-amoxiclav
Amoxycillin see Amoxicillin

Amphotericin B
(Abelcet*, AmBisome*, Amphocil*, Fungizone*) **POM**

Formulations: Injectable: 50 mg/vial powder for reconstitution.

Action: Binds to sterols in fungal cell membrane creating pores and allowing leakage of contents.

Use: Management of systemic fungal infections and leishmaniosis. Given the risk of severe toxicity it is advisable to reserve use for severe/potentially fatal fungal infections only. Abelcet, AmBisome,

Amphocil are lipid formulations that are less toxic. Physically incompatible with electrolyte solutions. Lipid formulations are far less toxic than conventional formulations for i.v. use because the drug is targeted to macrophages, but these preparations are far more expensive. Solutions are usually given i.v. but if regular venous catheterization is problematic then an s.c. alternative has been used for cryptococcosis and could potentially be used for other systemic mycoses. Renal values and electrolytes should be monitored pre and post each treatment; urinalysis and liver function tests weekly. If considering use in patients with pre-existing renal insufficiency (where other treatment options have failed and benefits outweigh risks), consider lipid formulations, concurrent saline administration and dose reduction.

Safety and handling: Keep in dark, although loss of drug activity is negligible for at least 8 hours in room light. After initial reconstitution (but not further dilution), the drug is stable for 1 week if refrigerated and stored in the dark. Do not dilute in saline. Pre-treatment heating of the reconstituted concentrated solution to 70°C for 20 min produces superaggregates which are less nephrotoxic. To produce a lipid-formulated product if not commercially available mix 40 ml sterile saline, 10 ml of lipid infusion (q.v.) and 50 mg of the reconstituted concentrated solution.

Contraindications: Do not use in renal or hepatic failure.

Adverse reactions: Include hypokalaemia, leading to cardiac arrhythmias, phlebitis, hepatic failure, renal failure, vomiting, diarrhoea, pyrexia, muscle and joint pain, anorexia and anaphylactoid reactions. Nephrotoxicity is a major concern; do not use other nephrotoxic drugs concurrently. Nephrotoxicity may be reduced by saline infusion (20 ml/kg over 60 minutes) prior to administration of amphotericin B. Fever and vomiting may be decreased by pre-treating with aspirin, diphenhydramine or an antiemetic. Amphotericin B is toxic to birds when administered systemically; administer fluids and monitor carefully if giving i.v.

Drug interactions: Amphotericin may increase the toxic effects of fluorouracil, doxorubicin and methotrexate. Flucytosine is synergistic with amphotericin B *in vitro* against *Candida*, *Cryptococcus* and *Aspergillus*.

DOSES
Dogs: Systemic mycoses: 0.25–1 mg/kg i.v. q48h. Administer slowly over 4–6 hours. Reconstitute vial with 10 ml water giving 5 mg/ml solution; dilute further 1:50 with 5% dextrose to give 0.1 mg/ml solution. Alternatively, 0.25–1 mg/kg may be dissolved in 10–60 ml 5% dextrose given over 10 min i.v. 3 times a week. Start at the lower end of the dose range and increase gradually as the patient tolerates therapy. Several months of therapy are often necessary. A total cumulative dose of 4–8 mg/kg is recommended by some authors.
Cats: Systemic mycoses: 0.1–0.25 i.v. q48h. For details on administration, see doses for dogs.

A B C D E F G H I J K L M N O P Q R S T U V W X Y Z

Dogs, Cats:
- Lipid formulations (general guidelines): 1 mg/kg q48h to cumulative dose of 12 mg/kg. Higher doses are tolerated (e.g. 1–2.5 mg/kg i.v. q48h for 4 wks/to cumulative dose of 24–30 mg/kg).
- Cryptococcosis (subcutaneous alternative): 0.5–0.8 mg/kg added to 400–500 ml of 0.45% saline/2.5% dextrose. This total volume is then administered s.c. 2 to 3 times a week to a cumulative level of 8–26 mg/kg in dogs and 10–15 mg/kg in cats. Do not inject solutions more concentrated than 20 mg/l as they will cause subcutaneous abscesses. Intralesional injection (1 mg/kg q7d) in combination with oral itraconazole.
- Leishmaniosis (lipid-formulated products): 1–2.5 mg/kg i.v. twice weekly for 8 injections. Increase dose rate gradually. A total cumulative dose of at least 10 mg/kg is required but treatment may be continued long term depending on clinical response. Use in this context is discouraged to avoid resistance developing to therapy for humans.
- Irrigation of bladder: 30–50 mg in 50–100 ml of sterile water infused at a rate of 5–10 ml/kg into the bladder lumen daily for 5–15 days.

Small mammals: Ferrets: 0.4–0.8 mg/kg i.v. q7d for treatment of blastomycosis; Rabbits: 1 mg/kg i.v. q24h; Guinea pigs: 1.25–2.5 mg/kg s.c. q24h for cryptococcosis; Mice: 0.11 mg/kg s.c. q24h, 0.43 mg/kg p.o. q24h.

Birds: Systemic fungal infections: 1–1.5 mg/kg i.v. q8–12h for 3–5 days (give with 10–15 ml/kg saline) or 1 mg/kg in 2 ml sterile water intratracheally q8–12h for 12 days then q48h for 5 weeks; Parrots: 100–300 mg/kg p.o. q12–24h for *Macrorhabdus* infection; Passerines: 100,000 IU/kg p.o. q8–12h or 1–5 g/l drinking water) or 1 mg/ml in saline nebulized for 15 min q12h.

Reptiles: 0.5–1 mg/kg i.v., intracoelomically q24–72h for 2–4 weeks; for respiratory infections nebulize 5 mg in 150 ml saline for 30–60 min; may also use topically on lesions q12h.

Ampicillin
(Amfipen, Ampicaps, Ampicare, Duphacillin) **POM-V**

Formulations: Injectable: Ampicillin sodium 250 mg, 500 mg powders for reconstitution (human licensed product only); 150 mg/ml suspension, 100 mg/ml long-acting preparation. Oral: 500 mg tablets; 250 mg capsule.

Action: Binds to penicillin-binding proteins involved in bacterial cell wall synthesis, thereby decreasing cell wall strength and rigidity, affecting cell division, growth and septum formation. It acts in a time-dependent bactericidal fashion.

Use: Active against many Gram-positive and Gram-negative aerobic organisms and obligate anaerobes, but not against those that produce penicillinases (beta-lactamases), e.g. *Escherichia coli*,

Staphylococcus aureus. The difficult Gram-negative organisms such as *Pseudomonas aeruginosa* and *Klebsiella* are usually resistant. Ampicillin is excreted well in bile and urine. Maintaining levels above the MIC is critical for efficacy and thereby prolonged dosage intervals or missed doses can compromise therapeutic response. Dose and dosing interval is determined by infection site, severity and organism. Oral bioavailability is reduced in the presence of food. The predominant bacterial infections in reptiles are Gram-negative and many are resistant to penicillins.

Safety and handling: After reconstitution the sodium salt will retain adequate potency for up to 8 hours if refrigerated, but use within 2 hours if kept at room temperature.

Contraindications: Avoid the use of oral antibiotic agents in critically ill patients, as absorption from the GI tract may be unreliable. Do not administer penicillins to hamsters, guinea pigs, chinchillas or rabbits. Use with caution in gerbils and only when indicated by sensitivity testing.

Adverse reactions: Nausea, diarrhoea and skin rashes are the commonest adverse effects.

Drug interactions: Avoid the concurrent use of ampicillin with bacteriostatic antibiotics (e.g. tetracycline, erythromycin, chloramphenicol). Do not mix in the same syringe as aminoglycosides. A synergistic effect is seen when beta-lactam and aminoglycoside antimicrobials are used concurrently.

DOSES
See Appendix for guidelines on responsible antibacterial use.
Dogs: Routine infections: 10–20 mg/kg i.v., i.m., s.c., p.o. q6–8h. CNS or serious bacterial infections: up to 40 mg/kg i.v. q6h has been recommended.
Cats: 10–20 mg/kg i.v., i.m., s.c., p.o. q6–8h.
Small mammals: Ferrets: 5–30 mg/kg i.m., s.c. q12h; Rabbits, Chinchillas, Guinea pigs, Hamsters: do not use; Gerbils: 20–100 mg/kg s.c. q8h, 6–30 mg/kg p.o. q8h; Rats, Mice: 25 mg/kg i.m., s.c. q12h, 50–200 mg/kg p.o. q12h.
Birds: 50–100 mg/kg i.v., i.m. q8–12h, 150–200 mg/kg p.o. q8–12h, 1–2 g/l drinking water, 2–3 g/kg soft feed.
Reptiles: 20 mg/kg s.c., i.m. q24h at 26°C.

Amprolium
(Coxoid) **AVM-GSL**

Formulations: Oral: 3.84% solution for dilution in water.

Action: Thiamine analogue that disrupts protozoal metabolism.

Use: Coccidiosis in homing/racing pigeons. Has been used for coccidiosis in dogs and cats. Limit duration of therapy to 2 weeks.

Safety and handling: Normal precautions should be observed.

Contraindications: No information available.

Adverse reactions: Anorexia, diarrhoea and depression in dogs. Prolonged high doses can cause thiamine deficiency.

Drug interactions: No information available.

DOSES
Dogs: 300–400 mg/dog p.o. q24h for 5 days. Use lower end of dose in puppies.
Cats: 300–400 mg/cat p.o. q24h.
Small mammals: Ferrets: 19 mg/kg p.o. q72h; Rabbits: 20 mg/kg p.o. q24h for 2–4 weeks; Chinchillas: 10–15 mg/kg p.o. total daily dose divided q8–24h; Gerbils, Hamsters, Rats, Mice: 10–20 mg/kg p.o. total daily dose divided q8–24h.
Birds: Pigeons: 28 ml of the concentrate in 4.5 l of drinking water for 7 days; in severe outbreaks continue with half-strength solution for a further 7 days; medicated water should be discarded after 24 hours. Passerines: 50–100 mg/l drinking water for 5 days or longer.
Reptiles: No information available.

Antivenom (European Adder)
POM

Formulations: Injectable: 10 ml vial for injection.

Action: Immunoglobulin raised against venom inhibits toxic effects.

Use: Used in the management of snake bites by the European Adder (Viper). The current supplier can be found on the internet and a special dispensation from the VMD allows supply, purchase and use prior to STC approval (contact the Pharmaceuticals and Feed Additive Section at the VMD). The value of antivenom decreases with time following the bite. There are no published studies on efficacy in small animals. This antivenom is unlikely to work for other snake bites and specialist help should be urgently sought for such bites.

Safety and handling: Normal precautions should be observed.

Contraindications: No information available.

Adverse reactions: Anaphylactic reactions may develop.

Drug interactions: No information available.

DOSES
Dogs, Cats: 10 ml per animal (regardless of size). Consider giving 0.5 ml i.v. first and then wait 20 minutes to test for anaphylaxis.
Small mammals, Birds, Reptiles: No information available.

Apomorphine

(Apometic, Apomorphine, APO-go*) **POM, POM-V**

Formulations: Injectable: 10 mg/ml solution in 2 ml or 5 ml ampoules; 5 mg/ml, 10 mg/ml solutions in 10 ml pre-filled syringes.

Action: Stimulates emesis through D2 dopamine receptors in the chemoreceptor trigger zone.

Use: Induction of self-limiting emesis within a few minutes of administration in dogs where vomiting is desirable, e.g. following the ingestion of toxic, non-caustic foreign material. Emesis generally occurs rapidly and within a maximum of 10 min. Further doses depress the vomiting centre and may not result in any further vomiting.

Safety and handling: Normal precautions should be observed.

Contraindications: Induction of emesis is contraindicated if strong acid or alkali has been ingested, due to the risk of further damage to the oesophagus. Induction of vomiting is contraindicated if the dog is unconscious, fitting, or has a reduced cough reflex, or if the poison has been ingested for >2 hours, or if the ingesta contains paraffin, petroleum products or other oily or volatile organic products, due to the risk of inhalation. Contraindicated in rabbits as they are unable to vomit. Contraindicated in rodents as their stomach walls lack the strength to tolerate forced emesis.

Adverse reactions: Apomorphine may induce excessive vomiting, respiratory depression and sedation.

Drug interactions: In the absence of compatibility studies, apomorphine must not be mixed with other products. Antiemetic drugs, particularly antidopaminergics (e.g. phenothiazines) may reduce the emetic effects of apomorphine. Additive CNS or respiratory depression may occur when apomorphine is used with opiates or other CNS or respiratory depressants.

DOSES

Dogs: 20-40 µg (micrograms)/kg i.v., 40–100 µg/kg s.c., i.m. (i.v. route most effective, i.m. least effective).
Cats: Not recommended; xylazine is a potent emetic in cats and at least as safe.
Small mammals: Do not use.
Birds, Reptiles: No information available.

Appeasines see Dog appeasing pheromone

Apraclonidine
(Iopidine*) **POM**

Formulations: Ophthalmic: 0.5% solution (5 ml bottle); preservative-free 1% solution (single-dose vials).

Action: Topical alpha-2-selective agonist that decreases aqueous humour production by inhibition of adenylate cyclase activity in the ciliary body.

Use: Reducing intraocular pressure in glaucoma. However, effect in dogs is inconsistent and it is unlikely to be effective as the sole agent in most forms of canine glaucoma. It may be most useful in alleviating pressure rises after intraocular surgery. It is prudent to monitor heart rate before and after topical application of apraclonidine, particularly with initial use and in small dogs.

Safety and handling: Normal precautions should be observed.

Contraindications: Commercial preparations are considered too toxic for use in cats. Do not use in dogs with uncontrolled cardiac disease.

Adverse reactions: Causes blanching of conjunctival vessels and bradycardia in dogs and cats. Causes mydriasis in dogs, miosis and severe vomiting in cats.

Drug interactions: No information available.

DOSES
Dogs: 1 drop per eye q8–12h for short-term use only.
Cats: Do not use.
Small mammals, Birds, Reptiles: No information available.

Ara-C see Cytarabine

Arginine (L-Arginine)
(Numerous trade names) **GSL**

Formulations: Oral: various strength tablets and powder.

Action: Arginine is an essential amino acid in cats. It is an intermediate of the hepatic urea cycle, which is involved in the detoxification of ammonia. Reduced dietary arginine intake in starvation or in the face of low protein diets may result in hyperammonaemia and signs of hepatic encephalopathy.

Use: Adjunctive dietary supplementation in cats with liver disease, especially hepatic lipidosis. Arginine may also have beneficial effects on wound healing.

Safety and handling: Normal precautions should be observed.

Contraindications: No information available.

Adverse reactions: Can cause pancreatitis in rats.

Drug interactions: None reported.

DOSES
Cats: 1000 mg/cat p.o. q24h.
Dogs, Small mammals, Birds, Reptiles: No information available.

Arnica
(Arnicare*) **GSL**

Formulations: *Arnica montana* tincture 0.9% w/v.

Action: *Arnica montana* is an alpine plant that contains helenalin, which has anti-inflammatory properties.

Use: First aid application for bruises resulting from a number of causes but especially those resulting from extravasation of non-toxic fluids from intravenous catheters. Also useful for peri-surgical bruising. Arnica has been found to be as effective as some NSAIDs (e.g. ibuprofen) in humans with hand arthritis and in reducing bruising following facelift surgery. However, some studies have shown no effect over placebo. No anti-infective properties; therefore skin infections require other specific therapy.

Safety and handling: Wear gloves when applying cream as contact with the plant can cause skin irritation in some individuals.

Contraindications: Do not apply to broken skin.

Adverse reactions: Ingestion of large amounts of the plant can be poisonous. There are no reports of problems associated with the cream.

Drug interactions: No information available.

DOSES
Dogs, Cats: Apply sparingly to site of bruising twice daily.
Small mammals, Birds: As for dogs and cats; appears effective, with no recorded side effects.
Reptiles: No information available.

Ascorbic acid see Vitamin C
Asparaginase, L-Asparginase see Crisantaspase

Aspirin (Acetylsalicyclic acid)
(Aspirin BP* and component of many others) **P** **CIL**

Formulations: Oral: 75 mg, 300 mg tablets.

Action: Produces irreversible inhibition of cyclo-oxygenase (COX) by acetylation, thereby preventing the production of both prostaglandins and thromboxanes from membrane phospholipids.

Use: Prevention of arterial thromboembolism. Also can be used to control mild to moderate pain, although NSAIDs that are more selective for the COX-2 enzyme have a better safety profile; not an NSAID of choice for analgesia in dogs or cats. In one study the use of ultralow dose aspirin (0.5 mg/kg q12h) may have improved the short-term and long-term survival in dogs with immune-mediated haemolytic anaemia when combined with glucocorticoid and azothioprine therapy. Administration of aspirin to animals with renal disease must be carefully evaluated. It is advisable to stop aspirin before surgery (at least 2 weeks) to allow recovery of normal platelet function and prevent excessive bleeding.

Safety and handling: Normal precautions should be observed.

Contraindications: Do not give aspirin to dehydrated, hypovolaemic or hypotensive patients or those with GI disease. Do not give to pregnant animals or animals <6 weeks.

Adverse reactions: GI ulceration and irritation are common side effects of all NSAIDs. It is advisable to stop therapy if diarrhoea or nausea persists beyond 1–2 days. Stop therapy immediately if GI bleeding is suspected and begin symptomatic treatment. There is a small risk that NSAIDs may precipitate cardiac failure in animals with cardiovascular disease. All NSAIDs carry a risk of renal papillary necrosis due to reduced renal perfusion caused by a reduction in the production of renal prostaglandins. This risk is greatest when NSAIDs are given to animals that are hypotensive or animals with pre-existing renal disease.

Drug interactions: Do not administer concurrently or within 24 hours of other NSAIDs and glucocorticoids. Do not administer with other potentially nephrotoxic agents, e.g. aminoglycosides.

DOSES
Dogs: Doses are anecdotal and range from 10 mg/kg to 20 mg/kg p.o. q12h. The safety and efficacy of this dose has not been established. Ultralow dose used in IMHA is 0.5 mg/kg p.o. q12h.

Cats: Doses of 10–25 mg/kg p.o. q48h have been suggested for the prevention of thromboembolism; this equates to $1/4$ of a 300 mg tablet for an average sized cat 3 days a week. Some authors suggest a very low dose (0.5 mg/kg p.o. q24h) to inhibit platelet COX without preventing the beneficial effects of prostacyclin production. The safety and efficacy of these different doses have not been evaluated in clinical or experimental studies.

Small mammals: Ferrets: 10–20 mg/kg p.o. q24h; Rabbits: 100 mg/kg p.o. q12–24h; Rodents: 50–150 mg/kg p.o. q4–8h.

Birds: Parrots: 5 mg/kg p.o. q8h, 325 mg/250 ml drinking water.

Reptiles: No information available.

Atenolol

CIL · A

(Atenolol*, Tenormin*) **POM**

Formulations: Oral: 25 mg, 50 mg, 100 mg tablets; 5 mg/ml syrup. Injectable: 0.5 mg/ml.

Action: Cardioselective beta-adrenergic blocker. It is relatively specific for beta-1 adrenergic receptors but can antagonize beta-2 receptors at high doses. Blocks the chronotropic and inotropic effects of beta-1 adrenergic stimulation on the heart, thereby reducing myocardial oxygen demand. Bronchoconstrictor, vasodilatory and hypoglycaemic effects are less marked due to its cardioselective nature.

Use: Cardiac tachyarrhythmias, hyperthyroidism, hypertrophic cardiomyopathy (cats), obstructive cardiac disease (severe aortic or pulmonic stenosis) and systemic hypertension. Commonly used in combination with mexiletine for ventricular arrhythmias. Less effective when used alone for ventricular arrhythmias unless the arrhythmia is mediated by sympathetic tone. It is recommended to withdraw therapy gradually in patients who have been receiving the drug chronically.

Safety and handling: Normal precautions should be observed.

Contraindications: Patients with bradyarrhythmias, acute or decompensated congestive heart failure. Relatively contraindicated in animals with medically controlled congestive heart failure as is poorly tolerated.

Adverse reactions: Most frequently seen in geriatric patients with chronic heart disease or in patients with acute or decompensated heart failure. Include bradycardia, AV block, myocardial depression, heart failure, syncope, hypotension, hypoglycaemia, bronchospasm and diarrhoea. Depression and lethargy may occur as a result of atenolol's high lipid solubility and its penetration into the CNS.

Drug interactions: Do not administer concurrently with alpha-adrenergic agonists (e.g. phenylpropanolamine). The hypotensive effect of atenolol is enhanced by many agents that depress myocardial activity including anaesthetic agents, phenothiazines, antihypertensive drugs, diuretics and diazepam. There is an increased risk of bradycardia, severe hypotension, heart failure and AV block if atenolol is used concurrently with calcium-channel blockers. Concurrent digoxin administration potentiates bradycardia. The metabolism of atenolol is accelerated by thyroid hormones; thus the dose of atenolol may need to be decreased when initiating carbimazole therapy. Atenolol enhances the effects of muscle relaxants (e.g. suxamethonium, tubocurarine). Hepatic enzyme induction by phenobarbital may increase the rate of metabolism of atenolol. The bronchodilatory effects of theophylline may be blocked by atenolol. Atenolol may enhance the hypoglycaemic effect of insulin.

DOSES

Dogs: 0.2–2 mg/kg p.o. q12h; a lower dose is often used initially with gradual titration upwards if necessary.

Cats: 6.25–12.5 mg/cat p.o. q12–24h; a lower dose is often used initially with gradual titration upwards if necessary.

Small mammals: Ferrets: 3.125–6.25 mg/ferret p.o. q24h; Rabbits: 0.5–2 mg/kg p.o. q24h; Mice: 2–10 mg/kg i.v., i.p. q24h.

Birds, Reptiles: No information available.

Atipamezole

(Alzane, Antisedan, Atipam, Revertor, Sedastop) **POM-V**

Formulations: Injectable: 5 mg/ml solution.

Action: Selective alpha-2 adrenoreceptor antagonist.

Use: Reverses the sedative effects of medetomidine or dexmedetomidine; will also reverse other alpha-2 agonists to provide a quick recovery from anaesthesia and sedation. It also reverses other effects such as the analgesic, cardiovascular and respiratory effects of alpha-2 agonists. Atipamezole does not alter the metabolism of medetomidine or dexmedetomidine but occupies the alpha-2 receptor preventing binding of the drug. The duration of action of atipamezole and medetomidine or dexmedetomidine are similar, so re-sedation is uncommon. Atipamezole should not be administered until at least 30 minutes after medetomidine/ketamine combinations have been given to cats, to avoid CNS excitation in recovery. Routine administration of atipamezole i.v. is not recommended because the rapid recovery from sedation is usually associated with excitation, though i.v. administration may be indicated in an emergency (e.g. excessive sedation from medetomidine or dexmedetomidine or cardiovascular complications).

Safety and handling: Normal precautions should be observed.

Contraindications: Atipamezole has been administered to a limited number of pregnant dogs and cats and therefore cannot be recommended in pregnancy.

Adverse reactions: Transient over-alertness and tachycardia may be observed after overdosage. This is best handled by minimizing external stimuli and allowing the animal to recover quietly.

Drug interactions: No information available.

DOSES

Dogs:
- Five times the previous medetomidine or dexmedetomidine dose i.m. (i.e. equal volume of solution to medetomidine or dexmedetomidine). When medetomidine or dexmedetomidine has been administered at least an hour before, dose of atipamezole can be reduced by half (i.e. half the volume of medetomidine or dexmedetomidine) and repeated if recovery is slow.

- Amitraz toxicity: 25 µg (micrograms)/kg i.m. but if there is no benefit within half an hour this can be repeated or incrementally increased every 30 minutes up to 200 µg/kg.

Cats: Two and a half times the previous medetomidine or dexmedetomidine dose i.m. (i.e. half the volume of medetomidine or dexmedetomidine given).

Small mammals: Ferrets, Rodents: Five times the previous medetomidine dose s.c., i.m.; Rabbits: Two and a half times the previous medetomidine dose.

Birds: 0.065–0.25 mg/kg i.m.

Reptiles: Five times the previous medetomidine or dexmedetomidine dose i.m., i.v.

Atracurium

(Tracrium*) **POM**

Formulations: Injectable: 10 mg/ml solution.

Action: Inhibits the actions of acetylcholine at the neuromuscular junction by binding competitively to the nicotinic acetylcholine receptor on the post-junctional membrane.

Use: Neuromuscular blockade during anaesthesia. This may be to improve surgical access through muscle relaxation, to facilitate positive pressure ventilation or for intraocular surgery. Atracurium has an intermediate duration of action (15–35 min) and is non-cumulative due to non-enzymatic (Hofmann) elimination. It is therefore suitable for administration to animals with renal or hepatic disease. Monitoring (using a nerve stimulator) and reversal of the neuromuscular blockade is recommended to ensure complete recovery before the end of anaesthesia. Hypothermia, acidosis and hypokalaemia will prolong the duration of action of neuromuscular blockade. Use the low end of the dose range in patients with myasthenia gravis and ensure that neuromuscular function is monitored during the period of the blockade and recovery using standard techniques.

Safety and handling: Store in refrigerator.

Contraindications: Do not administer unless the animal is adequately anaesthetized and facilities to provide positive pressure ventilation are available.

Adverse reactions: Can precipitate the release of histamine after rapid i.v. administration, resulting in bronchospasm and hypotension. Diluting the drug in normal saline and giving the drug slowly i.v. minimizes these effects.

Drug interactions: Neuromuscular blockade is more prolonged when atracurium is given in combination with volatile anaesthetics, aminoglycosides, clindamycin or lincomycin.

DOSES

Dogs, Cats: 0.5 mg/kg i.v. initially, followed by increments of 0.2 mg/kg.

Small mammals, Birds, Reptiles: No information available.

A

Atropine
(Atrocare) **POM-V**

B
C

Formulations: Injectable: 0.6 mg/ml. Ophthalmic: 0.5%, 1% solution in single-use vials, 5 ml bottle; 1% ointment.

D

Action: Blocks the action of acetylcholine at muscarinic receptors at the terminal ends of the parasympathetic nervous system, reversing parasympathetic effects and producing mydriasis, tachycardia, bronchodilation and general inhibition of GI function.

E
F

Use: Prevent or correct bradycardia and bradyarrhythmias, to dilate pupils, in the management of organophosphate and carbamate toxicities, and in conjunction with anticholinesterase drugs during antagonism of neuromuscular block. Routine administration prior to anaesthesia as part of premedication is no longer recommended; it is better to monitor heart rate and give atropine to manage a low heart rate if necessary. Atropine has a slow onset of action (10 min i.m., 2–3 min i.v.), therefore it is important to wait for an adequate period of time for the desired effect before redosing. The ophthalmic solution tastes very bitter and can cause hypersalivation in cats (and a few dogs); therefore the ophthalmic ointment preparation is preferred.

G
H
I
J
K

Safety and handling: The solution does not contain any antimicrobial preservative, therefore any remaining solution in the vial should be discarded after use. The solution should be protected from light.

L
M

Contraindications: Glaucoma, lens luxation, keratoconjunctivitis sicca.

N

Adverse reactions: Include sinus tachycardia (usually of short duration after i.v. administration), blurred vision from mydriasis, which may worsen recovery from anaesthesia, and drying of bronchial secretions. Atropine increases intraocular pressure and reduces tear production. Ventricular arrhythmias may be treated with lidocaine if severe. Other GI side effects such as ileus and vomiting are rare in small animals.

O
P
Q

Drug interactions: Atropine is compatible (for at least 15 min) mixed with various medications but not with bromides, iodides, sodium bicarbonate, other alkalis or noradrenaline. The following may enhance the activity of atropine: antihistamines, quinidine, pethidine, benzodiazepines, phenothiazines, thiazide diuretics and sympathomimetics. Combining atropine and alpha-2 agonists is not recommended. Atropine may aggravate some signs seen with amitraz toxicity, leading to hypertension and gut stasis.

R
S
T
U
V
W

DOSES
Dogs, Cats:
- Ophthalmic: 1 drop or a small amount of ointment in the affected eye q8–12h to cause mydriasis, then once q24–72h to maintain mydriasis.
- Bradyarrhythmias: 0.01–0.03 mg/kg i.v. Low doses may exacerbate bradycardia; repetition of the dose will usually

X
Y
Z

promote an increase in heart rate. 0.03–0.04 mg/kg i.m. can be given to prevent development of bradycardia during administration of potent opioids such as fentanyl.
- Organophosphate poisoning: dose 0.2–0.5 mg/kg ($1/4$ dose i.v., $3/4$ i.m., s.c.) to effect; repeat as necessary; or 0.1–0.2 mg/kg ($1/2$ i.v., $1/2$ i.m.) then i.m. q6h.
- Neuromuscular blockade antagonism: 0.04 mg/kg i.v. with edrophonium (0.5–1.0 mg/kg).

Small mammals: Ferrets: 0.04 mg/kg s.c., i.m., i.v.; Others: 0.04–0.1 mg/kg i.m., s.c.; Rabbits: endogenous atropinase levels may make repeated injections q10–15min necessary; Rodents: OP poisoning may require up to 10 mg/kg q20min.

Birds:
- Organophosphate poisoning: 0.04–0.5 mg/kg i.v., i.m. q4h.
- Supraventricular bradycardia: 0.01–0.02 mg/kg i.v. once.

Reptiles: 0.01–0.04 mg/kg i.m., i.v.

Azathioprine CIL

(Azathioprine*, Imuran*) **POM**

Formulations: Oral: 25 mg, 50 mg tablets.

Action: Inhibits purine synthesis, which is necessary for cell proliferation especially of leucocytes and lymphocytes. It suppresses cell-mediated immunity, alters antibody production and inhibits cell growth.

Use: Management of immune-mediated diseases. Often used in conjunction with corticosteroids. Routine haematology (including platelets) should be monitored closely: initially every 1–2 weeks; and every 1–2 months when on maintenance therapy. Use with caution in patients with hepatic disease. In animals with renal impairment, dosing interval should be extended. Clinical responses can take up to 6 weeks. Mycophenolic acid may be preferred if a more rapid response is required.

Safety and handling: Cytotoxic drug; see Appendix and specialist texts for further advice on chemotherapeutic agents. Azathioprine tablets should be stored at room temperature in well closed containers and protected from light.

Contraindications: Do not use in patients with bone marrow suppression or those at high risk of infection. Not recommended for use in cats.

Adverse reactions: Bone marrow suppression is the most serious adverse effect. This may be influenced by the activity of thiopurine *s*-methyltransferase, which is involved in the metabolism of the drug and which can vary between individuals due to genetic polymorphism. GI upset/anorexia, poor hair growth, acute pancreatitis and hepatotoxicity have been seen in dogs. Cats in particular often develop a severe, non-responsive fatal leucopenia and thrombocytopenia. Avoid rapid withdrawal.

A

Drug interactions: Enhanced effects and increased azathioprine toxicity when used with allopurinol. Increased risk of azathioprine toxicity with aminosalicylates and corticosteroids.

DOSES
See Appendix for immunosuppression protocols.
Dogs: 2 mg/kg p.o. q24h until remission achieved, then 0.5–2 mg/kg q48h.
Cats: Not recommended.
Small mammals: Ferrets: 0.5 mg/kg p.o. q48h to 5 mg/kg p.o. q24h for eosinophilic gastroenteritis (limited evidence); 0.9 mg/kg p.o. q24–72h with prednisolone and dietary management for inflammatory bowel disease.
Birds, Reptiles: No information available.

Azidothymidine see Zidovudine

Azithromycin
(Zithromax*) **POM**

Formulations: Oral: 250 mg capsule; 200 mg/5 ml suspension (reconstitute with water).

Action: Binds to the 50S bacterial ribosome (like erythromycin), inhibiting peptide bond formation and has bactericidal or bacteriostatic activity depending on the susceptibility of the organism. Azithromycin has a longer tissue half-life than erythromycin, shows better oral absorption and is better tolerated in humans.

Use: Alternative to penicillin in allergic individuals as it has a similar, although not identical, antibacterial spectrum. It is active against Gram-positive cocci (some *Staphylococcus* species are resistant), Gram-positive bacilli, some Gram-negative bacilli (*Haemophilus*, *Pasteurella*), mycobacteria, obligate anaerobes, *Chlamydophila*, *Mycoplasma* and *Toxoplasma*. Some strains of *Actinomyces*, *Nocardia* and *Rickettsia* are also inhibited. Most strains of the Enterobacteriaceae (*Pseudomonas*, *Escherichia coli*, *Klebsiella*) are resistant. Useful in the management of respiratory tract, mild to moderate skin and soft tissue, and non-tubercular mycobacterial infections. Is used to treat chlamydophilosis in birds, but it has not proved possible to eliminate *Chlamydophila felis* from chronically infected cats using azithromycin, even with once daily administration. Little information is available on the use of this drug in animals and drug pharmacokinetics have not been studied closely in the dog and cat. Doses are empirical and subject to change as experience with the drug is gained. More work is needed to optimize the clinically effective dose rate. Azithromycin activity is enhanced in an alkaline pH; administer on an empty stomach.

Safety and handling: Normal precautions should be observed.

Contraindications: Avoid in renal and hepatic failure in all species.

Adverse reactions: In humans similar adverse effects to those of erythromycin are seen, i.e. vomiting, cholestatic hepatitis, stomatitis and glossitis, but the effects are generally less marked than with erythromycin.

Drug interactions: Azithromycin may increase the serum levels of methylprednisolone, theophylline and terfenadine. The absorption of digoxin may be enhanced.

DOSES
See Appendix for guidelines on responsible antibacterial use.

Dogs: 5–10 mg/kg p.o. q24h. May increase dosing interval to q48h after 3–5 days of treatment.

Cats: Various regimes are suggested: 5–10 mg/kg p.o q24h for 3–5 days; 5 mg/kg p.o. q24h for 2 days then every 3–5 days up to a total of 5 doses; for upper respiratory tract disease: 5–10 mg/kg p.o. q24h for 5 days then q72h. Specialist texts should be consulted.

Small mammals: Ferrets: 5 mg/kg p.o. q24h for 5 days as part of a protocol for treatment of *Helicobacter*; Rabbits: 4–5 mg/kg i.m. q48h for 7 days is effective against syphilis; Prairie dogs: 15–30 mg/kg p.o. q24h for 15 days; Rats: 10–20 mg/kg p.o. q12h for 14 days.

Birds: 40 mg/kg p.o. q24–48h for up to 45 days (chlamydophilosis); *Mycoplasma*: 50–80 mg/kg p.o. q24h for 3 days, then 4 days off; repeat for up to 3 weeks.

Reptiles: 10 mg/kg p.o. q3d for skin infections; q5d for respiratory tract infections; q7d for liver and kidney infections.

AZT see **Zidovudine**

A
B
C
D
E
F
G
H
I
J
K
L
M
N
O
P
Q
R
S
T
U
V
W
X
Y
Z

Benazepril
(Benefortin, Cardalis, Fortekor, Nelio, Prilben, Vetpril)
POM-V

Formulations: Oral: 2.5 mg, 5 mg, 20 mg tablets. Available in a compound preparation with spironolactone (Cardalis tablets) in the following formulations: 2.5 mg benazepril/20 mg spironolactone, 5 mg benazepril/40 mg spironolactone, 10 mg benazepril/80 mg spironolactone.

Action: Angiotensin converting enzyme (ACE) inhibitor. It inhibits conversion of angiotensin I to angiotensin II and inhibits the breakdown of bradykinin. Overall effect is a reduction in preload and afterload via venodilation and arteriodilation, decreased salt and water retention via reduced aldosterone production and inhibition of the angiotensin-aldosterone-mediated cardiac and vascular remodelling. Efferent arteriolar dilation in the kidney can reduce intraglomerular pressure and therefore glomerular filtration. This may decrease proteinuria.

Use: Treatment of congestive heart failure in dogs and cats and chronic renal insufficiency in cats. Often used in conjunction with diuretics when heart failure is present as most effective when used in these cases. Can be used in combination with other drugs to treat heart failure (e.g. pimobendan, spironolactone, digoxin). Beneficial in cases of chronic renal insufficiency in cats, particularly protein-losing nephropathies. May reduce blood pressure in hypertension. Less potent in reducing blood pressure compared with amlodipine in cats but sometimes used together. Benazepril undergoes significant hepatic metabolism and may not need dose adjustment in renal failure. ACE inhibitors are more likely to cause or exacerbate prerenal azotaemia in hypotensive animals and those with poor renal perfusion (e.g. acute, oliguric renal failure). Use cautiously if hypotension, hyponatraemia or outflow tract obstruction are present. Regular monitoring of blood pressure, serum creatinine, urea and electrolytes is strongly recommended with ACE inhibitor treatment. Hypotension, azotaemia and hyperkalaemia are all indications to stop or reduce ACE inhibitor treatment in rabbits. The use of ACE inhibitors in cats with cardiac disease stems from extrapolation from theoretical benefits and studies showing a benefit in other species with heart failure and different cardiac diseases (mainly dogs and humans).

Safety and handling: Normal precautions should be observed.

Contraindications: Do not use in cases of cardiac output failure.

Adverse reactions: Potential adverse effects include hypotension, hyperkalaemia and azotaemia. Monitor blood pressure, serum creatinine and electrolytes when used in cases of heart failure. Dosage should be reduced if there are signs of hypotension (weakness, disorientation). Anorexia, vomiting and diarrhoea are rare. In pre-clinical trials there were no serious reactions when the drug was given to normal dogs at 200 times the label dose. It is not recommended for breeding, or pregnant or lactating dogs and cats, as safety has not been established. The safety of benazepril has not been established in cats <2.5 kg. In rabbits, treatment with ACE inhibitors can be associated with an increase in azotaemia.

Drug interactions: Concomitant usage with potassium-sparing diuretics (e.g. spironolactone) or potassium supplements could result in hyperkalaemia. However, in practice, spironolactone and ACE inhibitors appear safe to use concurrently. There may be an increased risk of nephrotoxicity and decreased clinical efficacy when used with NSAIDs. There is a risk of hypotension with concomitant administration of diuretics, vasodilators (e.g. anaesthetic agents, antihypertensive agents) or negative inotropes (e.g. beta-blockers).

DOSES
Dogs: Heart failure: 0.25–0.5 mg/kg p.o. q24h.
Cats: Chronic renal insufficiency: 0.5–1.0 mg/kg p.o. q24h.
Small mammals: Rabbits, Guinea pigs: Starting dose 0.05 mg/kg p.o. q24h. Dose may be increased to a maximum of 0.1 mg/kg.
Birds, Reptiles: No information available.

Benzoyl peroxide
(Paxcutol) **POM-V**

Formulations: Topical: 2.5% shampoo.

Action: Antimicrobial and keratolytic.

Use: Topical treatment of bacterial skin infections in dogs. Concurrent systemic antibacterial therapy is generally advised. Leave in contact with the skin for 5–10 min prior to washing off.

Safety and handling: Normal precautions should be observed. Impervious gloves should be worn at all times when applying and using the shampoo.

Contraindications: No information available.

Adverse reactions: May irritate mucous membranes. Can bleach some fabrics.

Drug interactions: No information available.

DOSES
Dogs: To be used as a shampoo 2–3 times weekly. May be used less frequently once infection is controlled.
Cats, Small mammals, Birds, Reptiles: No information available.

Benzyl penicillin see **Penicillin G**

Betamethasone

(Fuciderm, Norbet, Otomax, Betnesol*, Maxidex*) **POM-V, POM**

Formulations: Injectable: 4 mg/ml solution for i.v. or i.m. use. Oral: 0.25 mg tablet. Topical: 0.1% cream with 0.5% fusidic acid. Ophthalmic/Otic: 0.1% solution; 0.88% mg/ml suspension with clotrimazole and gentamicin. Betamethasone is also present in varying concentrations in several topical preparations with or without antibacterials.

Action: Alters the transcription of DNA, leading to alterations in cellular metabolism which causes reduction in inflammatory responses. Has high glucocorticoid but low mineralocorticoid activity. Betamethasone also antagonizes insulin and ADH.

Use: Short-term relief of many inflammatory but non-infectious conditions. Long duration of activity and therefore not suitable for long-term daily or alternate-day use. On a dose basis, 0.12 mg betamethasone is equivalent to 1 mg prednisolone. Prolonged use of glucocorticoids suppresses the hypothalamic-pituitary axis, resulting in adrenal atrophy. Animals on chronic corticosteroid therapy should be given tapered decreasing doses when discontinuing the drug. The use of long-acting steroids in most cases of shock is of no benefit, and may be detrimental. Use glucocorticoids with care in rabbits as they are very sensitive to these drugs.

Safety and handling: Wear gloves when applying cream.

Contraindications: Do not use in pregnant animals. Systemic corticosteroids are generally contraindicated in patients with renal disease and diabetes mellitus. Topical corticosteroids are contraindicated in ulcerative keratitis.

Adverse reactions: Catabolic effects of glucocorticoids lead to weight loss and cutaneous atrophy. Iatrogenic hyperadrenocorticism may develop. Vomiting, diarrhoea and GI ulceration may develop. Glucocorticoids may increase glucose levels and decrease serum T3 and T4 values. Impaired wound healing and delayed recovery from infections may be seen. Corticosteroids should be used with care in birds as there is a high risk of immunosuppression and side effects, such as hepatopathy and a diabetes mellitus-like syndrome. In rabbits, even small single doses can cause severe adverse reactions.

Drug interactions: There is an increased risk of GI ulceration if used concurrently with NSAIDs. Glucocorticoids antagonize the effect of insulin. Phenobarbital may accelerate the metabolism of corticosteroids and antifungals (e.g. itraconazole) may decrease it. There is an increased risk of hypokalaemia when used concurrently with acetazolamide, amphotericin and potassium-depleting diuretics (furosemide, thiazides).

DOSES
Dogs:
- Otic: 4 drops of polypharmaceutical to affected ear q12h.
- Ocular: 1 drop of ophthalmic solution to affected eye q6–8h.
- Skin: Apply cream to affected area q8–12h.
- Anti-inflammatory: 0.04 mg/kg i.v., i.m. q3w prn for up to 4 injections, 0.025 mg/kg p.o. q24h.

Cats:
- Ocular: dose as for dogs.
- Skin: dose as for dogs.
- Anti-inflammatory: 0.04 mg/kg i.v. q3w prn for up to 4 injections.

Small mammals: 0.1 mg/kg s.c. q24h.
Birds, Reptiles: No information available.

Betaxolol
(Betoptic*) **POM**

Formulations: Ophthalmic: 0.25%, 0.5% solution; 0.25% suspension in single-use vials.

Action: Betaxolol is a beta-1 selective beta-blocker that decreases aqueous humour production via beta-adrenoreceptor blockade in the ciliary body.

Use: Management of glaucoma. It can be used alone or in combination with other topical glaucoma drugs, such as a topical carbonic anhydrase inhibitor. Betaxolol can be used in the prophylactic management of glaucoma in the other eye of dogs with unilateral primary closed angle glaucoma.

Safety and handling: Normal precautions should be observed.

Contraindications: Avoid in uncontrolled heart failure and asthma.

Adverse reactions: Ocular adverse effects include miosis, conjunctival hyperaemia and local irritation.

Drug interactions: Additive adverse effects may develop if given concurrently with oral beta-blockers. Concomitant administration of timolol with verapamil may cause a bradycardia and asystole. Prolonged atrioventricular conduction times may result if used with calcium antagonists or digoxin.

DOSES
Dogs: 1 drop per eye q12h.
Cats, Small mammals, Birds, Reptiles: No information available.

Bethanecol
(Myotonine*) **POM**

Formulations: Oral: 10 mg tablets.

Action: A muscarinic agonist (cholinergic or parasympathomimetic) that increases urinary bladder detrusor muscle tone and contraction.

Use: Management of urinary retention with reduced detrusor tone. It does not initiate a detrusor reflex and is ineffective if the bladder is areflexic. Best given on an empty stomach to avoid GI distress.

Safety and handling: Normal precautions should be observed.

Contraindications: Do not use when urethral resistance is increased unless in combination with agents that reduce urethral outflow pressure (e.g. phenoxybenzamine).

Adverse reactions: Vomiting, diarrhoea, GI cramping, anorexia, salivation and bradycardia (with overdosage). Treat overdoses with atropine.

Drug interactions: No information available.

DOSES
Dogs: 1.25–25 mg/dog p.o. q8h. Titrate dose upwards to avoid side effects.
Cats: 0.625–5 mg/cat or 0.1–0.2 mg/kg p.o. q8h. Titrate dose upwards to avoid side effects.
Small mammals: Rabbits: 2.5–5 mg/kg p.o. q12h.
Birds, Reptiles: No information available.

Bisacodyl
(Dulcolax*) **P, GSL**

Formulations: Oral: 5 mg yellow, enteric-coated tablet. Rectal: 10 mg suppository.

Action: Mild stimulant laxative that increases intestinal motility, but inhibits absorption of water. It is locally active with <5% systemic absorption.

Use: Constipation. Doses are empirical; none have been defined in the veterinary literature. Single doses given the night before the procedure can also be used for preparation for colonoscopy in dogs and cats.

Safety and handling: Normal precautions should be observed.

Contraindications: Must not be used in patients with ileus, intestinal obstruction or dehydration.

Adverse reactions: Abdominal discomfort and diarrhoea.

Drug interactions: No information available.

DOSES
Dogs: 5–20 mg/dog prn.
Cats: 2–5 mg/cat prn.
Small mammals, Birds, Reptiles: No information available.

Bismuth salts (Bismuth carbonate, subnitrate and subsalicylate: tri-potassium di-citrato bismuthate (bismuth chelate))
(De-Noltab*, Pepto-Bismol*) **AVM-GSL, P**

Formulations: Oral: De-Noltab: tablets containing the equivalent of 120 mg bismuth oxide. Pepto-Bismol: bismuth subsalicylate suspension.

Action: Bismuth is a gastric cytoprotectant with activity against spiral bacteria. Bismuth chelate is effective in healing gastric and duodenal ulcers in humans, due to its direct toxic effects on gastric *Helicobacter pylori* and by stimulating mucosal prostaglandin and bicarbonate secretion. It is often used in conjunction with an H2 receptor antagonist. Bismuth subsalicylate has a mild anti-inflammatory effect. Pepto-Bismol should be used with caution in cats due to its subsalicylate content.

Use: Acute oral poisoning, gastric ulceration and flatulent diarrhoea. Doses are empirical; none have been defined in dogs and cats.

Safety and handling: Normal precautions should be observed.

Contraindications: Do not use where specific oral antidotes are being administered in cases of poisoning. Do not use if the patient is unconscious, fitting, or has a reduced cough reflex, or in cases of intestinal obstruction, or where enterotomy or enterectomy is to be performed.

Adverse reactions: Avoid long-term use (except chelates) as absorbed bismuth is neurotoxic. Bismuth chelate is contraindicated in renal impairment. Nausea and vomiting reported in humans.

Drug interactions: Absorption of tetracyclines is reduced by bismuth and specific antidotes may also be affected.

DOSES
Dogs: De-Noltab: 1/2 tab p.o. q6h (dogs up to 30 kg), 1 tab p.o. q6h (>30 kg). Pepto-Bismol: 1 ml/kg p.o. q4–6h.
Cats: De-Noltab: 1/2 tab p.o. q6h. Pepto-Bismol: 1 ml/kg p.o. q4–6h – use with caution.
Small mammals: Ferrets: Pepto-Bismol: 17.6 mg/kg or 0.25–1.0 ml/kg p.o. q4–8h. Rabbits: Pepto-Bismol 0.3-0.6 ml/kg p.o. q4–6h.
Birds, Reptiles: No information available.

Bowel cleansing solutions
(Polyethylene glycol, Macrogol)
(Dulcobalance*, Klean-Prep*, Moviprep*) **P**

Formulations: Oral: Powder for reconstitution.

Action: Bowel cleansing solutions contain polyethylene glycol as an osmotic laxative and balanced electrolytes to maintain isotonicity and prevent net fluid loss or gain. When administered orally they rapidly empty the bowel.

Use: Bowel preparation before colonoscopy or radiographic examination; some authorities do not use in cats before colonoscopy. May also be used for constipation. Powder may take several minutes to dissolve, and reconstitution is best performed by adding warm water to the powder.

Safety and handling: Normal precautions should be observed.

Contraindications: GI obstruction or perforation. Do not administer to heavily sedated patients or animals with a reduced gag reflex.

Adverse reactions: Diarrhoea is an expected outcome. Occasional vomiting is seen, especially if the maximum volume is administered. Inhalation can cause severe, and even fatal, aspiration pneumonia.

Drug interactions: Oral medication should not be taken within 1 hour of administration as it may be flushed from the GI tract and not absorbed.

DOSES
Dogs: Prior to lower GI examination: 22–33 ml/kg p.o. by stomach tube, two or three times, at least 4h apart.
Cats: Prior to lower GI examination: 22–33 ml/kg p.o. by naso-oesophageal tube.
Small mammals, Birds, Reptiles: No information available.

Brinzolamide
(Azarga*, Azopt*) **POM**

Formulations: Ophthalmic drops: 10 mg/ml (1%) in 5 ml bottle (Azopt); 1% brinzolamide + 0.5% timolol in 5 ml bottle (Azarga).

Action: Reduces intraocular pressure by reducing the rate of aqueous humour production by inhibition of the formation of bicarbonate ions within the ciliary body epithelium.

Use: In the control of all types of glaucoma in dogs, either alone or in combination with other topical drugs. It may be better tolerated than dorzolamide because of its more physiological pH of 7.5. The concurrent use of a topical or systemic carbonic anhydrase inhibitor is not beneficial as there is no additional decrease in intraocular pressure compared with either route alone. Brinzolamide is ineffective in normal cats; by contrast dorzolamide is effective in both dogs and cats.

Safety and handling: Normal precautions should be observed.

Contraindications: Severe hepatic or renal impairment.

Adverse reactions: Local irritation. Brinzolamide may cause less ocular irritation than dorzolamide. Brinzolamide/timolol causes miosis and is therefore not the drug of choice in uveitis or anterior lens luxation.

Drug interactions: No information available.

DOSES
Dogs: 1 drop per eye q8–12h.
Cats: Not applicable.
Small mammals, Birds, Reptiles: No information available.

British anti-lewisite see **Dimercaprol**

Bromhexine
(Bisolvon) **POM-V**

Formulations: Injectable: 3 mg/ml solution. Oral: 10 mg/g powder.

Action: A bronchial secretolytic that disrupts the structure of acid mucopolysaccharide fibres in mucoid sputum and produces a less viscous mucus, which is easier to expectorate.

Use: To aid the management of respiratory diseases.

Safety and handling: Normal precautions should be observed.

Contraindications: No information available.

Adverse reactions: No information available.

Drug interactions: No information available.

DOSES
Dogs: 3–15 mg/dog i.m. q12h; 2 mg/kg p.o. q12h.
Cats: 3 mg/cat i.m. q24h; 1 mg/kg p.o. q24h.
Small mammals: 0.3 mg/animal p.o. q24h or via nebulizer as 0.15 mg/ml for 20–30 minutes, 1–3 times daily.
Birds: 1.5 mg/kg i.m., p.o. q12–24h.
Reptiles: 0.1–0.2 mg/kg q24h.

Budesonide   `CIL`
(Budenofalk*, Budenofalk Rectal Foam*, Entocort*, Pulmicort*) **POM**

Formulations: Oral: 3 mg gastroresistant capsule, 3 mg capsule containing gastroresistant slow-release granules. Rectal: 2 mg (total dose) rectal foam, 0.02 mg/ml enema.

Action: Anti-inflammatory and immunosuppressive steroid.

Use: A novel steroid that is metabolized on its first pass through the liver in humans and therefore might be expected to have reduced systemic side effects. It has been suggested that it is moderately effective as a monotherapy in dogs with inflammatory bowel disease when compared with other steroids (such as prednisolone). Systemic side effects were still seen in some patients. The dosing of this drug is unclear as it comes in a capsule of 0.3 mg and the dose is extrapolated from humans (no real pharamcokinetic data/hepatic metabolism data available in small animals). The uncoated powder for inhalant use in people (for which no information is available in small animals) should not be used for oral administration because of hydrolysis by gastric acid.

Safety and handling: Normal precautions should be observed.

Contraindications: Intestinal perforation; severe hepatic impairment.

Adverse reactions: In theory, the rapid metabolism should give minimal systemic adverse effects. However, signs of iatrogenic hyperadrenocorticism (hair loss, muscle wastage, elevation in liver enzymes, hepatomegaly, lethargy, polyphagia and polyuria/polydipsia) may develop. Adrenal suppression has been documented in dogs and iatrogenic hypocortisolaemia is a potential risk if budesonide is withdrawn rapidly following prolonged use. In theory sudden transfer from other steroid therapy might result in signs related to reductions in steroid levels. Corticosteroids can cause severe immunosuppression in rabbits; use with care.

Drug interactions: Additive effect if given with other corticosteroids. The metabolism of corticosteroids may be decrease by antifungals. Avoid using antacids, erythromycin, cimetidine, itraconazole and other drugs that inhibit the liver enzymes that metabolize budesonide.

DOSES
Dogs: Doses ranging from 0.05 to 0.99 mg/kg/day. The total dose should probably not exceed 3 mg p.o. q8h.
Cats: Total dose should probably not exceed 1 mg p.o. q8h.
Small mammals: Ferrets: Doses of up to 1 mg/ferret q24h have been suggested for the management of IBD.
Birds, Reptiles: No information available.

Bupivacaine
(Marcain*, Sensorcaine*) **POM**

Formulations: Injectable: 2.5, 5.0, 7.5 mg/ml solutions, 2.5, 5.0 mg/ml solution with 1:200,000 adrenaline.

Action: Reversible blockade of the sodium channel in nerve fibres produces local anaesthesia.

Use: Provision of analgesia by perineural nerve blocks, regional and epidural techniques. Onset of action is significantly slower than lidocaine (20–30 min for epidural analgesia) but duration of action is relatively prolonged (6–8 h). Lower doses should be used when

A
B
C
D
E
F
G
H
I
J
K
L
M
N
O
P
Q
R
S
T
U
V
W
X
Y
Z

systemic absorption is likely to be high (e.g. intrapleural analgesia). Small volumes of bupivacaine can be diluted with normal saline to enable wider distribution of the drug for perineural blockade. Doses of bupivacaine up to 2 mg/kg q8h are unlikely to be associated with systemic side effects if injected perineurally, epidurally or intrapleurally. Combining bupivacaine with lidocaine can prolong the duration of the sensory block whilst limiting the duration of the motor block compared with administration of bupivacaine alone.

Safety and handling: Normal precautions should be observed.

Contraindications: Do not give i.v. or use for i.v. regional anaesthesia. Use of bupivacaine with adrenaline is not recommended when local vasoconstriction is undesirable (e.g. end arterial sites) or when a significant degree of systemic absorption is likely.

Adverse reactions: Inadvertent intravascular injection may precipitate severe cardiac arrhythmias that are refractory to treatment.

Drug interactions: All local anaesthetics share similar side effects, therefore the dose of bupivacaine should be reduced when used in combination with other local anaesthetics.

DOSES
Dogs:
- Perineural: volume of injection depends on the site of placement and size of the animal. As a guide: 0.1 ml/kg for femoral, radial and sciatic nerve block; 0.15 ml/kg for combined ulnar, musculocutaneous, median and ulnar nerve blocks; 0.3 ml/kg for brachial plexus nerve block; 0.25–1 ml total volume for blockade of the infraorbital, mental, maxillary and mandibular nerves. Choose an appropriate concentration of bupivacaine to achieve a 1–2 mg/kg dose within these volume guidelines.
- Epidural: 1.6 mg/kg (analgesia to level of L4), 2.3 mg/kg (analgesia to level of T11–T13); 1 mg/kg bupivacaine combined with preservative-free morphine 0.1 mg/kg. Limit the total volume of solution injected into the epidural space to 1 ml/4.5 kg up to a maximum volume of 6 ml in order to limit the cranial distribution of drugs in the epidural space and prevent adverse pressure effects.
- Interpleural: 1 mg/kg diluted with normal saline to a total volume of 5–20 ml depending on the size of the animal. The solution can be instilled via a thoracotomy tube. Dilution reduces pain on injection due to the acidity of bupivacaine.

Cats: Doses as for dogs. Accurate dosing in cats is essential to prevent overdose.

Small mammals: Ferrets: 2 mg/kg local infusion; Rabbits: 1 mg/kg local infusion, do not exceed 2 mg/kg; Guinea pigs: 1–2 mg/kg for specific nerve blocks (may require dilution with saline for local infusion); Rats: 1–2 mg/kg local infusion or intradermally once.

Birds: <2 mg/kg – local infusion; may mix with dimethylsulfoxide (DMSO) for topical application preoperatively in bumblefoot.

Reptiles: 1–2 mg/kg q4–12h.

Buprenorphine

(Buprecare, Buprenodale, Vetergesic) **POM-V CD SCHEDULE 3**

Formulations: Injectable: 0.3 mg/ml solution; available in 1 ml vials that do not contain a preservative, or in 10 ml multidose bottle that contains chlorocresol as preservative.

Action: Analgesia through high affinity, low intrinsic activity and slow dissociation with the mu receptor.

Use: Relief of mild to moderate perioperative pain. As a partial agonist it antagonizes the effects of full opioid agonists (e.g. methadone, fentanyl), although the clinical relevance of interactions between full mu agonists and buprenorphine has recently been questioned. However, in practice it is not recommended to administer buprenorphine when the subsequent administration of full mu agonists is likely. If analgesia is inadequate after buprenorphine, a full mu agonist may be administered without delay. Buprenorphine may be mixed with acepromazine or dexmedetomidine to provide sedation for minor procedures or pre-anaesthetic medication. Response to all opioids is variable between individuals; therefore assessment of pain after administration is imperative. Onset of action of buprenorphine may be slower than methadone (>15 min). Duration of effect is approximately 6 hours in cats and is likely to be similar in dogs. Buprenorphine is metabolized in the liver; some prolongation of effect may be seen with impaired liver function. The multidose preparation is unpalatable given sublingually due to the preservative. There is emerging evidence that analgesic efficacy of buprenorphine s.c. may be less than similar doses of buprenorphine administered i.m. or i.v. to cats, therefore, this route is not recommended in cats or dogs. Be careful of species differences in effect in birds. Appears active for 2–5 hours in birds.

Safety and handling: Normal precautions should be observed.

Contraindications: Combination with full mu agonists is not recommended for analgesia; therefore, do not use for premedication when administration of potent opioids during surgery is anticipated.

Adverse reactions: As a partial mu agonist, side effects are rare after clinical doses. Buprenorphine crosses the placenta and may exert sedative effects in neonates born to bitches treated prior to parturition. Pain on i.m. injection of the multidose preparation has been anecdotally reported.

Drug interactions: In common with other opioids, buprenorphine will reduce the doses of other drugs required for induction and maintenance of anaesthesia.

DOSES

When used for sedation is generally given as part of a combination. See Appendix for sedation protocols in all species.

Dogs: Analgesia: 0.02 mg/kg i.v., i.m., s.c. q6h. High doses (120 µg/kg) administered by the oral transmucosal route will provide analgesia in dogs, although this route is less practical in dogs than cats due to the large volume.

Cats: Analgesia: 0.02–0.03 mg/kg i.v., i.m., s.c. q6h. Also well tolerated and effective when given oral transmucosally.

Small mammals: Analgesia: Ferrets: 0.01–0.10 mg/kg s.c., i.m., i.v. q8–12h; Rabbits: 0.01–0.05 mg/kg s.c., i.m., i.v. q6–12h (doses <0.03 mg/kg have very limited analgesic effects but still have some sedative effects); Guinea pigs, Gerbils, Hamsters, Rats: 0.01–0.05 mg/kg i.m., s.c. q6–12h; Mice: 0.05-0.1 mg/kg i.m., s.c. q6–12h. Anecdotally, oral transmucosal delivery appears effective in rabbits and chinchillas.

Birds: Analgesia: 0.01–0.05 mg/kg i.v., i.m q8–12h. African Grey Parrots: 0.25 mg/kg i.m.; Chickens: 0.25–0.5 mg/kg i.m.

Reptiles: Analgesia: 0.01–0.02 mg/kg i.m. q24–48h.

Buserelin
(Receptal) **POM-V**

Formulations: Injectable: 4 µg (micrograms)/ml solution. Authorized for use in rabbits and certain large animal species.

Action: Synthetic GnRH (gonadotrophin releasing hormone) analogue that stimulates LH and FSH production, thus causing oestrus to develop and progress.

Use: To supplement natural LH in cases of ovulation failure or delay. Will also induce lactation postpartum. In males, it may stimulate testosterone secretion and is indicated in the management of genital hypoplasia and reduced libido. In ferrets it may be used in the management of signs of oestrus. In rabbits it is used to induce ovulation postpartum for insemination and to improve conception rates. Used in birds for chronic egg laying (must be combined with husbandry changes).

Safety and handling: Normal precautions should be observed.

Contraindications: No information available.

Adverse reactions: Anaphylactic reactions may occasionally occur.

Drug interactions: No information available.

DOSES
Dogs: 4 µg (micrograms)/dog i.m. q24–48h.
Cats: 2 µg (micrograms)/cat i.m. once.
Small mammals: Ferrets: 1.5 µg (micrograms)/ferret i.m. q24h for 2 days; Rabbits: 0.8 µg (micrograms)/rabbit s.c. at time of insemination or mating; Guinea pigs: 25 µg (micrograms)/guinea pig, repeat in 2 weeks.
Birds: 0.5–1.0 µg (micrograms)/kg q48h, up to 3 times.
Reptiles: No information available.

Busulfan (Busulphan)
(Busilvex*, Myleran*) **POM**

CIL

Formulations: Oral: 2 mg tablet.

Action: An alkylating agent that interacts with cellular thio groups and nucleic acid to form DNA-DNA and DNA-protein crosslinks, resulting in inhibition of DNA synthesis and function. Cell cycle non-specific.

Use: Management of chronic granulocytic leukaemia and polycythaemia vera. Rarely used in veterinary patients.

Safety and handling: Cytotoxic drug; see Appendix and specialist texts for further advice on chemotherapeutic agents.

Contraindications: Bone marrow suppression, animals at high risk of infection.

Adverse reactions: Frequent haematological assessment is required, as excessive myelosuppression may result in irreversible bone marrow aplasia. Hyperpigmentation of the skin, progressive pulmonary fibrosis and hepatotoxicity may occur. May raise serum uric acid levels; drugs such as allopurinol may be required to control hyperuricaemia. Oral ulceration, nausea and vomiting are seen in humans.

Drug interactions: Phenytoin increases busulfan metabolism in the liver. Paracetamol and cyclophosphamide may reduce drug clearance.

DOSES
See Appendix for chemotherapy protocols and conversion of body weight to body surface area.
Dogs, Cats: 2–4 mg/m^2 p.o. q24h initially until remission achieved, then at a reduced dosage/frequency as required to maintain remission.
Small mammals, Birds, Reptiles: No information available.

Butorphanol
(Alvegesic, Dolorex, Torbugesic, Torbutrol, Torphasol) **POM-V**

Formulations: Injectable: 10 mg/ml solution. Oral: 5 mg, 10 mg tablets.

Action: Analgesia resulting from affinity for the kappa opioid receptor. Also has mu receptor antagonist properties and an antitussive action resulting from central depression of the cough mechanism.

Use: Management of mild perioperative pain. Provision of sedation through combination with acepromazine or alpha-2 agonists. Potent antitussive agent indicated for the relief of acute or chronic non-productive cough associated with tracheobronchitis, tracheitis, tonsillitis or laryngitis resulting from inflammatory conditions of the upper respiratory tract. Butorphanol has a very rapid and relatively short duration of action; in different models analgesia has been shown to last between 45 minutes and 4 hours. Butorphanol is metabolized in the liver and some prolongation of effect may be seen with impaired liver function. Butorphanol crosses the placenta and may exert sedative effects in neonates born to bitches treated prior to parturition. Butorphanol is unlikely to be adequate for the management of severe pain. Higher doses of full mu agonists may be needed to provide additional analgesia after butorphanol but it is not necessary to wait 4h after butorphanol administration to give other opioids. Response to all opioids appears to be very variable between individuals; therefore assessment of pain after administration is imperative. Be careful of species differences in effect in birds.

Safety and handling: Protect from light.

Contraindications: Animals with diseases of the lower respiratory tract associated with copious mucous production. Premedication when administration of potent opioids during surgery is anticipated.

Adverse reactions: As a kappa agonist/mu antagonist, side effects such as respiratory depression, bradycardia and vomiting are rare after clinical doses. Cough suppression following torbugesic tablets may be associated with mild sedation.

Drug interactions: In common with other opioids, butorphanol will reduce the doses of other drugs required for induction and maintenance of anaesthesia. Combination with full mu agonists is not recommended for analgesia, addition of butorphanol will reduce analgesia produced from the full mu agonist.

DOSES
When used for sedation is generally given as part of a combination. See Appendix for sedation protocols in all species.
Dogs:
- Analgesia: 0.2–0.5 mg/kg i.v., i.m., s.c.
- Antitussive: 0.05–0.1 mg/kg i.v., i.m., s.c., 0.5–1 mg/kg p.o q6–12h.
Cats: Analgesia: 0.2–0.5 mg/kg i.v., i.m., s.c.
Small mammals: Analgesia: Ferrets: 0.25–0.4 mg/kg s.c. q4–6h; Rabbits: 0.1–0.5 mg/kg s.c q4h; Chinchilla: 0.5–2 mg/kg s.c. q4h; Guinea pigs: 0.2–2 mg/kg s.c. q4h; Gerbils, Hamsters, Rats, Mice: 1–5 mg/kg s.c. q4h.
Birds: Analgesia: 0.3–4 mg/kg i.m., i.v. q6–12h.
Reptiles: Analgesia: 0.5–2 mg/kg i.m.

Butylscopolamine (Hyoscine)
(Buscopan) **POM-V, P**

Formulations: Injectable: 4 mg/ml butylscopolamine + 500 mg/ml metamizole in 100 ml multidose bottle (Buscopan Compositum);

20 mg/ml butylscopolamine only, in 2 ml ampoules. Oral: 10 mg tablet containing butylscopolamine only.

Action: Inhibits M1 muscarinic acetylcholine receptors in the GI and urinary tracts causing smooth muscle relaxation but does not cross blood-brain barrier.

Use: Control of diarrhoea in dogs, particularly when pain or abdominal discomfort is present. Control of pain associated with urinary obstruction in dogs. Should be used in combination with investigations into the cause of abdominal pain or definitive relief of urinary obstruction.

Safety and handling: Avoid self-injection: metamizole can cause reversible but potentially serious agranulocytosis and skin allergies. Protect solution from light.

Contraindications: Intestinal obstruction. Contraindicated for the treatment of gastrointestinal ileus in rabbits.

Adverse reactions: Dry mouth, blurred vision, hesitant micturition and constipation at doses acting as gut neuromuscular relaxants. The i.m. route may cause a local reaction. See also Metamizole.

Drug interactions: Metamizole should not be given to dogs that have been treated with a phenothiazine, as hypothermia may result. Effects may be potentiated by concurrent use of other anticholinergic or analgesic drugs.

DOSES
Dogs: 0.1 ml/kg i.v., i.m. q12h; 0.5 mg/kg i.m., p.o. q12h.
Cats: Do not use.
Small mammals: Rabbits: 0.1 ml/kg i.v., i.m. q12h (Buscopan Compositum) as analgesic/antispasmolytic.
Birds, Reptiles: No information available.

Cabergoline
(Galastop) **POM-V**

Formulations: Oral: 50 μg/ml solution.

Action: Potent selective inhibition of prolactin.

Use: Induction of oestrus, control of false pregnancy in the bitch, including associated behavioural problems, and galactostasis in lactating bitches. May also be used to induce abortion in bitches and queens. Has been used for pituitary adenomas in rats. May have beneficial effect in birds with chronic egg laying and other hormonal disorders when combined with management changes. Generally ineffective if given for short periods in rabbits due to lack of clearly defined oestrus.

Safety and handling: Normal precautions should be observed.

Contraindications: Do not use in pregnant bitches unless abortion is desired. Should not be used in combination with hypotensive drugs or in animals in a hypotensive state.

Adverse reactions: Vomiting or anorexia may occur after the first one or two doses in a small proportion of cases; there is no need to discontinue treatment unless vomiting is severe or it persists beyond the second dose. In some animals a degree of drowsiness may be seen in the first 2 days of dosing. May induce transient hypotension.

Drug interactions: Metoclopramide antagonizes the effects on prolactin.

DOSES
Dogs: 5 μg (micrograms)/kg p.o. q24h for 4–6 days. Control of aggression-related signs may require dosing for 2 weeks. To induce abortion: 15 μg/kg p.o. between days 30 and 42.
Cats: To induce abortion: 15 μg (micrograms)/kg p.o. between days 30 and 42.
Small mammals: Rats: 10–50 μg (micrograms)/kg q12–24h.
Birds: 10–50 μg (micrograms)/kg p.o. q24h.
Reptiles: No information available.

CaEDTA see Edetate calcium disodium

Calcium acetate
(Phosex*, PhosLo*) **POM**

Formulations: Oral: 1 g tablet; 667 mg capsule (calcium 169 mg, Ca^{2+} 4.2 mmol).

Action: Binds phosphorus in GI tract, thus lowering serum phosphate levels over a wider range of pH than calcium carbonate.

Use: Phosphate reduction in chronic renal failure. Phosphate-binding agents are usually only used if low phosphate diets are unsuccessful. Monitor serum phosphate levels at 10–14 day intervals and adjust dosage accordingly if trying to normalize serum concentrations.

Safety and handling: Normal precautions should be observed.

Contraindications: Hypercalcaemia and calcium urolithiasis. Generally contraindicated in rabbits due to tendency to increase calcium content of urine.

Adverse reactions: Risk of increasing the calcium:phosphate ratio and thus the incidence of soft tissue and vascular calcification.

Drug interactions: May affect absorption of tetracycline and fluoroquinolone antibiotics. Increased risk of hypercalcaemia with concurrent calcitriol administration.

DOSES
Dogs, Cats: 20–40 mg/kg p.o. with each meal.
Small mammals: Rabbits: see above.
Birds, Reptiles: No information available.

Calcium salts (Calcium borogluconate, Calcium carbonate, Calcium chloride, Calcium gluconate, Calcium lactate)

((Calcichew*) Many cattle preparations, e.g. Calcibor. Minor component of Aqupharm No.9 and No.11. Several generic formulations.) **POM-V**

Formulations: There are many formulations available; a selection is given here.
- Injectable: 200 mg/ml calcium borogluconate solution equivalent to 15 mg/ml calcium formed from 168 mg/ml of calcium gluconate and 34 mg/ml boric acid (Calcibor 20); 100 mg/ml (10%) calcium chloride solution containing 27.3 mg/ml elemental calcium (= 1.36 mEq calcium/ml = 680 μmol/ml); 100 mg/ml calcium gluconate solution 10 ml ampoules containing 9 mg elemental calcium/ml (= mEq calcium/ml).
- Oral: 600 mg calcium gluconate tablets (= 53.4 mg elemental calcium); 1250 mg chewable calcium carbonate tablets (Calcichew) (= 500 mg elemental calcium).
- Note on other formulations: 11.2 mg calcium gluconate, 13.3 mg calcium borogluconate, 7.7 mg calcium lactate, 3.6 mg calcium chloride; each contains 1 mg elemental calcium = 0.5 mEq calcium.

Action: Calcium is an essential element involved in maintenance of numerous homeostatic roles and key reactions including activation of key enzymes, cell membrane potentials and nerve and musculoskeletal function.

Use: Management of hypocalcaemia and hyperkalaemic cardiotoxicity associated with urinary obstruction. Calcium gluconate and borogluconate are preferred for this. Serum calcium levels and renal function tests should be assessed before starting therapy. ECG monitoring during i.v. infusions is advised. Avoid using mixed electrolyte solutions intended for cattle use if possible. Treatment of hyperkalaemic cardiotoxicity with calcium rapidly corrects arrhythmias but effects are short-lived (5–10 min to effect) and i.v. glucose 0.5–1 g/kg ± insulin may be needed to decrease serum potassium. Parenteral calcium should be used very cautiously in patients receiving digitalis glycosides or those with cardiac or renal disease.

Safety and handling: Normal precautions should be observed.

Contraindications: Ventricular fibrillation or hypercalcaemia. Calcium should be avoided in pregnancy unless there is a deficient state. Hyperkalaemia associated with hypoadrenocorticism is often associated with hypercalcaemia and therefore additional calcium is not recommended in those cases.

Adverse reactions: Hypercalcaemia can occur, especially in renal impairment or cardiac disease. Tissue irritation is common and can occur with injectable preparation regardless of route. Rapid injection may cause hypotension, cardiac arrhythmias and cardiac arrest. Perivascular administration is treated by stopping the infusion, infiltrating the tissue with normal saline and topical application of corticosteroids. Use i.v. in dehydrated reptiles and birds may precipitate gout.

Drug interactions: Patients on digitalis glycosides are more prone to develop arrhythmias if given i.v. calcium. All calcium salts may antagonize verapamil and other calcium-channel blockers. Calcium borogluconate is compatible with most i.v. fluids except those containing other divalent cations or phosphorus. Calcium borogluconate is reportedly compatible with lidocaine, adrenaline and hydrocortisone. Calcium chloride is incompatible with amphotericin B, cefalotin sodium and chlorphenamine. Calcium gluconate is incompatible with many drugs, including lipid emulsions, propofol, amphotericin B, cefamandole, naftate, cefalotin sodium, dobutamine, methylprednisolone sodium succinate and metoclopramide. Consult manufacturers' data sheets for incompatibilities with other solutions.

DOSES

Dogs:
- Parenteral: 50–150 mg/kg calcium (boro)gluconate = 0.5–1.5 ml/kg of a 10% solution i.v. over 20–30 min (equivalent to 3.8–11.4 mg/kg calcium borogluconate or 4.5–14 mg/kg calcium gluconate). Alternatively 5–10 mg/kg calcium chloride or 0.05–0.1 ml/kg of a 10% solution i.v. (equivalent to 0.068–0.136 mEq/kg). Additional doses to a maximum of 1–1.5 g/kg calcium boro(gluconate) may need to be administered i.v. over the next 24 hours. Adjust dose by monitoring serum calcium and phosphorus levels.

- Oral treatment of hypocalcaemia: 5–22 mg of elemental calcium/kg p.o. q8h; adjust dose by monitoring serum calcium and phosphorus levels.

Cats:
- Parenteral: 95–140 mg calcium gluconate/kg slowly i.v. to effect. Using 10% calcium gluconate this is equivalent to 1–1.5 ml/kg slowly i.v. over 10–20 min. Monitor ECG if possible. If bradycardia, or Q–T interval shortening occurs, slow rate or temporarily discontinue. Once life-threatening signs are resolved, add calcium gluconate to i.v. fluids and administer slowly at 60–90 mg/kg/day elemental calcium. This converts to 2.5 ml/kg of 10% calcium gluconate q6–8h or the equivalent as a constant rate infusion over 24h. Monitor serum calcium and adjust as needed.
- Oral: Begin oral therapy at 10–25 mg elemental calcium/kg q6–8h; adjust dose by monitoring serum calcium and phosphorus levels.

Small mammals: Chinchillas, Guinea pigs: 100 mg/kg i.m., i.p.

Birds: Egg retention, hypocalcaemia: 150–200 mg/kg calcium borogluconate i.m., s.c.; Hypocalcaemia: 5–10 mg/kg calcium gluconate i.m. q12h.

Reptiles: Egg retention, hypocalcaemia: 100 mg/kg calcium borogluconate i.v., i.m., s.c. or 50–100 mg/kg calcium gluconate i.m., s.c. Use before oxytocin for egg retention. Dilute both 1 in 10 with water for injection or dextrose-saline before use.

Carbimazole
(Vidalta) POM-V

Formulations: Oral: 10 mg, 15 mg tablets in a sustained release formulation.

Action: Carbimazole is metabolized to the active drug methimazole, which interferes with the synthesis of thyroid hormones.

Use: Control of thyroid hormone levels in cats with hyperthyroidism. Has also been used in canine hyperthyroidism. There are no data on the use of the sustained release formulation in dogs.

Safety and handling: Normal precautions should be observed.

Contraindications: No information available.

Adverse reactions: Vomiting and inappetence/anorexia may be seen but are often transient. Jaundice, cytopenias, immune-mediated diseases and dermatological changes (pruritus, alopecia and self-induced trauma) are reported but rarely seen. Treatment of hyperthyroidism can decrease glomerular filtration rate, thereby raising serum urea and creatinine values, and can occasionally unmask occult renal failure. Animals that have an adverse reaction to methimazole are likely also to have an adverse reaction to carbimazole.

Drug interactions: Carbimazole should be discontinued before iodine-131 treatment. Do not use with low iodine prescription diets.

DOSES
Dogs, Cats: Starting dose 15 mg/animal p.o. q24h unless total thyroxine concentrations are <100 nmol/l in which case starting dose is 10 mg p.o. q24h. Adjust dose in 5 mg increments but do not break tablets.
Small mammals, Birds, Reptiles: No information available.

Carbomer 980
(Lubrithal) **P, general sale**

Formulations: Ophthalmic: 0.2% (10 g tube, single-use vial), 0.25% (10 g tube) gel. This formulation is marketed specifically for small animals. Other formulations are widely available for general sale.

Action: Mucinomimetic, replacing both aqueous and mucin components of the tear film.

Use: Tear replacement and beneficial for management of quantitative (keratoconjunctivitis sicca (KCS) or dry eye) and qualitative tear film disorders. It has longer corneal contact time than the aqueous tear substitutes.

Safety and handling: Normal precautions should be observed.

Contraindications: No information available.

Adverse reactions: It is tolerated well and ocular irritation is unusual.

Drug interactions: No information available.

DOSES
Dogs, Cats, Small mammals: 1 drop per eye q4–6h.
Birds, Reptiles: No information available.

Carboplatin
(Carboplatin*, Paraplatin*) **POM**

Formulations: Injectable: 10 mg/ml solution.

Action: Binds to DNA to form intra- and interstrand crosslinks and DNA-protein crosslinks, resulting in inhibition of DNA synthesis and function.

Use: May be of use in a number of neoplastic diseases including anal adenocarcinoma, squamous cell carcinoma, ovarian carcinoma, mediastinal carcinoma, pleural adenocarcinoma, nasal carcinoma and thyroid adenocarcinoma. Improves survival times when used as an adjunct to amputation in dogs with appendicular osteosarcoma. The drug is highly irritant and must be administered via a preplaced i.v. catheter. Do not use needles or i.v. sets containing aluminium as precipitation of the drug may occur. This drug is generally now preterred over cisplatin due to reduced GI and renal toxicity. Use with caution in patients with abnormal renal function, active infections, hearing impairment or pre-existing hepatic disease. Has been used in renal adenocarcinoma in Budgerigars and squamous cell carcinoma (mixed with bird's own plasma for intralesional use) and bile duct carcinoma in Amazon parrots. The health risks to owners of (particularly indoor) birds from such treatments need to be considered carefully before recommending chemotherapy in birds.

Safety and handling: Potent cytotoxic drug that should only be prepared and administered by trained personnel. See Appendix and specialist texts for further advice on chemotherapeutic agents.

Contraindications: No information available.

Adverse reactions: Include myelosuppression, nephrotoxicity, ototoxicity, nausea, vomiting, electrolyte abnormalities, neurotoxicity and anaphylactic reactions. However, produces fewer adverse reactions than cisplatin.

Drug interactions: Concomitant use of aminoglycosides or other nephrotoxic agents may increase risk of nephrotoxicity. May adversely affect the safety and efficacy of vaccinations.

DOSES
See Appendix for chemotherapy protocols and conversion of body weight to body surface area.
Dogs: 300 mg/m^2 i.v. q3–4wk injected into the side port of a freely running i.v. infusion of 0.9% NaCl over a 10–15 min period.
Cats: 200 mg/m^2 i.v. q3–4wk injected into the side port of a freely running i.v. infusion of 0.9% NaCl over a 10–15 min period.
Small mammals: No information available.
Birds: 5 mg/kg i.v., i.o. over 3 minutes; 5 mg/kg intralesional use (mixed with plasma to make a concentration of 10 mg/ml) for squamous cell carcinoma.
Reptiles: No information available.

Carnidazole
(Spartix*) **AVM-GSL**

Formulations: Oral: 10 mg tablet.

Action: Coccidiocidal; mode of action not known.

Use: Pigeon canker (*Trichomonas columbae*); treat all birds in loft simultaneously. It should be used in conjunction with good loft hygiene, including disinfection of feed and water bowls.

Safety and handling: Direct contact with the product must be avoided. Wear impermeable gloves when handling.

Contraindications: Not to be used in birds intended for human consumption.

Adverse reactions: No information available.

Drug interactions: None known.

DOSES

Birds: Pigeons: 12.5–25 mg p.o. once; Raptors: 25–30 mg/kg p.o., one dose normally sufficient but can be repeated next day if needed; Psittacids: 30–50 mg/kg p.o., repeat after 2 wk; Other birds: 20–30 mg/kg p.o. once.

Dogs, Cats, Small mammals, Reptiles: No information available.

Carprofen

(Canidryl, Carprodyl, Dolagis, Rimadyl, Rimifin) **POM-V**

Formulations: Injectable: 50 mg/ml. Oral: 20 mg, 50 mg, 100 mg tablets (in plain and palatable formulations).

Action: Preferentially inhibits COX-2 enzyme, thereby limiting the production of prostaglandins involved in inflammation. Other non-COX-mediated mechanisms are suspected to contribute to the anti-inflammatory effect but these have not yet been identified.

Use: Control of postoperative pain and inflammation following surgery and reduction of chronic inflammation, e.g. degenerative joint disease, osteoarthritis. In cats carprofen is only licensed as a single perioperative dose for the control of postoperative pain. Carprofen also has antipyretic effects. All NSAIDs should be administered cautiously in the perioperative period. Although carprofen preferentially inhibits COX-2, it may still adversely affect renal perfusion during periods of hypotension. If hypotension during anaesthesia is anticipated, delay carprofen administration until the animal is fully recovered from anaesthesia and normotensive. Liver disease will prolong the metabolism of carprofen, leading to the potential for drug accumulation and overdose with repeated dosing. Prolonged long-term treatment should be under veterinary supervision. In cats, due to the longer half-life and narrower therapeutic index, particular care should be taken not to exceed the recommended dose and the use of a 1 ml graduated syringe is recommended to measure the dose accurately. Tablets are not authorized for use in cats. Use with caution in birds with dehydration, shock and renal dysfunction.

Safety and handling: Formulations that use palatable tablets can be extremely palatable. Animals have been reported to eat tablets spontaneously, resulting in overdose. Ensure that tablets are stored out of animal reach. Store injectable solution in the refrigerator; once broached the product is stable for use at temperatures up to 25°C for 28 days.

Contraindications: Do not give to dehydrated, hypovolaemic or hypotensive patients or those with GI disease or blood clotting abnormalities. Administration of carprofen to animals with renal disease must be carefully evaluated and is not advisable in the perioperative period. Do not give to pregnant animals or animals <6 weeks old.

Adverse reactions: GI signs may occur in all animals after NSAID administration. Stop therapy if this persists beyond 1–2 days. Some animals develop signs with one NSAID and not another. A 1–2 wk wash-out period should be allowed before starting another NSAID after cessation of therapy. Stop therapy immediately if GI bleeding is suspected. There is a small risk that NSAIDs may precipitate cardiac failure in animals with cardiovascular disease.

Drug interactions: Different NSAIDs should not be administered within 24 hours of each other or glucocorticoids as they are more ulcerogenic when used concurrently. The nephrotoxic tendencies of all NSAIDs are significantly increased when administered concurrently with other nephrotoxic agents, e.g. aminoglycosides.

DOSES

Dogs: 4 mg/kg i.v., s.c. preoperatively or at time of anaesthetic induction; single dose should provide analgesia for up to 24h. Continued analgesia can be provided orally at 4 mg/kg/day, in single or divided dose for up to 5 days after injection. In dogs started on oral medication, subject to clinical response the dose may be reduced to 2 mg/kg/day, single dose, after 7 days.
Cats: 4 mg/kg i.v., s.c., single dose preoperatively or at time of anaesthetic induction.
Small mammals: Ferrets: 1 mg/kg p.o.; Rabbits: 2–4 mg/kg s.c. q24h, 1.5 mg/kg p.o.; Rodents: 2–5 mg/kg total daily dose i.v., i.m., s.c., p.o., in single or two divided doses; Others: 4 mg/kg i.v., i.m., s.c.
Birds: 1–5 mg/kg i.m., s.c., p.o. q12–24h (higher rate appears effective for 24 hours).
Reptiles: 4 mg/kg s.c., i.m., p.o. once, then 2 mg/kg s.c., i.m., p.o. q24h.

Carvedilol
(Cardevidol*, Eucardic*) **POM**

Formulations: Oral: 3.125 mg, 6.25 mg, 12.5 mg, 25 mg tablets.

Action: Non-selective beta-adrenergic blocker with the afterload reduction properties of an alpha-1 adrenergic blocker. Additional antioxidant properties may decrease the oxidant stress associated with heart failure.

Use: Has been advocated for use as an adjunctive therapy in the management of chronic heart failure due to valvular disease or DCM and as an antihypertensive drug in patients that do not respond to first-line therapy. Veterinary experience is limited and benefit has not been established. Limited data on pharmacokinetics and pharmacodynamics in dogs. Treatment should not be started until congestive heart failure has been stabilized for at least 2 weeks initially. Since it undergoes extensive hepatic metabolism, caution should be exercised in patients with hepatic insufficiency.

Safety and handling: Normal precautions should be observed.

Contraindications: Patients with bradyarrhythmias, acute or decompensated heart failure and bronchial disease. Do not administer concurrently with alpha-adrenergic agonists (e.g. adrenaline).

Adverse reactions: Potential side effects include lethargy, diarrhoea, bradycardia, AV block, myocardial depression, exacerbation of heart failure, syncope, hypotension and bronchospasm. A reduction in the glomerular filtration rate may exacerbate pre-existing renal impairment.

Drug interactions: The hypotensive effect of carvedilol is enhanced by many agents that depress myocardial activity including anaesthetic agents, phenothiazines, antihypertensive drugs, diuretics and diazepam. There is an increased risk of bradycardia, severe hypotension, heart failure and AV block if carvedilol is used concurrently with calcium-channel blockers. Hypotensive effect may be antagonized by NSAIDs. Concurrent digoxin administration potentiates bradycardia. Carvedilol may enhance the hypoglycaemic effect of insulin. Carvedilol increases plasma concentration of ciclosporin. Rifampin can decrease carvedilol plasma concentrations.

DOSES
Dogs: Start at 0.05–0.1 mg/kg p.o. q12h and gradually increase at 2-week intervals to target dose of 0.3–0.4 mg/kg p.o. q12h, if tolerated.
Cats: No information available.
Small mammals: Hamsters: 1–11 mg/kg p.o. q24h; Rats: 60 mg/kg p.o. q24h.
Birds, Reptiles: No information available.

CCNU see Lomustine

Cefalexin (Cephalexin)
(Cefaseptin, Cephacare, Ceporex, Rilexine, Therios)
POM-V

Formulations: Injectable: 180 mg/ml (18%) suspension. Oral: 50 mg, 75 mg, 120 mg, 250 mg, 300 mg, 500 mg, 600 mg, 750 mg tablets; granules which, when reconstituted, provide a 100 mg/ml oral syrup.

Action: Binds to proteins involved in bacterial cell wall synthesis, thereby decreasing cell wall strength and rigidity, and affecting cell division. Resistant to some bacterial beta-lactamases, particularly those produced by *Staphylococcus* spp. As for other beta-lactam antibacterials, works in a time-dependent fashion.

Use: Active against several Gram-positive and Gram-negative organisms (e.g. *Staphylococcus*, *Pasteurella* and *Escherichia coli*). *Pseudomonas* and *Proteus* are often resistant. Maintaining levels above the MIC is critical for efficacy and prolonged dosage intervals or missed doses can compromise therapeutic response. Dose and dosing interval is determined by infection site, severity and organism. In severe or acute conditions, doses may be doubled or given at more frequent intervals. Use in rabbits only when specifically indicated as can be toxic.

Safety and handling: Reconstituted oral drops should be stored in the refrigerator and discarded after 10 days.

Contraindications: Patients hypersensitive to penicillins may also be sensitive to cephalosporins (cross-hypersensitivity in <10% of human patients); avoid use in animals with reported sensitivity to other beta-lactam antimicrobials.

Adverse reactions: Vomiting and diarrhoea most common; administration with food may reduce these. Cefalexin may cause enterotoxaemia in rodents and lagomorphs. Oral administration in particular carries a significant risk of fatal enterotoxaemia. Injection may be painful.

Drug interactions: Bactericidal activity may be affected by concomitant use of bacteriostatic agents (e.g. erythromycin, oxytetracycline). May be an increased risk of nephrotoxicity if cephalosporins are used with amphotericin or loop diuretics (e.g. furosemide); monitor renal function. Do not mix in the same syringe as aminoglycosides.

DOSES
See Appendix for guidelines on responsible antibacterial use.
Dogs, Cats: 10–25 mg/kg p.o. q8–12h; i.m., s.c. q24h.
Small mammals: Ferrets: 15–30 mg/kg p.o. q8–12h; Rabbits: 15–20 mg/kg s.c. q12–24h; Guinea pigs: 25 mg/kg i.m. q12–24h; Others: 15–30 mg/kg i.m. q8–12h.
Birds: 35–100 mg/kg p.o., i.m. q6–8h.
Reptiles: 20–40 mg/kg p.o. q12h.

Cefotaxime
(Cefotaxime*) **POM**

Formulations: Injectable: 500 mg, 1 g, 2 g powders for reconstitution.

Action: A 3rd generation cephalosporin that binds to proteins involved in bacterial cell wall synthesis, thereby decreasing cell wall strength and rigidity, and affecting cell division. Resistant to many bacterial beta-lactamases, particularly those produced by *Staphylococcus* spp. As other beta-lactam antibacterials, works in a time-dependent fashion.

Use: Good activity against many Gram-negative organisms, especially Enterobacteriaceae (not *Pseudomonas*) but lower activity against many Gram-positive organisms than 1st and 2nd generation cephalosporins. It is important to maintain tissue concentrations above the MIC. Use should be reserved for: patients with acute sepsis or serious infections; where cultures are pending or culture and sensitivity testing shows sensitivity; or where other licensed preparations are not appropriate, and the animal is not a good candidate for intensive aminoglycoside therapy (e.g. pre-existing renal dysfunction). Use with care in patients with renal disease and consider increasing dose interval.

Safety and handling: The reconstituted solution is stable for 10 days when refrigerated.

Contraindications: Patients hypersensitive to penicillins may also be sensitive to cephalosporins (cross-hypersensitivity in <10% of human patients); avoid use in animals with reported sensitivity to other beta-lactam antimicrobials.

Adverse reactions: May produce pain on injection. GI disturbance and superinfection with resistant microorganisms is a potential risk.

Drug interactions: Bactericidal activity may be affected by concomitant use of bacteriostatic agents (e.g. oxytetracycline, erythromycin). The cephalosporins are synergistic with the aminoglycosides, but should not be mixed in the same syringe. May be increased risk of nephrotoxicity if cephalosporins are used with amphotericin or loop diuretics (e.g. furosemide); monitor renal function.

DOSES
See Appendix for guidelines on responsible antibacterial use.
Dogs, Cats: 20–40 mg/kg i.v., i.m., s.c. q8–12h. Some authors have suggested that lower doses of 10–20 mg/kg q12h have good clinical efficacy in the dog.
Small mammals: No information available.
Birds: 50–100 mg/kg i.m. q6–8h.
Reptiles: 20–40 mg/kg i.m. q24h.

Cefovecin
(Convenia) **POM-V**

Formulations: Injectable: Lyophilized powder which when reconstituted contains 80 mg/ml cefovecin.

Action: Binds to proteins involved in bacterial cell wall synthesis, thereby decreasing cell wall strength and rigidity, and affecting cell division. Resistant to some bacterial beta-lactamases. Assumed to work in a time-dependent fashion as other beta-lactam antibacterials.

Use: In line with rational antimicrobial use, cefovecin should not be considered if a 14 day course of antimicrobial would not ordinarily be required for the infection being treated. Specifically indicated for the prolonged treatment of skin and soft tissue infections and for infections of the urinary tract. Also used as part of the management of severe periodontal disease. Good efficacy against organisms commonly associated with these conditions (e.g. *Staphylococcus*,

Streptococcus, *Escherichia coli*, *Pasteurella multocida*, *Proteus*). Activity against anaerobes such as *Prevotella*, *Fusobacterium*, *Bacteroides* and *Clostridium* also appears to be good. Not active against *Pseudomonas*. Due to unique pharmacokinetic profile, cefovecin has an extremely long half-life and only requires administration every 14 days.

Safety and handling: Store in the refrigerator even prior to reconstitution; use reconstituted drug within 28 days.

Contraindications: Do not use in small herbivores such as rabbits, guinea pigs and rodents. Do not use in cats and dogs <8 weeks old. Avoid use during lactation and in pregnant animals, as safety has not been established.

Adverse reactions: Appears to be relatively safe but has not been assessed in renal disease. Reported adverse reactions include mild GI disturbance and transient swelling at the injection site.

Drug interactions: Highly bound to plasma proteins, therefore it would be prudent to exhibit caution when using in conjunction with other highly protein-bound drugs such as furosemide and NSAIDs.

DOSES
See Appendix for guidelines on responsible antibacterial use.
Dogs, Cats: 8 mg/kg s.c., equivalent to 1 ml/10 kg of reconstituted drug subcutaneously. May be repeated after 14 days up to three times.
Small mammals: Ferrets: 8 mg/kg s.c. every 2–3 days.
Birds: Initial data appear to show it is not practicable (half-life <2h in poultry). Further data show that the half-life in parrots is similar to that in chickens.
Reptiles: No information available.

Ceftazidime
(Fortum*, Kefadim*) **POM**

Formulations: Injectable: 500 mg, 1 g, 2 g, 3 g powders for reconstitution.

Action: A 3rd generation cephalosporin that binds to proteins involved in bacterial cell wall synthesis, thereby decreasing cell wall strength and rigidity, and affecting cell division. Resistant to some bacterial beta-lactamases. As other beta-lactam antibacterials, works in a time-dependent fashion.

Use: Higher activity against many Gram-negative organisms but lower activity against many Gram-positives when compared to 1st and 2nd generation cephalosporins. Very good activity against *Pseudomonas* in humans. Use should be limited to cases with a confirmed susceptibility and acute sepsis or serious infections where licensed preparations are found to be inappropriate. Limited information on clinical pharmacokinetics in animal species and doses given below are empirical. Important to maintain tissue concentrations above the MIC with regular doses.

Safety and handling: Normal precautions should be observed.

Contraindications: Patients hypersensitive to penicillins may also be sensitive to cephalosporins (cross-hypersensitivity in <10% of human patients); avoid use in animals with reported sensitivity to other beta-lactam antimicrobials.

Adverse reactions: GI disturbances associated with drug use in humans. Pain may be noted following injection.

Drug interactions: Bactericidal activity may be affected by concomitant use of bacteriostatic agents (e.g. oxytetracycline, erythromycin). May be an increased risk of nephrotoxicity if cephalosporins are used with amphotericin or loop diuretics (e.g. furosemide); monitor renal function. Do not mix in the same syringe as aminoglycosides. Ceftazidime is synergistic with the aminoglycoside antimicrobials *in vivo* (often used in humans for pseudomonal infection in neutropenic patients).

DOSES
See Appendix for guidelines on responsible antibacterial use.
Dogs, Cats: 20–50 mg/kg i.v. q8–12h.
Small mammals: Rabbits: 100 mg/kg i.m. q12h.
Birds: 75–200 mg/kg i.v., i.m. q6–12h.
Reptiles: Most species: 20 mg/kg i.m., s.c., i.v. q72h; Chameleons: 20 mg/kg i.m., s.c. q24–48h.

Ceftiofur
(Excenel) **POM-V**

Formulations: Injectable: 1 g, 4 g powder for reconstitution; 50 mg/ml suspension.

Action: Binds to proteins involved in bacterial cell wall synthesis, thereby decreasing cell wall strength and rigidity and affecting cell division. Resistant to many bacterial beta-lactamases, particularly those produced by *Staphylococcus* spp. Uniquely among the cephalosporins, ceftiofur is metabolized to desfuroylceftiofur which is an active metabolite. Action is time-dependent.

Use: Higher activity against many Gram-negative organisms, especially Enterobacteriaceae (not *Pseudomonas*) but lower activity against many Gram-positives than 1st and 2nd generation cephalosporins. Particularly useful for tortoises with bacterial respiratory tract infections (e.g. *Pasteurella* or Gram-negative bacteria). Use should be reserved for patients suffering from acute sepsis or serious infections where cultures are pending, other licensed preparations are not appropriate and the animal is not a good candidate for intensive aminoglycoside therapy (pre-existing renal dysfunction). Important to maintain tissue concentrations above the MIC. Authorized for use in dogs in other countries where the main indication for use is in the treatment of urinary tract infections. Use with care in patients with renal disease and consider increasing dose interval.

Safety and handling: Store powder in the refrigerator; once reconstituted store in the refrigerator and discard after 7 days or within 12 hours if stored at room temperature.

Contraindications: Patients hypersensitive to penicillins may also be sensitive to cephalosporins (cross-hypersensitivity in <10% of human patients); avoid use in animals with reported sensitivity to other beta-lactam antimicrobials.

Adverse reactions: May produce pain on injection. GI disturbance and superinfection with resistant microorganisms is a potential risk. May be an increased risk of nephrotoxicity if cephalosporins are used with amphotericin or loop diuretics (e.g. furosemide); monitor renal function. In dogs a dose- and duration-dependent anaemia and thrombocytopenia has been recorded, although this should not occur with recommended doses.

Drug interactions: Bactericidal activity may be affected by concomitant use of bacteriostatic agents (e.g. oxytetracycline, erythromycin). The cephalosporins are synergistic with the aminoglycosides, but should not be mixed in the same syringe.

DOSES
See Appendix for guidelines on responsible antibacterial use.
Dogs: 2.2 mg/kg s.c. q24h.
Cats, Small mammals: No information available.
Birds: Amazons: 10 mg/kg i.m. q8–12h; Cockatiels: 10 mg/kg i.m. q4h; in some cases, higher doses (up to 100 mg/kg) may be necessary.
Reptiles: Chelonians: 4 mg/kg i.m. q24h; Snakes: 2.2 mg/kg i.m. q48h.

Cefuroxime
(Zinacef*, Zinnat*) **POM**

Formulations: Injectable: 250 mg, 750 mg, 1.5 g powders for reconstitution (sodium salt). Oral (as cefuroxime axetil): 125 mg, 250 mg tablets; 125 mg/5 ml suspension.

Action: A 2nd generation cephalosporin that binds to proteins involved in bacterial cell wall synthesis, thereby decreasing cell wall strength and rigidity, and affecting cell division. Resistant to some bacterial beta-lactamases. As other beta-lactam antibacterials, works in a time-dependent fashion. Cefuroxime axetil is hydrolysed in intestinal mucosa and liver to yield active drug giving oral bioavailability.

Use: Higher activity against many Gram-negative organisms when compared to 1st generation cephalosporins. Good activity against a wider spectrum of Enterobacteriaceae (not *Pseudomonas*). Many obligate anaerobes also susceptible. It is a time-dependent antimicrobial, so maintaining levels above the MIC are important for efficacy. Limited applications in veterinary species and limited pharmacokinetic data make appropriate dose selection problematical. **See Appendix for further information on surgical prophylaxis.**

Safety and handling: Normal precautions should be observed.

Contraindications: Patients hypersensitive to penicillins may also be sensitive to cephalosporins (cross-hypersensitivity in <10% of human patients); avoid use in animals with reported sensitivity to other beta-lactam antimicrobials.

Adverse reactions: May cause pain on i.m. and s.c. injection. GI disturbance has been reported in humans, particularly associated with the oral axetil formulation.

Drug interactions: Bactericidal activity may be affected by concomitant use of bacteriostatic agents (e.g. oxytetracycline, erythromycin). May be an increased risk of nephrotoxicity if cephalosporins are used with amphotericin or loop diuretics (e.g. furosemide); monitor renal function. Synergistic with aminoglycosides, do not mix in the same syringe.

DOSES
See Appendix for guidelines on responsible antibacterial use.
Dogs, Cats: 10–15 mg/kg i.v. q8–12h.
Small mammals: No information available.
Birds: No information available.
Reptiles: 100 mg/kg i.m. q24h for 10 days at 30°C.

Cephalexin see **Cefalexin**

Cetirizine
(Piriteze*, Zirtec*) **GSL**

Formulations: Oral: 10 mg tablets; 5 mg/5 ml solution.

Action: Binds to H1 histamine receptors to prevent histamine from binding.

Use: Management of allergic disease and prevention and early treatment of anaphylaxis. Cetirizine is a metabolite of hydroxyzine. Less sedative effect in humans that chlorpheniramine.

Safety and handling: Normal precautions should be observed.

Contraindications: None reported.

Adverse reactions: May reduce seizure threshold.

Drug interactions: None reported.

DOSES

Dogs: 1 mg/kg p.o. q24h.
Cats: 5 mg/cat p.o. q24h.
Small mammals, Birds, Reptiles: No information available.

Charcoal (Activated charcoal)
(Actidose-Aqua*, Charcodote*, Liqui-Char*) AVM-GSL

Formulations: Oral: 50 g activated charcoal powder or premixed slurry (200 mg/ml).

Action: Absorbs toxins, fluids and gases in the GI tract. Activated charcoal has increased porosity and enhanced absorptive capacity.

Use: In acute poisoning with organophosphates, carbamates, chlorinated hydrocarbons, strychnine, ethylene glycol, inorganic and organic arsenical and mercurial compounds, polycyclic organic compounds (most pesticides), and dermal toxicants that may be ingested following grooming. As a general rule administer at a dose of at least 10 times the volume of intoxicant ingested. Repeat dosing as required if emesis or massive toxin ingestion occurs. Repeated dosing necessary if highly lipid-soluble toxins, which are likely to undergo enterohepatic recirculation, have been ingested.

Safety and handling: Activated charcoal powder floats, covering everything in the area; prepare very carefully as it will stain permanently.

Contraindications: Activated charcoal should not be used prior to the use of emetics.

Adverse reactions: Charcoal colours stools black, which is medically insignificant but may be alarming to the owner.

Drug interactions: Activated charcoal reduces the absorption and therefore efficacy of orally administered drugs.

DOSES

Dogs, Cats: 0.5–4 g p.o. of activated charcoal/kg as a slurry in water by stomach tube; usually followed by a saline cathartic 20–30 min later.
Small mammals: 0.5–5 g/kg p.o. (anecdotal).
Birds: No information available.
Reptiles: Chelonians: 2–8 g/kg by stomach tube.

Chitosan
(Ipakitine) GSL

Formulations: Oral: powder containing 8% chitosan, 10% calcium carbonate and 82% lactose.

Action: Adsorbent for intestinal uraemic toxins, including phosphate.

Use: The combination has been shown to reduce serum urea and phosphate in chronic renal disease in cats. Phosphate-binding agents are usually only used if low phosphate diets are unsuccessful. Monitor serum phosphate levels at 10–14 day intervals and adjust dosage accordingly if trying to normalize serum concentrations. As formulation contains lactose, use with care in diabetic and lactose-intolerant animals.

Safety and handling: Normal precautions should be observed.

Contraindications: Not advised in rabbits due to the risk of hypercalcuria.

Adverse reactions: Hypercalcaemia, possibly due to the calcium carbonate component.

Drug interactions: None noted.

DOSES
Dogs, Cats: 200 mg/kg p.o. q12h (mixed with food).
Small mammals: Ferrets: 0.5 mg/kg on food q12h (anecdotal).
Birds, Reptiles: No information available.

Chlorambucil

(Leukeran*) **POM**

Formulations: Oral: 2 mg tablet.

Action: Alkylating agent that inhibits DNA synthesis and function through cross-linking with cellular DNA. Cell cycle non-specific.

Use: Management of some malignancies, lymphoproliferative, myeloproliferative and immune-mediated diseases. Immunosuppressive effect is not well defined and therefore it should only be considered where more established therapies such as prednisolone and azathioprine have failed. May be useful in the treatment of feline pemphigus foliaceus and severe feline eosinophilic granuloma complex. Has been used in lymphosarcoma in cockatoos.

Safety and handling: Cytotoxic drug; see Appendix and specialist texts for further advice on chemotherapeutic agents. Tablets should be stored in a closed, light-protected container under refrigeration (2–8°C).

Contraindications: Bone marrow suppression, factors predisposing to infection.

Adverse reactions: Anorexia, nausea, vomiting, leucopenia, thrombocytopenia, anaemia (rarely), neurotoxicity (1 case reported in a cat), alopecia (rarely) and slow regrowth of clipped hair coat.

Drug interactions: Drugs that stimulate hepatic cytochrome P450 system increase cytotoxic effects. Prednisolone has a synergistic effect in the management of lymphoid neoplasia.

DOSES

See Appendix for chemotherapy protocols and conversion of body weight to body surface area.

Dogs:

- Chronic lymphocytic leukaemia: 2–6 mg/m² p.o. q24h initially until remission achieved, then at reduced dosage/frequency as required to maintain remission; or 0.2 mg/kg q24h for 7 days then 0.1 mg/kg q24h for maintenance; or 20 mg/m² every 1–2 weeks. Often used with prednisolone 40 mg/m² p.o. q24h for 7 days then 20 mg/m² q48h.
- Lymphoma: 15–20 mg/m² p.o. q2wk with prednisolone; or 2–6 mg/m² q24–48h. 1.4 mg/kg p.o. as single dose as substitute for cyclophosphamide in CHOP-type protocols.
- Pemphigus complex (in combination with corticosteroids): 0.1–0.2 mg/kg p.o. q24h initially until marked improvement of clinical signs; then alternate-day dosing, often for several weeks.
- Other immune-mediated diseases: 1–2 mg/m² p.o. q24h.

Cats:

- Immune-mediated disease: Cats >4 kg: 2 mg (total dose) p.o. q48h for 2–4 weeks, then tapered to lowest effective dose; cats <4 kg started at 2 mg (total dose) q72h.
- Chronic lymphocytic leukaemia: 2 mg/m2 p.o. q48h or 20 mg/m² q14d, with or without prednisolone.
- Feline pemphigus foliaceus or severe feline eosinophilic granuloma complex (in combination with corticosteroids): 0.1–0.2 mg/kg p.o. q24h until marked improvement of clinical signs; then alternate-day dosing, often for several weeks.

Small mammals: No information available.

Birds: Lymphosarcoma: 1–2 mg/kg p.o. twice weekly.

Reptiles: No information available.

Chloramphenicol

(Chloramphenicol*, Chloromycetin Ophthalmic Ointment*, Chloromycetin Redidrops*, Kemicetine*) **POM**

Formulations: Injectable: 1 g powder for reconstitution. Topical: Ophthalmic 1% ointment; 0.5% solution. Oral: 250 mg capsules.

Action: Bacteriostatic antimicrobial that acts by binding to the 50S ribosomal subunit of susceptible bacteria, preventing bacterial protein synthesis.

Use: Broad spectrum of activity against Gram-positive (e.g. *Streptococcus*, *Staphylococcus*), Gram-negative (e.g. *Brucella*, *Salmonella*, *Haemophilus*) and obligate anaerobic bacteria (e.g. *Clostridium*, *Bacteroides fragilis*). Other sensitive organisms include *Chlamydophila*, *Mycoplasma* (unreliable in treatment of ocular mycoplasmosis) and *Rickettsia*. Resistant organisms include *Nocardia* and *Mycobacterium*. Acquired resistance may occur in

Enterobacteriaceae. High lipid solubility makes it suitable for the treatment of intraocular infections. It will also access the CNS. However, due to concerns of resistance development and human toxicity use should be restricted to individual animals where there is a specific indication such as salmonellosis resistant to other antimicrobials or deep infections of the eye. Patients with hepatic or renal dysfunction may need adjustment to dose. Decrease dose or increase dosing interval in neonates. Use with caution or avoid in nursing bitches or queens, especially those with neonates, as crosses into milk.

Safety and handling: Humans exposed to chloramphenicol may have an increased risk of developing a fatal aplastic anaemia. Products should be handled with care; use impervious gloves and avoid skin contact.

Contraindications: No information available.

Adverse reactions: Dose-related reversible bone marrow suppression can develop in all species. Unlike humans, the development of irreversible aplastic anaemia in veterinary species does not appear to be a significant problem. The cat, which has a reduced capacity to metabolize chloramphenicol, is more susceptible to bone marrow suppression and this is associated with both dose size and duration of therapy. Other adverse effects include nausea, vomiting, diarrhoea and anaphylaxis.

Drug interactions: Irreversible inhibitor of a large number of hepatic cytochrome P450-dependent enzymes and so increases plasma levels of pentobarbital, phenobarbital and oral hypoglycaemic agents. Recovery requires synthesis of new liver enzymes and can take up to 3 weeks. Rifampin accelerates the metabolism of chloramphenicol, thus decreasing serum levels. Chloramphenicol may inhibit activity of bactericidal antimicrobials such as the aminoglycosides and beta-lactams. May also be an inhibitory effect if used in combination with macrolide or lincosamide antimicrobials.

DOSES
See Appendix for guidelines on responsible antibacterial use.
Dogs: Ophthalmic: 1 drop q4–8h; ointment q8–12h. Systemic: 25–50 mg/kg i.v., i.m., s.c., p.o. q8–12h. CNS infections: 10–15 mg/kg p.o. q4–6h is recommended in some texts.
Cats: Ophthalmic: 1 drop q4–8h; ointment q8–12h. Systemic: 15–25 mg/kg slow i.v., i.m., s.c., p.o. q12h.
Small mammals: Ferrets: 25–50 mg/kg p.o., s.c., i.m., i.v. q12h; Rabbits: 50 mg/kg p.o., s.c. (ophthalmic drops) q12–24h; Mice: 50 mg/kg i.m., p.o. q12h, 200 mg/kg p.o. q12h or 0.5 mg/ml drinking water; Other rodents: 30–50 mg/kg i.v., i.m., s.c., p.o. q8–12h or, in drinking water, 1 mg/ml for Guinea pigs, 0.83 mg/ml for Gerbils.
Birds: 50 mg/kg i.v., i.m. q8h; 75 mg/kg p.o. q8h; Pigeons: 25 mg/kg p.o. q12h.
Reptiles: 40–50 mg/kg i.m., s.c., p.o. q24h.

Chlorhexidine

(Hibiscrub, Malaseb, Microbex, Savlon, Chlorohex*, CLX wipes*, Otodine*, TrizChlor*, Viatop*) **POM-V, AVM-GSL**

Formulations: Topical shampoo: 2% chlorhexidine + 2% miconazole (Malaseb); 31.2 mg/ml chlorhexidine (Microbex); Cleansing solution: 1.5% chlorhexidine + cetrimide (Savlon); Surgical scrub solution: 4% chlorhexidine + isopropyl alcohol (Hibiscrub); Mouthwash: 0.12% chlorhexidine (Chlorohex); Topical gel: 0.06% chlorhexidine, aqua, raffinose, propylene glycol, saponins, triethanolamine, acrylates, phenoxyethanol, benzoic acid esters, allantoin (Viatop); Topical skin cleaner: Chlorhexidine, Tris-EDTA, zinc gluconate, glycerine, climbazole, benzyl alcohol, propylene glycol (CLX wipes); Ear cleaner: 0.15% chlorhexidine + EDTA (TrizChlor); Chlorhexidine, Tris-EDTA, lactic acid (Otodine).

Action: Chemical antiseptic that disrupts bacterial cell membrane.

Use: Topical treatment of bacterial, dermatophyte and *Malassezia* skin infections in dogs as a shampoo (Malaseb). Topical treatment of *Malassezia* infections (Microbex). Washing surgical instruments, routine antisepsis for surgical operations (Savlon, Hibiscrub) and dental hygiene (Chlorohex). Topical treatment of mild pruritus (Viatop). Concurrent systemic antibacterial therapy is generally advised when treating bacterial skin infections. Leave in contact with the skin for 5–10 minutes prior to washing off. Ear cleaners for cleansing and removal of cerumen. Chlorhexidine as a single agent is not consistently effective as an antifungal.

Safety and handling: Normal precautions should be observed.

Contraindications: Do not instil into ears where the integrity of the tympanum is unknown. Do not use on eyes.

Adverse reactions: Ototoxic. May irritate mucous membranes.

Drug interactions: Not known.

DOSES

Dogs, Cats: Shampoo 2–3 times weekly. May be used less frequently once infection is controlled.

Small mammals: Apply to affected area q8h at 0.5–2.0% concentrations. 0.05% solution in water can be used as a safe wound flush. When treating dermatophytosis continue treatment for 2 weeks after apparent clinical cure and negative fungal culture results. Otic: Dilute topical products to a 1.0% concentration and apply topically q8–12h.

Birds: Doses as for dogs and cats.

Reptiles: No information available.

Chlorphenamine (Chlorpheniramine) CIL
(Piriton*) **POM, GSL**

Formulations: Injectable: 10 mg/ml solution. Oral: 4 mg tablet, 0.4 mg/ml syrup.

Action: Binds to H1 histamine receptors to prevent histamine binding.

Use: Management of allergic disease and prevention and early treatment of anaphylaxis. Commonly used as premedication before transfusions and certain chemotherapeutic agents. Specific doses for dogs and cats have not been determined by pharmacokinetic studies. Use with caution in cases with urinary retention, angle-closure glaucoma and pyloroduodenal obstruction.

Safety and handling: Normal precautions should be observed.

Contraindications: No information available.

Adverse reactions: May cause mild sedation. May reduce seizure threshold.

Drug interactions: No information available.

DOSES
Dogs: 4–8 mg/dog p.o. q8h; 2.5–10 mg/dog i.m. or slow i.v.
Cats: 2–4 mg/cat p.o. q8–12h; 2–5 mg/cat i.m. or slow i.v.
Small mammals: Ferrets: 1–2 mg/kg p.o. q8–12h; Rabbits: 0.2–0.4 mg/kg p.o. q12h; Rodents: 0.6 mg/kg p.o. q24h.
Birds, Reptiles: No information available.

Cholestyramine see Colestyramine

Chorionic gonadotrophin (Human chorionic gonadotrophin, hCG)
(Chorulon) **POM-V**

Formulations: Injectable: 1500 IU powder for reconstitution.

Action: In females induces follicular maturation, ovulation and development of the corpus luteum. In males stimulates testosterone secretion.

Use: Used to supplement or replace LH in cases of ovulation failure or delay, to induce lactation post-partum, or in bitches who fail to hold to mating. Used in ferrets to treat persistent oestrus. In male animals it may increase libido; may also assist the treatment of cryptorchidism before surgical castration, provided inguinal canal remains patent and therapy is started early.

Safety and handling: Reconstituted vials do not contain any preservative and so should be discarded within 24 hours.

Contraindications: No information available.

Adverse reactions: Anaphylactic reactions may occasionally occur.

Drug interactions: No information available.

DOSES

Dogs:
- Delayed ovulation: 22 IU/kg i.m. q24–48h or 44 IU/kg i.m. once; mate on behavioural oestrus.
- Anoestrus: 500 IU/dog i.m. (following serum gonadotrophin 20 IU/kg s.c. q24h for 10 days).
- Deficient male libido, cryptorchidism: 100–500 IU/dog i.m. twice weekly for up to 6 weeks.

Cats: Not authorized for use in cats. Doses as for dogs.
Small mammals: Ferrets: 100 IU/ferret i.m.q14d for 2 doses; Guinea pigs: 100 IU/kg i.m. weekly for 3 doses.
Birds, Reptiles: No information available.

Ciclosporin (Cyclosporin(e))
(Atopica, Optimmune, Neoral*, Sandimmun*) **POM**

Formulations: Ophthalmic: 0.2% ointment (Optimmune). Oral: 10 mg, 25 mg, 50 mg, 100 mg capsules; 100 mg/ml solution. Injectable: 50 mg/ml solution.

Action: T lymphocyte inhibition.

Use: Authorized for veterinary use as topical ophthalmic preparation for immune-mediated keratoconjunctivitis sicca in dogs and as oral preparation for atopic dermatitis in dogs. May also be useful as an immunosuppressant in chronic superficial keratoconjunctivitis (pannus), perianal fistula, sebaceous adenitis and immune-mediated diseases. Also used for disseminated idiopathic myositis in ferrets. No evidence of systemic or ocular toxicity following ocular administration but systemic absorption has been reported. Recommended that bacterial and fungal infections are treated before use. Whilst the nephrotoxicity seen in human patients does not appear to be common in dogs, care should be taken in treating dogs with renal impairment, and creatinine levels should be monitored regularly. In dogs with atopic dermatitis, ciclosporin may reduce circulating levels of insulin and cause an increase in blood glucose and fructosamines. In the dogs with diabetes mellitus, the effect of treatment on glycaemia must be carefully monitored. Use with caution in patients with pre-existing infections (including FIV and FeLV) and monitor for opportunistic infections.

Safety and handling: Use gloves to prevent cutaneous absorption.

Contraindications: Systemic use is not recommended in dogs up to 6 months old or <2 kg. Do not use in progressive malignant disorders.

Do not give live vaccines during treatment or within a 2-week interval before or after treatment. The manufacturer does not recommend in diabetic dogs.

Adverse reactions: Hypertrichosis is common. Immediate discomfort on topical application (blepharospasm) has been reported in dogs. Transient vomiting and diarrhoea may follow systemic administration; these are usually mild and do not require cessation of treatment. Infrequently observed adverse effects include: anorexia; mild to moderate gingival hyperplasia; papillomatous lesions of the skin; red and swollen pinnae; muscle weakness; and muscle cramps. These effects resolve spontaneously after treatment is stopped. Systemic treatment may be associated with an increased risk of malignancy.

Drug interactions: The metabolism of ciclosporin is reduced, and thus serum levels increased, by various drugs that competitively inhibit or induce enzymes involved in its metabolism, particularly cytochrome P450, including diltiazem, doxycycline and imidazole antifungal drugs. Itraconazole at 5–10 mg/kg is known to increase the blood concentration of ciclosporin in dogs up to five-fold, which is considered to be clinically relevant. During concomitant use of itraconazole and ciclosporin consider halving the dose or doubling the treatment interval if dog is on daily treatment. In humans is increased risk of nephrotoxicity if ciclosporin is administered with aminoglycosides, NSAIDs, quinolones, or trimethoprim/sulphonamides; concomitant use of ciclosporin not recommended. Increased risk of hyperkalaemia if used with ACE inhibitors. As a substrate and inhibitor of the MDR 1 P-glycoprotein transporter, co-administration of ciclosporin with P-glycoprotein substrates such as macrocyclic lactones (e.g. ivermectin and milbemycin) could decrease the efflux of such drugs from blood–brain barrier cells, potentially resulting in signs of CNS toxicity. Ciclosporin has been shown to affect glucose metabolism and decrease the effects of insulin and to do so as much as low doses of glucocorticoids; therefore, use with caution in diabetic patients.

DOSES
See Appendix for immunosuppression protocols.
Dogs:
- Ocular disease: Apply approximately 0.5 cm of ointment to the affected eye q12h. It may take 2–4 weeks for improvement to occur (occasionally up to 12 weeks). Maintenance treatment should be continued with application q12h; in cases of excessive tear production (>20 mm/minute), application can be reduced to q24h but only with caution and long-term, regular monitoring of tear production.
- Atopic dermatitis: 5 mg/kg p.o. q24h until signs controlled, then q48h as a maintenance dose.
- Perianal fistula, sebaceous adenitis: 5 mg/kg p.o. q12–24h.
- Immune-mediated disease: 5 mg/kg p.o. q12–24h.

Cats: 7 mg/kg/day for atopic dermatitis.

Small mammals: Ferrets: 5 mg/kg p.o. q24h; Rabbits: 5 mg/kg p.o. q24h for idiopathic sebaceous adenitis; Rats: 10 mg/kg p.o. q24h.

Birds, Reptiles: No information available.

Cimetidine

(Zitac, Cimetidine*, Dyspamet*, Tagamet*) **POM-V, POM**

Formulations: Injectable: 100 mg/ml solution in 2 ml ampoule. Oral: 100 mg, 200 mg, 400 mg, 800 mg tablets; 40 mg/ml syrup.

Action: Histamine (H2) receptor antagonist, blocking histamine-induced gastric acid secretion. Rapidly absorbed with high bioavailability; undergoes hepatic metabolism and renal excretion. Plasma half-life is about an hour.

Use: Management of idiopathic, uraemic or drug-related erosive gastritis, gastric and duodenal ulcers, oesophagitis, and hypersecretory conditions secondary to gastrinoma mast cell neoplasia or short bowel syndrome. Efficacy against NSAID-induced ulcers is controversial. Reduction of vomiting due to gastritis and gastric ulceration is typically achieved in about 2 weeks but animals should be treated for at least 2 weeks after the remission of clinical signs, so minimum of 28 days recommended. If considered successful, medication can then be stopped. Rebound gastric acid secretion may be seen on cessation of cimetidine, so therapy should be tapered. A 2-week medication-free period should be allowed to see if vomiting occurs again. If the dog starts vomiting again after a medication-free period, treatment can be re-initiated, without risk for intolerance. Depending on the response, treatment can be adapted to the individual animal until the response is considered to be adequate and then continued at this level. Concomitant treatment with sucralfate may be helpful, and dietary measures should always be maintained. If used i.v., should be administered over 30 min to prevent cardiac arrhythmias and hypotension. Dosage should be reduced for animals with renal impairment. Less effective at reducing gastric acidity than more modern H2 blockers and proton pump inhibitors. Cimetidine has minimal prokinetic effects.

Safety and handling: Normal precautions should be observed.

Contraindications: No information available.

Adverse reactions: Rare, although hepatotoxicity and nephrotoxicity have been reported in humans. Adverse reactions are generally minor even at high doses, but thrombocytopenia has been reported in dogs. In humans cimetidine has been associated with headache, gynaecomastia and decreased libido.

Drug interactions: Retards oxidative hepatic drug metabolism by binding to the microsomal cytochrome P450. May increase plasma levels of beta-blockers (e.g. propranolol), calcium-channel blockers (e.g. verapamil), diazepam, lidocaine, metronidazole, pethidine and theophylline. When used with other agents that cause leucopenia may exacerbate the problem. Sucralfate may decrease bioavailability; although there is little evidence to suggest this is of clinical importance it may be a wise precaution to administer sucralfate at least 2 hours before cimetidine. Stagger oral doses by 2 hours when used with other antacids, digoxin, itraconazole or maropitant.

DOSES

Dogs: 5–10 mg/kg p.o., i.v., i.m. q8h.

Cats: 2.5–5 mg/kg p.o., i.v., i.m. q12h.

Small mammals: Ferrets: 5–10 mg/kg i.m., s.c., p.o. q8h; Rabbits: 5–10 mg/kg p.o. q6–8h; Rodents: 5–10 mg/kg p.o., s.c., i.m., i.v. q6–12h.

Birds: 5 mg/kg i.m., p.o. q8–12h.

Reptiles: 4 mg/kg i.m., p.o. q8h.

Cimicoxib

(Cimalgex) **POM-V**

Formulations: Oral: 8 mg, 30 mg, 80 mg chewable tablets.

Action: Selectively inhibits COX-2 enzyme, thereby limiting the production of prostaglandins involved in inflammation.

Use: For the treatment of pain and inflammation associated with osteoarthritis and the management of perioperative pain due to orthopaedic or soft tissue surgery in dogs. For perioperative use, one dose 2 hours before surgery, followed by 3–7 days of treatment, is indicated. For the relief of pain and inflammation associated with osteoarthritis, an initial treatment period of 6 months is indicated; this can be extended depending on clinical need for analgesic treatment. Unlike some NSAIDs, there is no specific contraindication to the administration of cimicoxib to dogs with stable mild to moderate renal disease (IRIS Stages I to II) but as with any long-term NSAID therapy, monitoring of renal parameters is recommended.

Safety and handling: Normal precautions should be observed.

Contraindications: Do not give to dogs <10 weeks of age; the safety of cimicoxib has not been determined in dogs <6 months of age, therefore, monitor dogs in this age group carefully for signs of NSAID-related adverse effects. Do not give to dehydrated, hypovolaemic or hypotensive patients, or those with GI disease or blood clotting problems. Do not give to pregnant or lactating bitches. Do not administer concurrently or within 24 hours of other NSAIDs and glucocorticoids.

Adverse reactions: GI signs are commonly reported but most cases are mild and recover without treatment. Stop therapy if signs persist beyond 1–2 days. Some animals develop signs with one NSAID and not another. A 1–2 week wash-out period should be allowed before starting therapy with another NSAID. Stop therapy immediately if GI bleeding is suspected. There is a small risk that NSAIDs may precipitate cardiac failure in animals with cardiovascular disease.

Drug interactions: No information available.

DOSES
Dogs: 2 mg/kg p.o. q24h administered with or without food.
Cats: Not authorized for cats.
Small mammals, Birds, Reptiles: No information available.

Cinchophen
(PLT tablets) **POM-V**

Formulations: Oral: 200 mg tablets in combination with prednisolone 1 mg.

Action: Anti-inflammatory agent via non-steroidal action.

Use: Management of osteoarthritis pain in dogs. Animals should be monitored for signs of GI ulceration and deterioration in liver function. At the end of treatment the dose should be reduced gradually as with any glucocorticoid.

Safety and handling: Normal precautions should be observed.

Contraindications: Only commercially available in tablets combined with prednisolone, therefore do not administer to animals that are receiving therapy with other steroids or with NSAIDs. Do not give in perioperative period or to animals that are shocked, hypotensive or have renal insufficiency. Do not give to animals with hepatic disease or with pre-existing GI ulceration. Do not use in cats or small mammals.

Adverse reactions: GI ulceration and irritation are common side effects of all NSAIDs and particularly so with cinchophen. Advisable to stop therapy if diarrhoea or nausea persists beyond 1–2 days. Stop therapy immediately if GI bleeding suspected and begin symptomatic treatment. There is a small risk that NSAIDs may precipitate cardiac failure in animals with cardiovascular disease. Cinchophen has been associated with liver damage in dogs after prolonged oral administration (6 weeks).

Drug interactions: Increased risk of GI ulceration if administered concurrently or within 24 hours of other NSAIDs and glucocorticoids. Increased risk of nephrotoxicity if administered with other potentially nephrotoxic agents, e.g. aminoglycosides.

DOSES
Dogs: 12.5 mg/kg p.o. q12h.
Cats, Small mammals: Do not use.
Birds, Reptiles: No information available.

Ciprofloxacin
(Ciloxan*, Ciproxin*) **POM**

Formulations: Oral: 100 mg, 250 mg and 500 mg tablets; 50 mg/ml suspension. Injectable: 2 mg/ml for i.v. infusion. Ophthalmic: 0.3% solution in 5 ml bottle; 0.3% ointment in 3.5 g tube.

Action: Bactericidal through inhibition of bacterial DNA gyrase.

Use: Ideally fluoroquinolone use should be reserved for infections where culture and sensitivity testing predicts a clinical response and where first- and second-line antimicrobials would not be effective. Broad-spectrum activity against wide range of Gram-negative and some Gram-positive aerobes; some activity against *Mycoplasma* and *Chlamydophila*. Active against many ocular pathogens, including *Staphylococcus* and *Pseudomonas aeruginosa*, although there is increasing resistance amongst staphylococci and streptococci. The eye drop formulation is also used in reptiles for the topical management of wounds.

Safety and handling: Normal precautions should be observed.

Contraindications: No information available.

Adverse reactions: May cause local irritation after application. In humans the following are reported: local burning and itching; lid margin crusting; hyperaemia; taste disturbances; corneal staining, keratitis, lid oedema, lacrimation, photophobia, corneal infiltrates; nausea; and visual disturbances.

Drug interactions: No information available.

DOSES
See Appendix for guidelines on responsible antibacterial use.
Dogs, Cats: 1 drop to affected eye q6h; loading dose can be used 1 drop to affected eye q15min for 4 doses.
Small mammals: Ferrets: 10–30 mg/kg p.o. q24h; Rabbits: 10–20 mg/kg p.o. q24h or 1 drop to affected eye q6h; loading dose can be used 1 drop to affected eye q15min for 4 doses; Chinchillas, Guinea pigs: 5–25 mg/kg p.o. q12h; Hamsters: 10–20 mg/kg p.o. q12h; Other rodents: 7–25 mg/kg p.o. q12h.
Birds: 5–20 mg/kg i.v., i.m., p.o. q12h.
Reptiles: Topical: 1 drop to affected eyes or in wounds. Systemic: 5–10 mg/kg p.o., s.c., i.m. q24h.

Cisapride
(Cisapride) **POM-V**

Formulations: Various formulations (including tablets and suspensions) available as a veterinary special depending on requirements.

Action: Gastrointestinal prokinetic agent related to metoclopramide but has no central antiemetic activity.

Use: Primarily used in feline idiopathic megacolon and in GI stasis in rabbits and herbivorous rodents (e.g. guinea pigs, chinchillas). Its license for humans was withdrawn due to potentially fatal cardiac arrhythmias and it is solely available to the veterinary profession on a named patient or named veterinary surgeon 'special basis'.

Safety and handling: Normal precautions should be observed.

Contraindications: It should not be given within 2 hours of metoclopramide or ranitidine.

Adverse reactions: Abdominal cramps and diarrhoea may develop, especially at higher doses or if used alongside other prokinetic agents. Fatal cardiac arrhythmias have not been reported in cats, rabbits or rodents.

Drug interactions: Opioid analgesics and antimuscarinics (e.g. atropine) may antagonize the effects of cisapride. In humans, it is known that drugs inhibiting the cytochrome P450 3A4 enzymes which metabolize cisapride (clarithromycin, erythromycin, itraconazole) when taken alongside cisapride have led to fatal arrhythmias.

DOSES
Dogs: Rarely used.
Cats: 0.1–1.0 mg/kg (typically 0.5 mg/kg) q8–12h.
Small mammals: Rabbits, Guinea pigs, Chinchillas: 0.1–1.0 mg/kg (typically 0.5 mg/kg) q8–12h.
Birds, Reptiles: No information available.

Cisatracurium
(Nimbex*) **POM**

Formulations: Injectable: 2 mg/ml, 10 mg/ml solutions.

Action: Inhibits actions of acetylcholine at neuromuscular junction by binding competitively to nicotinic acetylcholine receptor on post-junctional membrane.

Use: Provision of neuromuscular blockade during anaesthesia. This may be to improve surgical access through muscle relaxation, to facilitate positive pressure ventilation or for intraocular surgery. Cisatracurium is one of the isomers that comprise atracurium; it is 3–5 times more potent than atracurium in dogs. This means that the plasma concentrations of the epileptogenic byproduct laudanosine are lower and there is less histamine release. Monitoring (using a nerve stimulator) and reversal of the neuromuscular blockade is recommended to ensure complete recovery before the end of anaesthesia. Hypothermia, acidosis and hypokalaemia will prolong the duration of action of neuromuscular blockade. There are no published clinical studies describing the use of cisatracurium in cats; limited experimental studies suggest that cisatracurium has similar characteristics in cats to those described for dogs.

Safety and handling: Store in refrigerator.

Contraindications: Do not administer unless the animal is adequately anaesthetized and facilities to provide positive pressure ventilation are available.

Adverse reactions: Can precipitate the release of histamine after rapid i.v. administration, resulting in bronchospasm and hypotension. Diluting the drug in normal saline and giving the drug slowly i.v. minimizes these effects.

Drug interactions: Neuromuscular blockade is more prolonged when given in combination with volatile anaesthetics, aminoglycosides, clindamycin and lincomycin.

DOSES
Dogs: 0.1 mg/kg i.v. followed by additional doses of 0.03 mg/kg as required (based on monitoring of neuromuscular blockade).
Cats, Small mammals, Birds, Reptiles: No information available.

Clarithromycin
(Klaricid*) **POM**

Formulations: Oral: 250 mg, 500 mg tablets; 125 mg/5 ml suspension; 250 mg/5 ml suspension; 250 mg granules sachet (to be dissolved in water). Injectable: 500 mg vial for reconstitution.

Action: Derived from erythromycin and with greater activity. Bactericidal (time-dependent) or bacteriostatic properties, depending on concentration and susceptibility. Binds to the 50S ribosome, inhibiting peptide bond formation.

Use: Alternative to penicillin in penicillin-allergic humans as it has a similar, although not identical, antibacterial spectrum. Active against Gram-positive cocci (some *Staphylococcus* spp. resistant), Gram-positive bacilli, some Gram-negative bacilli (e.g. *Pasteurella*) and some spirochaetes (e.g. *Helicobacter*). Some strains of *Actinomyces*, *Nocardia*, *Chlamydophila* and *Rickettsia* also inhibited. Most strains of Enterobacteriaceae (*Pseudomonas*, *Escherichia coli*, *Klebsiella*) are resistant. Highly lipid-soluble and useful against intracellular pathogens. Particularly useful in management of respiratory tract infections, mild to moderate skin and soft tissue infections, and non-tubercular mycobacterial infections. For the latter used in combination with enrofloxacin and rifampin. Activity is enhanced in an alkaline pH; administer on an empty stomach. There is limited information regarding use in animals. Use with caution in animals with hepatic dysfunction. Reduce dose in animals with renal impairment. In ferrets it has been used successfully to treat pneumonia due to *Mycobacterium abscessus* and it can be used in combination with omeprazole or ranitidine and bismuth plus amoxicillin or metronidazole for treatment of *Helicobacter mustelae*.

Safety and handling: Normal precautions should be observed.

Contraindications: No information available.

Adverse reactions: In humans similar adverse effects to those of erythromycin are seen, i.e. vomiting, cholestatic hepatitis, stomatitis and glossitis.

Drug interactions: May increase serum levels of several drugs, including methylprednisolone, theophylline, omeprazole and itraconazole. The absorption of digoxin may be enhanced.

DOSES
See Appendix for guidelines on responsible antibacterial use.
Dogs: 4–12 mg/kg i.v. infusion, p.o. q12h. Doses of 15–25 mg/kg p.o. q8–12h are recommended in the treatment of leproid granuloma syndrome. These doses are empirical and are based on a very few reports.
Cats: 5–10 mg/kg i.v. infusion, p.o. q12h or 62.5 mg/cat p.o. These doses are empirical and are based on a very few reports.
Small mammals: Ferrets: 50 mg/kg p.o. q12–14h; Rats: 3.5–10 mg/kg p.o. q8–12h.
Birds: 85 mg/kg p.o. q24h.
Reptiles: 15 mg/kg p.o. q48–72h.

Clazuril
(Appertex) **AVM-GSL**

Formulations: Oral: 2.5 mg tablet.

Action: Coccidiocidal; mode of action unclear.

Use: Treatment and control of coccidiosis (*Eimeria labbeana*, *E. columbarum*) in homing and show pigeons. Birds should be treated following transportation to shows or races where they may have been exposed to coccidia.

Safety and handling: Normal precautions should be observed.

Contraindications: Do not use in birds intended for human consumption.

Adverse reactions: No information available.

Drug interactions: Do not administer with drugs that may cause vomiting.

DOSES
Birds: Raptors: 30 mg/kg once; Pigeons: 5–10 mg/kg once (treat all birds in loft simultaneously); Psittacines: 7 mg/kg p.o q2d for 2 doses.
Dogs, Cats, Small mammals, Reptiles: No information available.

Clemastine
(Tavegil*) **GSL**

Formulations: Oral: 1 mg tablet.

Action: Binds to H1 histamine receptors and prevents histamine from binding.

Use: Management of allergic disease. Specific doses for cats have not been determined by pharmokinetic studies and in dogs therapeutic levels are not usually achieved by oral administration. Use with caution in cases with urinary retention, angle-closure glaucoma and pyloroduodenal obstruction.

Safety and handling: Normal precautions should be observed.

Contraindications: No information available.

Adverse reactions: May cause mild sedation. May reduce seizure threshold.

Drug interactions: No information available.

DOSES
Dogs: 0.05–0.1mg/kg p.o. q12h.
Cats: 0.1 mg/kg p.o. q12h.
Small mammals, Birds, Reptiles: No information available.

Clindamycin

(Antirobe, Clinacin, Clindacyl, Clindaseptin) **POM-V**

Formulations: Oral: 25 mg, 75 mg, 150 mg, 300 mg capsules and tablets; 25 mg/ml solution.

Action: Lincosamide antibiotic that binds to the 50S ribosomal subunit, inhibiting peptide bond formation. May be bactericidal or bacteriostatic depending on susceptibility.

Use: Bone and joint infections associated with Gram-positive bacteria; pyoderma; toxoplasmosis; and infections associated with the oral cavity. Active against Gram-positive cocci (including penicillin-resistant staphylococci), many obligate anaerobes, mycoplasmas and *Toxoplasma gondii*. Attains high concentrations in bone and bile. Being a weak base, it becomes ion-trapped (and therefore concentrated) in fluids that are more acidic than plasma, such as prostatic fluid, milk and intracellular fluid. There is complete cross resistance between lincomycin and clindamycin, and partial cross resistance with erythromycin. Use with care in individuals with hepatic or renal impairment.

Safety and handling: Normal precautions should be observed.

Contraindications: Do not use in rabbits, guinea pigs, chinchillas or hamsters.

Adverse reactions: Colitis, vomiting and diarrhoea are reported. Although not a major problem in dogs and cats, discontinue drug if diarrhoea develops. In cats may be associated with oesophagitis and oesophageal stricture; therefore consider following tablet administration with a small water or food bolus. Lincosamides cause a potentially fatal clostridial enterotoxaemia in rabbits, guinea pigs, chinchillas and hamsters.

Drug interactions: May enhance the effect of non-depolarizing muscle relaxants (e.g. tubocurarine) and may antagonize the effects of neostigmine and pyridostigmine. Do not administer with macrolide, chloramphenicol or other lincosamide antimicrobials as these combinations are antagonistic.

DOSES
See Appendix for guidelines on responsible antibacterial use.
Dogs: 5.5 mg/kg p.o. q12h or 11 mg/kg q24h; in severe infection can increase to 11 mg/kg q12h. Toxoplasmosis: 25 mg/kg p.o. daily in divided doses.
Cats: 5.5 mg/kg p.o. q12h or 11mg/kg q24h. Toxoplasmosis: 25 mg/kg p.o. daily in divided doses.
Small mammals: Ferrets: 5.5–11 mg/kg p.o. q12h (toxoplasmosis: 12.5–25 mg/kg p.o. q12h). Rabbits, Rodents: Do not use.
Birds: 25 mg/kg p.o. q8h or 50 mg/kg p.o. q12h or 100 mg/kg p.o. q24h.
Reptiles: 2.5–5 mg/kg p.o. q24h.

Clodronate
(Bonefos*, Loron*) **POM**

Formulations: Oral: 400 mg capsule.

Action: Adsorbed on to hydroxyapatite crystals and ingested by osteoclasts. Metabolized in the cell to compounds that compete with ATP, leading to apoptosis of the cell and thus slowing the rate of bone destruction. This class of drugs may also decrease intestinal absorption of calcium and influence vitamin D3 metabolism.

Use: Treatment of acute moderate to severe hypercalcaemia when other therapies are ineffective, or in the long-term therapy of chronic hypercalcaemia. Few reports of use in dogs and no reports of use in cats or other veterinary species. Excretion reduced in chronic renal failure; dose adjustment may be required. Aledronate is similar to clodronate but experience is limited.

Safety and handling: Normal precautions should be observed.

Contraindications: No information available.

Adverse reactions: Nausea, diarrhoea, hypocalcaemia, hypophosphataemia, hypomagnesaemia and hypersensitivity reactions.

Drug interactions: Reduced absorption if administered with antacids, calcium and iron salts; administer 2 hours apart. Concurrent use of aminoglycosides may result in severe hypocalcaemia.

DOSES
Dogs: 5–14 mg/kg slow i.v. over a minimum of 2 hours (diluted according to the manufacturer's instructions) or 10–30 mg/kg p.o. q8–12h.
Cats, Small mammals, Birds, Reptiles: No information available.

Clofazimine
(Clofazimine*) **POM**

Formulations: Oral: 100 mg capsule.

Action: Not entirely clear but appears to be bactericidal and has membrane disrupting properties.

Use: Mycobacterial infections including feline leprosy. Limited information available, most derived from human medicine. For feline mycobacterial infection long-term treatment is required and combination therapy is utilized, e.g. with clarithromycin and doxycycline. Monitor hepatic and renal function during treatment. Use with caution in hepatic and renal impairment.

Safety and handling: Normal precautions should be observed.

Contraindications: No information available.

Adverse reactions: In humans the major adverse effects are nausea, diarrhoea and renal and hepatic impairment (monitor functions during therapy). Skin discoloration has been reported in the cat.

Drug interactions: No information available.

DOSES
See Appendix for guidelines on responsible antibacterial use.
Dogs, Cats: 2–12 mg/kg p.o. q24h for 2–6 months.
Small mammals, Birds, Reptiles: No information available.

Clomipramine
(Clomicalm) **POM**

Formulations: Oral: 5 mg, 20 mg, 80 mg tablets.

Action: Both clomipramine and its primary metabolite desmethylclomipramine are active in blocking serotonin and noradrenaline re-uptake in the brain, with resultant anxiolytic, antidepressant and anticompulsive effects.

Use: Licensed for use in association with a behaviour modification plan for the management of separation-related disorders in dogs. Also used in management of a wider range of anxiety-related disorders in dogs and cats, including 'compulsive behaviours', noise fears and urine spraying. Care required before use in animals with a history of constipation, epilepsy, glaucoma, urinary retention or arrhythmias. Used in birds for feather plucking, especially if due to separation anxiety; should be used in association with a behaviour modification plan. Can be used with benzodiazepines.

Safety and handling: Normal precautions should be observed.

Contraindications: Patients sensitive to tricyclic antidepressants. Do not give with, or within 2 weeks of, monoamine oxidase inhibitors (e.g. selegiline). Not recommended for use in male breeding animals, as testicular hypoplasia may occur.

Adverse reactions: May cause sporadic vomiting, changes in appetite or lethargy. Vomiting may be reduced by co-administration with a small quantity of food.

Drug interactions: May potentiate the effects of the antiarrhythmic drug quinidine, anticholinergic agents (e.g. atropine), other CNS active drugs (e.g. barbiturates, benzodiazepines, general anaesthetics, neuroleptics), sympathomimetics (e.g. adrenaline) and coumarin derivatives. Simultaneous administration with cimetidine may lead to increased plasma levels of clomipramine. Plasma levels of certain antiepileptic drugs, e.g. phenytoin and carbamazepine, may be increased by coadministration with clomipramine.

DOSES
Dogs: 1–2 mg/kg p.o. q12h.
Cats: 0.25–1 mg/kg p.o. q24h.
Small mammals: Rats: 16–32 mg/kg p.o. q12h.
Birds: 0.5–1 mg/kg p.o. q6–8h.
Reptiles: No information available.

Clonazepam
(Klonopin*, Linotril*, Rivotril*) **POM**

Formulations: Oral: 0.25 mg, 0.5 mg, 1.0 mg, 2 mg tablets.

Action: Long-acting benzodiazepine with anticonvulsant, muscle relaxant and anxiolytic properties. Enhances activity of gamma-aminobutyric acid (GABA), through binding at the benzodiazepine site of the $GABA_A$ receptor. In addition, affects glutamate decarboxylase activity.

Use: Management of muscular hypertonicity (episodic falling) in the Cavalier King Charles Spaniel and refractory epileptic seizures in cats. More suitable medications for the management of refractory epilepsy in cats are available, including phenobarbital, imepitoin (although at the time of publication no reports on the use of imepitoin in cats have been published), levetiracetam and diazepam. Tolerance may develop following prolonged therapy, with reduction in clinical effect. Care is required when withdrawing clonazepam after prolonged therapy and the dose should be tapered off.

Safety and handling: Normal precautions should be observed.

Contraindications: Avoid use in patients with marked CNS depression, respiratory depression, severe muscle weakness or hepatic impairment (may worsen hepatic encephalopathy).

Adverse reactions: Generally mild; sedation and respiratory suppression at higher doses most important. In cats potential adverse effects include acute hepatic necrosis, sedation and ataxia.

Drug interactions: Drugs that result in hepatic enzyme induction, e.g. phenobarbital and phenytoin, may accelerate metabolism of clonazepam.

DOSES
Dogs: 0.5 mg/kg p.o. q8–12h.
Cats: 0.5 mg/cat p.o. q12–24h (starting dose).
Small mammals, Birds, Reptiles: No information available.

Clonidine
(Catapres*) **POM**

Formulations: Injectable: 150 µg/ml solution.

Action: Stimulates the secretion of growth hormone releasing hormone (GHRH) from the hypothalamus.

Use: To assess the pituitary's ability to produce growth hormone (GH). The dose required to elicit a response has not been well established in dogs and not at all in other veterinary species. Specialist texts should be consulted if attempting a clonidine stimulation test. Assessment of plasma insulin-like growth factor-1 (IGF-1) concentration in a single sample is a useful screening test for growth hormone disorders. Also used in dogs to control panic responses and high arousal frustration responses. Effect develops in about 30 min and lasts for 3–4h, so often needs to be used tactically. Can be used over longer term but may take 1–2wks to see full response. Withdrawal must be done gradually to avoid hypertension.

Safety and handling: Normal precautions should be observed.

Contraindications: Due to effects on blood glucose, use in diabetic animals is not recommended.

Adverse reactions: Transient sedation and bradycardia may develop.

Drug interactions: Care should be exercised when using with drugs that also lower blood pressure or heart rate. Should not be used concurrently with barbiturates, opiates or hypotensive agents (e.g. beta-blockers).

DOSES
Dogs:
- Growth hormone stimulation: 3–10 µg (micrograms)/kg i.v. once.
- Behavioural modification: 0.05 mg/kg q12h (often with food).
Cats, Small mammals, Birds, Reptiles: No information available.

Clopidogrel

CIL

(Plavix*) **POM**

Formulations: Oral: 75 mg tablets.

Action: By binding to an ADP receptor on platelets, clopidogrel prevents the inhibition of adenylate cyclase. This maintains cAMP levels and therefore inhibits platelet aggregation.

Use: Thromboprophylaxis in cats and dogs. Commonly used to reduce the risk of thrombus formation in cats with advanced cardiac disease, to reduce the risk of thromboembolism in cats with a pre-existing thrombus or recurrence of embolism in cats with a previous arterial thromboembolic event. There are few published data on the usage of this drug in animals to date. May be used in cats in conjunction with aspirin (as the drugs act on different parts of the platelet activation cycle). May be substituted for aspirin if aspirin is not tolerated. Use with care in patients with renal or hepatic impairment.

Safety and handling: Normal precautions should be observed.

Contraindications: Bleeding disorders, GI ulceration.

Adverse reactions: Tablet formulations for humans are film-coated, which needs to be broken for appropriate dosing in cats. Many cats dislike the taste of the tablets when the film-coating is broken. In humans skin reactions have been reported. Overdoses will be expected to lead to bleeding disorders.

Drug interactions: High risk of bleeding complications if used with anticoagulants.

DOSES

Dogs: 2–4 mg/kg p.o. q24h.
Cats: 18.75 mg/cat p.o. q24h.
Small mammals, Birds, Reptiles: No information available.

Clotrimazole

(Canesten*, Clotrimazole*, Lotriderm*) **POM**

Formulations: Topical: 1% cream; 1% solution. Many other products available; some contain corticosteroids.

Action: Topical imidazole with an inhibitory action on the growth of pathogenic dermatophytes, *Aspergillus* and yeasts by inhibiting cytochrome P450-dependent ergosterol synthesis.

Use: Superficial fungal infections. Naso-sinal infections including aspergillosis.

Safety and handling: Normal precautions should be observed.

Contraindications: No information available.

Adverse reactions: No information available.

Drug interactions: No information available.

DOSES

Dogs, Cats:
- Otic: Instil 3–5 drops in ear q12h.
- Topical: Apply to affected area and massage in gently q12h; if no improvement in 4 weeks re-evaluate therapy or diagnosis.
- Nasal: Instil 10 g (dogs up to 10 kg) or 20 g (dogs >10 kg) of 1% cream in each frontal sinus via trephine holes. Alternatively, instil 30 ml (in dogs up to 10 kg) or 60 ml (in dogs >10 kg) of a 1% solution in polyethylene glycol into each nasal cavity, with nares and nasopharynx sealed by Foley catheters and turning every 15 min. A combination of both approaches may be used. Do not use this route if cribiform plate not intact.

Small mammals: Rabbits: Otic: Instil 3–5 drops in ear q12h; Topical: Apply to affected area and massage in gently q12h; if no improvement in 4 weeks re-evaluate therapy or diagnosis; Chinchillas, Guinea pigs, Hamsters, Rats: Topical application to defined lesions q12h for 3–6 weeks (anecdotal).

Birds: Endoscopic: 10 mg/kg applied directly to fungal lesions. Nasal flush: 10 mg/ml (flush volume 20 ml/kg). Intratracheal: 2–3 ml of a 1% solution nebulized for periods of 1 hour q24h or topically.

Reptiles: Apply topically to lesion q12h.

Cloxacillin
(Opticlox, Orbenin) **POM-V**

Formulations: Ophthalmic: Cloxacillin benzathine ester 16.7% suspension.

Action: Beta-lactamase-resistant penicillin which is bactericidal and works in a time-dependent fashion. Binds to penicillin-binding proteins involved in cell wall synthesis, thereby decreasing bacterial cell wall strength and rigidity, and affecting cell division, growth and septum formation.

Use: Narrow spectrum antimicrobial. Less active than penicillin G or V against *Streptococcus*. Specifically indicated for ocular infections with beta-lactamase-producing *Staphylococcus*.

Safety and handling: Normal precautions should be observed.

Contraindications: Do not administer penicillins to hamsters, gerbils, guinea pigs, chinchillas or rabbits.

Adverse reactions: No information available.

Drug interactions: Avoid the concomitant use of bacteriostatic antibiotics (chloramphenicol, erythromycin, tetracycline).

DOSES
See Appendix for guidelines on responsible antibacterial use.

Dogs, Cats, Birds: Apply 1/10th of a tube (0.3 g) q24h.
Small mammals: Rabbits, Chinchillas, Guinea pigs, Hamsters, Gerbils: do not use.
Reptiles: No information available.

Co-amoxiclav (Amoxicillin/Clavulanate, Amoxycillin/Clavulanic acid)
(Clavabactin, Clavaseptin, Clavucil, Clavudale, Combisyn, Kesium, Nisamox, Noroclav, Synulox, Augmentin*)
POM-V, POM

Formulations: Injectable: 175 mg/ml suspension (140 mg amoxicillin, 35 mg clavulanate); 600 mg powder (500 mg amoxicillin, 100 mg clavulanate); 1.2 g powder (1 g amoxicillin, 200 mg clavulanate) for reconstitution (Augmentin). Oral: 50 mg, 250 mg, 500 mg tablets each containing amoxicillin and clavulanate in a ratio of 4:1. Palatable drops which when reconstituted with water provide 40 mg amoxicillin and 10 mg clavulanic acid per ml.

Action: Amoxicillin binds to penicillin-binding proteins involved in bacterial cell wall synthesis, thereby decreasing cell wall strength and rigidity, affecting cell division, growth and septum formation. The addition of the beta-lactamase inhibitor clavulanate increases the antimicrobial spectrum against those organisms that produce beta-lactamase, such as *Staphylococcus* and *Escherichia coli*.

Use: Active against Gram-positive and Gram-negative aerobic organisms and many obligate anaerobes. Penicillinase-producing *Escherichia coli* and *Staphylococcus* are susceptible, but difficult Gram-negative organisms such as *Pseudomonas aeruginosa* and *Klebsiella* are often resistant. Dose and dosing interval will be determined by infection site, severity and organism. The predominant bacterial infections in reptiles are Gram-negative and many are resistant to penicillins.

Safety and handling: Tablets are wrapped in foil moisture-resistant packaging; do not remove until to be administered. Refrigerate oral suspension and i.v. solution after reconstitution. Discard oral suspension and i.v. formulation if they become dark or after 10 days. A small amount of discoloration of the i.v. solution is acceptable.

Contraindications: Avoid oral antibiotic agents in critically ill patients, as absorption from the GI tract may be unreliable; such patients may require i.v. formulation. Avoid use in animals which have displayed hypersensitivity reactions to other antimicrobials within the beta-lactam family (which includes cephalosporins). Do not administer to hamsters, guinea pigs, gerbils, chinchillas and rabbits.

Adverse reactions: Nausea, diarrhoea and skin rashes are the commonest adverse effects.

Drug interactions: Avoid the concurrent use of amoxicillin with bacteriostatic antibiotics (e.g. tetracycline, erythromycin). Do not mix in the same syringe as aminoglycosides. Do not use with allopurinol in birds. Synergism may occur between the beta-lactam and aminoglycoside antimicrobials *in vivo*.

DOSES
See Appendix for guidelines on responsible antibacterial use.
Dogs, Cats: Parenteral: 8.75 mg/kg (combined) i.v. q8h, i.m., s.c. q24h. Oral: 12.5–25 mg/kg (combined) p.o. q8–12h. (Doses up to 25 mg/kg i.v. q8h are used to treat serious infections in humans.)
Small mammals: Ferrets: 12.5–20 mg/kg i.m., s.c. q12h; Rats, Mice: 100 mg/kg q12h.
Birds: 125–150 mg/kg p.o., i.v. q12h; 125–150 mg/kg i.m. q24h.
Reptiles: No information available.

Co-danthramer, Co-danthrusate see Dantron

Codeine
(Pardale-V, Codeine*) **POM**

Formulations: Oral: 3 mg/5 ml paediatric linctus; 3 mg/ml linctus; 5 mg/ml syrup; 15 mg, 30 mg, 60 mg tablets.

Action: Opioid analgesic.

Use: Cough suppression, analgesia and diarrhoea. Pardale-V is a veterinary formulation with 400 mg paracetamol + 9 mg codeine. However, to deliver the dose of codeine listed below would result in a very high dose of paracetamol and therefore Pardale-V tablets cannot be recommended as a source of codeine for general usage.

Safety and handling: Normal precautions should be observed.

Contraindications: Renal insufficiency, hypoadrenocorticism, increased intracranial pressure, hypothyroidism. Care with severe respiratory compromise. Never administer Pardale-V to cats.

Adverse reactions: Sedation, ataxia, respiratory depression and constipation.

Drug interactions: No information available.

DOSES
Dogs: 0.5–2 mg/kg p.o. q12h. Do not use Pardale-V for codeine at this dose rate.
Cats: 0.5–2 mg/kg p.o. q12h. Do not use formulation with paracetamol.
Small mammals, Birds, Reptiles: No information available.

Colchicine

CIL

(Colchicine*) **POM**

Formulations: Oral: 0.5 mg tablet.

Action: Colchicine inhibits collagen synthesis, may enhance collagenase activity and blocks the synthesis and secretion of serum amyloid A.

Use: Management of fibrotic hepatic and pulmonary diseases, oesophageal stricture and renal amyloidosis (including that caused by 'Shar pei fever'). In birds, used for gout and hepatic cirrhosis/fibrosis. Only very limited and anecdotal evidence for its efficacy as an antifibrotic in dogs. Due to the relatively high incidence of adverse reactions, this drug should be used with caution. No evidence for its efficacy as an antifibrotic in cats. Prophylactic use in Shar pei fever cannot be recommended at this time.

Safety and handling: Protect from light.

Contraindications: Pregnancy.

Adverse reactions: Commoner adverse effects include vomiting, abdominal pain and diarrhoea. Rarely, renal damage, bone marrow suppression, myopathy and peripheral neuropathy may develop. Colchicine may increase serum ALP, decrease platelet counts and cause false-positive results when testing urine for RBCs and haemoglobin. Overdoses can be fatal.

Drug interactions: Possible increased risk of nephrotoxicity and myotoxicity when colchicine given with ciclosporin. NSAIDs, especially phenylbutazone, may increase the risks of thrombocytopenia, leucopenia or bone marrow depression when used concurrently with colchicine. Many anticancer chemotherapeutics may cause additive myelosuppressive effects when used with colchicine.

DOSES

Dogs: 0.03 mg/kg p.o. q24h.
Cats, Small mammals: No information available.
Birds: 0.04 mg/kg q12h.
Reptiles: No information available.

Colestyramine (Cholestyramine)

(Questran*) **POM**

Formulations: Oral: 4 g powder/sachet.

Action: Ion exchange resin.

Use: In rabbits for absorbing toxins produced in the GI tract following the development of overgrowth of *Clostridium*. In dogs for the reduction of serum cholesterol in idiopathic hypercholesterolaemia and for bile acid sequestration (may help alleviate diarrhoea in cases of fat malabsorption). May be used in digoxin overdose in dogs.

Safety and handling: Normal precautions should be observed.

Contraindications: No information available.

Adverse reactions: Constipation may develop. May cause taurine depletion in cats.

Drug interactions: Colestyramine reduces the absorption of digoxin, anticoagulants, diuretics and thyroxine.

DOSES
Dogs: 1–2 g/dog p.o. q12h.
Cats: No information available.
Small mammals: Rabbits: 2 g/rabbit p.o. syringed gently with 20 ml water; Guinea pigs: 1 g/guinea pig mixed with water p.o. q24h.
Birds, Reptiles: No information available.

Cordycepic acid see **Mannitol**

Crisantaspase (Asparaginase, L-Asparginase)
(Asparginase*, Elspar*, Erwinase*) **POM**

Formulations: Injectable: vials of 5,000 or 10,000 IU powder for reconstitution.

Action: Lymphoid tumour cells are not able to synthesize asparagine and are dependent upon supply from the extracellular fluid. Crisantaspase deprives malignant cells of this amino acid, which results in cessation of protein synthesis and cell death.

Use: Main indication is treatment of lymphoid malignancies.

Safety and handling: Cytotoxic drug; see Appendix and specialist texts for further advice on chemotherapeutic agents. Store in a refrigerator.

Contraindications: Patients with active pancreatitis or a history of pancreatitis. History of anaphylaxis associated with previous administration.

Adverse reactions: Anaphylaxis may follow administration, especially if repeated. Premedication with an antihistamine is recommended before administration. Haemorrhagic pancreatitis has been reported in dogs. Gastrointestinal disturbances, hepatotoxicity and coagulation deficits may also be observed.

Drug interactions: Administration with or before vincristine may reduce clearance of vincristine and increase toxicity; thus, if used in combination the vincristine should be given 12–24 hours before the enzyme.

DOSES

See Appendix for chemotherapy protocols and conversion of body weight to body surface area.

Dogs, Cats: 10,000 IU/m^2 or 400 IU/kg i.m. or s.c. q7d or less frequently.

Small mammals: Ferrets: 10,000 IU/m^2 s.c. weekly for the first 3 weeks as part of a chemotherapeutic protocol; Guinea pigs: 10,000 IU/m^2 s.c., i.m. q3wk.

Birds, Reptiles: No information available.

Cyclophosphamide   CIL
(Cyclophosphamide*, Endoxana*) **POM**

Formulations: Injectable: 100 mg, 200 mg, 500 mg, 1000 mg powder for reconstitution. Oral: 50 mg tablets.

Action: Metabolites crosslink DNA resulting in inhibition of DNA synthesis and function.

Use: Treatment of lymphoproliferative diseases, myeloproliferative disease and immune-mediated diseases. The use of cyclophosphamide in immune-mediated haemolytic anaemia is controversial and therefore it is not recommended as an immunosuppressant in the management of this disease. May have a role in management of certain sarcomas and carcinomas. Use with caution in patients with renal failure; dose reduction may be required. Has been used in lymphosarcoma in cockatoos.

Safety and handling: Cytotoxic drug; see Appendix and specialist texts for further advice on chemotherapeutic agents.

Contraindications: No information available.

Adverse reactions: Myelosuppression, with the nadir usually occurring 7–14 days after the start of therapy; regular monitoring of WBCs recommended. A metabolite of cyclophosphamide (acrolein) may cause a sterile haemorrhagic cystitis. The cystitis may be persistent. This risk may be reduced by increasing water consumption or by giving furosemide to ensure adequate urine production. Other effects include vomiting, diarrhoea, hepatotoxicity, nephrotoxicity and a reduction in hair growth rate.

Drug interactions: Increased risk of myelosuppression if thiazide diuretics given concomitantly. Absorption of orally administered digoxin may be decreased, may occur several days after dosing. Barbiturates increase cyclophosphamide toxicity due to increased rate of conversion to metabolites. Phenothiazines and chloramphenicol reduce cyclophosphamide efficacy. If administered with doxorubicin there is an increased risk of cardiotoxicity. Insulin requirements are altered by concurrent cyclophosphamide.

DOSES
See Appendix for chemotherapy protocols and conversion of body weight to body surface area.
Dogs:
- Lymphoid neoplasia: generally 50 mg/m^2 p.o. q48h or 4 consecutive days/week; or 200–250 mg/m^2 i.v. q3 weeks.
- Multiple myeloma in patients refractory to melphalan: 1 mg/kg p.o. q24h.
- Macroglobulinaemia in patients refractory to chlorambucil: 1 mg/kg p.o. q24h.
- Immune-mediated disease: 50 mg/m^2 p.o. or 1.5 mg/kg p.o. (dogs >25 kg); 2 mg/kg p.o. (dogs 5–25 kg); 2.5 mg/kg p.o. (dogs <5 kg). Give for 4 consecutive days/week or q48h.

Cats:
- Lymphoid neoplasia: as for dogs, except 200–300 mg/m^2 in 'high dose' COP regimes.
- Immune-mediated disease: 2.5 mg/kg p.o. q24h (or equivalent).

Small mammals: Ferrets: Lymphoma: 10 mg/kg p.o., s.c. as part of chemotherapy protocols similar to those in cats and dogs.
Birds: Lymphosarcoma: 200 mg/m^2 i.o. q7d.
Reptiles: No information available.

Cyclosporin(e) see Ciclosporin

Cyproheptadine
(Periactin*) **POM**

Formulations: Oral: 4 mg tablet.

Action: Binds to and blocks the activation of H1 histamine and serotonin receptors.

Use: Management of allergic disease and appetite stimulation. Also used in cats with aortic thromboembolism as serotonin, along with other mediators, is involved in collateral vasoconstriction. Maintenance of this collateral supply is important in recovery. Use with caution in cases with urinary retention, angle-closure glaucoma and pyloroduodenal obstruction. Specific doses for dogs and cats have not been determined by pharmokinetic studies and clinical effectiveness has not been established.

Safety and handling: Normal precautions should be observed.

Contraindications: No information available.

Adverse reactions: May cause mild sedation, polyphagia, weight gain. May reduce seizure threshold.

Drug interactions: No information available.

DOSES

Dogs, Cats: 0.1–0.5 mg/kg p.o. q8–12h.
Small mammals: Ferrets, Chinchillas, Guinea pigs: 0.5 mg p.o. q12h.
Birds, Reptiles: No information available.

Cytarabine (Cytosine arabinoside, Ara-C)
(Cytarabine*, Cytosar-U*) **POM**

Formulations: Injectable: 100 mg, 500 mg powders for reconstitution.

Action: The active nucleotide metabolite ara-CTP is incorporated into DNA and inhibits pyrimidine and DNA synthesis. Cytarabine is therefore S phase-specific.

Use: Management of lymphoproliferative and myeloproliferative disorders. For dogs diagnosed with lymphoma and bone marrow involvement, addition of cytarabine into a VCAA combination protocol may improve survival time. Cytarabine is widely used for the treatment of granulomatous meningoencephalitis (GME) and other suspected immune-mediated encephalitides in the dog. There is currently no general agreement on the best treatment protocol, but combination therapy of prednisolone and cytarabine is widely reported.

Safety and handling: Cytotoxic drug; see Appendix and specialist texts for further advice on chemotherapeutic agents. After reconstitution, store at room temperature and discard after 48 hours or if a slight haze develops.

Contraindications: Do not use if there is evidence of bone marrow suppression or substantial hepatic impairment.

Adverse reactions: Vomiting, diarrhoea, leucopenia. As it is a myelosuppressant, careful haematological monitoring is required. Conjunctivitis, oral ulceration, hepatotoxicity and fever have also been seen.

Drug interactions: Oral absorption of digoxin is decreased. Activity of gentamicin may be antagonized. Simultaneous administration of methotrexate increases the effect of cytarabine.

DOSES

See Appendix for chemotherapy protocols and conversion of body weight to body surface area.
Dogs, Cats:
- Lymphoproliferative disease: 100 mg/m^2 i.v. q24h for 2–4 days, or 100 mg/m^2 by i.v. infusion over 24–96h, or 20 mg/m^2 intrathecally q1–5d.
- MUA/GME: 50 mg/m^2 s.c. q12h for 4 doses. Repeat at 3, 7, 11, 16, 21, 27 and 33 weeks (if clinical benefit seen), then stop.

Small mammals: Ferrets: 1 mg per ferret p.o., s.c. q24h for 2 days.
Birds, Reptiles: No information available.

Dacarbazine
(Imidazole, Carboxamide*, Dacarbazine*, DTIC*) **POM**

Formulations: Injectable: 100 mg, 200 mg, 500 mg powders for reconstitution.

Action: Methylates nucleic acids and inhibits DNA, RNA and protein synthesis.

Use: Management of lymphoproliferative diseases (e.g. relapsed lymphoma), melanoma and soft tissue sarcoma. Use with caution in patients with renal or hepatic insufficiency. Can cause severe pain and extensive tissue damage with extravasation, and therefore must be administered via a preplaced i.v. catheter.

Safety and handling: Cytotoxic drug; see Appendix and specialist texts for further advice on chemotherapeutic agents.

Contraindications: Bone marrow suppression. Not recommended in cats, as unknown whether they can metabolize it adequately.

Adverse reactions: May be severe; include myelosuppression, intense nausea and vomiting.

Drug interactions: Phenobarbital increases the metabolic activation of dacarbazine. Do not use with other myelosuppressive drugs.

DOSES
See Appendix for chemotherapy protocols and conversion of body weight to body surface area.
Dogs: 200–250 mg/m^2 i.v. q24h on days 1–5. Repeat cycle q21–28d. Or, dependent upon the chemotherapy protocol, 800–1000 mg/m^2 i.v. over an 8h period, may repeat q21d provided the bone marrow has recovered.
Cats: Not recommended.
Small mammals, Birds, Reptiles: No information available.

Dactinomycin (Actinomycin-D)
(Cosmegen*, Dactinomycin*, Lyovac*) **POM**

Formulations: Injectable: 0.5 mg powder for reconstitution.

Action: An antibiotic antineoplastic that inhibits DNA synthesis and function. Inhibition of RNA and protein synthesis may also contribute to cytotoxic effects.

Use: Has been used in rescue protocols for canine lymphoma and also in some sarcomas and carcinomas. Use with caution with pre-existing bone marrow depression, hepatic dysfunction or infection. The drug is vesicant and tissue damage will result from extravasation, and therefore must be administered via a preplaced catheter.

Safety and handling: Potent cytotoxic drug that should only be prepared and administered by trained personnel. See Appendix and specialist texts for further advice on chemotherapeutic agents.

Contraindications: No information available.

Adverse reactions: Myelosuppression is the main dose-limiting toxicity. GI and hepatic toxicity may also occur. Can increase the risk of urate stone formation in susceptible breeds.

Drug interactions: No information available.

DOSES
See Appendix for chemotherapy protocols and conversion of body weight to body surface area.
Dogs: 0.5–0.75 mg/m^2 slow i.v. (over 20 mins) q2–3wk.
Cats, Small mammals, Birds, Reptiles: No information available.

Danazol
(Danazol*, Danol*) **POM**

Formulations: Oral: 100 mg, 200 mg capsules.

Action: Danazol is a synthetic androgen with weak androgenic properties that produces immunosuppression thought to be mediated through a reduction in macrophage cell surface immunoglobulin receptors and a decrease in the amount of antibody on target cells. May alter insulin requirements in animals with diabetes mellitus.

Use: Adjunct therapy for canine immune-mediated haemolytic anaemia and thrombocytopenia. The onset of action may be slow, with the effects taking several weeks to become apparent. Not commonly used due to unpredictable efficacy.

Safety and handling: Should be handled with gloves as it is teratogenic.

Contraindications: Avoid use in patients with cardiac, renal or hepatic impairment. Do not use in pregnant animals.

Adverse reactions: Teratogenic. May cause hepatotoxicity. Other effects result from suppression of the pituitary-ovarian axis and direct androgenic actions: virilization in females, increased muscle mass, testicular atrophy, alopecia.

Drug interactions: Synergistic action with corticosteroids. Inhibits metabolism of ciclosporin. Do not administer with anticoagulants as may decrease synthesis of coagulation factors in the liver. May decrease total serum T4 and increase T3 uptake.

DOSES
See Appendix for immunosuppression protocols.

Dogs: 4–10 mg/kg p.o. q12h, although an initial dose of 5 mg/kg q8–12h is suggested.
Cats: 5 mg/kg p.o. q12h.
Small mammals, Birds, Reptiles: No information available.

Danthron see Dantron

Dantrolene
(Dantrium*) POM

`CIL`

Formulations: Oral: 25 mg, 100 mg capsules. Injectable: Vials of 20 mg dantrolene powder, 3 g mannitol and sodium hydroxide for reconstitution.

Action: Uncouples the excitation contraction process by preventing the release of calcium ions from the sarcoplasmic reticulum in striated muscle. As vascular smooth muscle and cardiac muscle are not primarily dependent on calcium release for contraction they are not usually affected.

Use: Management of muscle spasms (e.g. urethral muscle spasm, tetanus). Prevention (oral) or treatment (i.v.) of malignant hyperthermia. Each vial should be reconstituted with 60 ml of water. Before administration the solution must be clear and without visible particles. The prepared solution must be protected from light and used within 6 hours.

Safety and handling: Normal precautions should be observed.

Contraindications: No information available.

Adverse reactions: Injectable preparation has pH 9.5 and is highly irritant when extravasated. Ideally administer via a large vein or inject into a fast running infusion to reduce the likelihood of thrombophlebitis. A diuresis follows i.v. administration, reflecting its formulation with mannitol. Chronic use is associated with hepatitis and pleural effusion; monitor liver function during therapy. Generalized muscle weakness, including the respiratory muscles, has been reported after overdose; initiate symptomatic supportive therapy and monitor the patient carefully, particularly with respect to efficacy of respiration.

Drug interactions: Do not combine with calcium-channel blockers.

DOSES
Dogs: Malignant hyperthermia: 2–5 mg/kg i.v.; Other indications: 0.5–2 mg/kg p.o. q12h.
Cats: 0.5–2 mg/kg p.o. q12h.
Small mammals, Birds, Reptiles: No information available.

Dantron (Danthron, Co-danthramer, Co-danthrusate)

(Co-danthramer*, Co-danthrusate Suspension*, Normax*) **POM**

Formulations: Dantron is only marketed in combination products. Oral: Co-danthramer: dantron/poloxamer 188 suspension 25/200 mg + 37.5/500 mg capsules; 5 mg/ml dantron + 40 mg/ml poloxamer suspension. Co-danthrusate: 50 mg dantron + 60 mg docusate capsule.

Action: Stimulates mild peristaltic effect in the lower bowel. Docusate and poloxamer are softening agents.

Use: Faecal softener/stimulant used to treat constipation in older patients.

Safety and handling: Normal precautions should be observed.

Contraindications: Do not use if GI obstruction present, or during pregnancy or lactation.

Adverse reactions: Dantron is potentially hepatotoxic and carcinogenic in experimental animals and therefore use in humans is restricted to aged or terminally ill patients. However, chronic toxicity has not been seen in dogs.

Drug interactions: No information available.

DOSES
Dogs: 2.5–5.0 ml p.o. q12h.
Cats: 1.0–2.5 ml p.o. q12h.
Small mammals, Birds, Reptiles: No information available.

DAP see Dog appeasing pheromone

Dapsone

(Dapsone*) **POM**

Formulations: Oral: 25 mg, 100 mg tablets.

Action: Proposed mechanisms include inhibition of the neutrophilic-cytotoxic system and interference with the alternate complement pathway. Also decreases antibody production and lysozymal enzyme synthesis. As an antibacterial, inhibits dihydropteroate synthase in susceptible organisms.

Use: Treatment of subcorneal pustular dermatitis, vasculitis and pemphigus. There is a lag phase of 4–8 weeks after starting treatment before effects are seen. Monitoring complete blood and platelet counts, chemistry analyses and urinalyses every 2–3 weeks for the first 4 months is recommended, at which point the frequency of monitoring can be reduced to every 3–4 months.

Safety and handling: Normal precautions should be observed.

Contraindications: No information available.

Adverse reactions: Side effects include anaemia, neutropenia, thrombocytopenia and hepatotoxicities. Cats have a greater sensitivity to dapsone, with a higher incidence of haemolytic anaemia and neurotoxicity.

Drug interactions: No information available.

DOSES
Dogs: 1 mg/kg q8–24h.
Cats: Do not use.
Small mammals, Birds, Reptiles: No information available.

Darbepoetin
(Aranesp) **POM**

CIL

Formulations: Injectable: 10–500 μg pre-filled syringes for injection.

Action: Stimulates division and differentiation of red blood cells. Darbepoetin is a derivative of human erythropoietin, which has been chemically modified to prolong its half-life. It may be less prone to produce anti-EPO antibodies than other rhEPO.

Use: Treatment of anaemia associated with chronic renal failure, although it is also used to treat anaemic human patients with cancer and rheumatoid arthritis, and cats with FeLV-associated anaemia. Monitoring and/or supplementation of iron may be necessary, especially if the response to treatment is poor.

Safety and handling: Normal precautions should be observed.

Contraindications: Conditions where high serum concentrations of erythropoietin already exist (e.g. haemolytic anaemia, anaemia due to blood loss), where anaemia is due to iron deficiency or where systemic hypertension is present.

Adverse reactions: Local and systemic allergic reactions may rarely develop (skin rash at the injection site, pyrexia, arthralgia and mucocutaneous ulcers).

Drug interactions: No information available.

DOSES
Dogs, Cats: 0.25–0.5 μg (micrograms)/kg s.c. weekly until PCV is normal, then increasing dose interval for maintenance. Doses of at least 1 μg/kg/week were more effective in one feline study.
Small mammals, Birds, Reptiles: No information available.

A B C D E F G H I J K L M N O P Q R S T U V W X Y Z

Deferoxamine (Desferrioxamine)
(Desferal*) POM

Formulations: Injectable: 500 mg vial for reconstitution.

Action: Deferoxamine chelates iron, and the complex is excreted in the urine.

Use: To remove iron from the body following poisoning. Also used for haemochromatosis (common in toucans, hornbills and softbills, though unusual in other birds).

Safety and handling: Normal precautions should be observed.

Contraindications: Avoid in severe renal disease.

Adverse reactions: Administration i.m. is painful. Anaphylactic reactions and hypotension may develop if administered rapidly i.v.

Drug interactions: No information available.

DOSES
Dogs, Cats: 10 mg/kg i.m., slow i.v. q4–8h or 15 mg/kg/h i.v. infusion. Maximum 80 mg/kg or 6 g in 24 hours.
Small mammals: No information available.
Birds: Various doses proposed, ranging from 20 mg/kg p.o. q4h to 40 mg/kg i.m. q24h (mynahs) to 100 mg/kg p.o., s.c., i.m. q24h for up to 14 weeks.
Reptiles: No information available.

Delmadinone
(Tardak) POM-V

Formulations: Injectable: 10 mg/ml suspension.

Action: Progestogens suppress FSH and LH production.

Use: Used in the treatment of hypersexuality (male dog and cat), prostatic hypertrophy, anal adenomas and hormonally driven canine aggression. In birds it may be useful for behavioural regurgitation or behaviour associated with sexual frustration. Dogs that show a reduced level of aggression when treated with delmadinone will not automatically show the same behavioural response to surgical castration because the drug also has a central calming effect. In situations of fear- or anxiety-related aggressive behaviour, the surgical approach can exacerbate the behaviour.

Safety and handling: Normal precautions should be observed.

Contraindications: No information available.

Adverse reactions: Possible adverse effects include a transient reduction in fertility and libido, polyuria and polydipsia, an increased appetite and hair colour change at the site of injection.

Drug interactions: Cortisol response to ACTH stimulation is significantly suppressed after just one dose of delmadinone.

DOSES

Dogs: 1.5–2 mg/kg (dogs <10 kg); 1–1.5 mg/kg (10-20 kg); 1 mg/kg (>20 kg) i.m., s.c. repeated after 8 days if no response. Animals that respond to treatment may need further treatment after 3–4 weeks.
Cats: 1.5 mg/kg repeated after 8 days if no response. Animals that respond to treatment may need further treatment after 3–4 weeks.
Small mammals: No information available.
Birds: 1 mg/kg i.m. once.
Reptiles: No information available.

Deltamethrin
(Scalibor) **NFA-VPS**

Formulations: Topical: 4% deltamethrin collar: 0.76 g (for small and medium dogs), 1.0 g (for large dogs).

Action: Acts as a sodium 'open channel blocker' resulting in muscular convulsions and death in arthropods. It also repels ticks and insects.

Use: Control of tick infestation (*Ixodes ricinus*, *Rhipicephalus sanguineus*) and prevention of feeding by sandflies and mosquitoes on dogs. May have additional repellant activity against fleas but should not be relied on for flea control.

Safety and handling: Wash hands after fitting the collar. Avoid letting children, in particular those under 2 years old, touch the collar, play with it or put it into their mouth.

Contraindications: Do not use on dogs <7 weeks old. Avoid use in dogs with skin lesions. Do not use on cats.

Adverse reactions: Highly toxic to aquatic animals and bees. Toxic to birds.

Drug interactions: No information available.

DOSES
Dogs: One collar q5–6months.
Cats: Do not use.
Small mammals, Birds, Reptiles: No information available.

L-Deprenyl see Selegiline
Desferrioxamine see Deferoxamine

Deslorelin
(Suprelorin) **POM-V**

Formulations: Implant containing 4.7 mg of active product.

Action: Desensitizes GnRH receptors, thereby decreasing release of LH and FSH. This leads to reduction in testosterone and sperm production.

Use: Chemical castration. There is a 14-day surge in testosterone followed by lowering of levels. Infertility is achieved from 6 weeks up to at least 6 months after initial treatment. Treated dogs should therefore still be kept away from bitches in heat within the first 6 weeks following initial treatment. Rarely, matings may occur during the 6 months but no pregnancy results. Any mating that occurs more than 6 months after the administration of the product may result in pregnancy. However, it is not necessary to keep bitches away from treated dogs following subsequent implantations, provided that the product is administered every 6 months. The ability of dogs to sire offspring following their return to normal plasma testosterone levels, after the administration of the product, has not been investigated. Dogs <10 kg may not recover their testosterone concentrations for 18 months. Disinfection of the site should be undertaken prior to implantation to avoid introduction of infection. If the hair is long, a small area should be clipped, if required. The product should be implanted subcutaneously in the loose skin on the back between the lower neck and the lumbar area. Avoid injection of the implant into fat, as release of the active substance might be impaired in areas of low vascularization. The biocompatible implant does not require removal. However, should it be necessary to end treatment, implants may be surgically removed. Implants can be located using ultrasonography. Deslorelin implants effectively prevent reproduction and the musky odour of intact male and female ferrets, and is therefore considered a suitable alternative for surgical neutering in these animals. Surgical neutering of ferrets has been implicated as an aetiological factor in the development of hyperadrenocorticism in this species. Deslorelin implants can be given to neutered ferrets to decrease the development or progression of adrenocortical disease. One implant per ferret may last 8.5–20.5 months. Anecdotally useful for some types of cystic ovarian disease in guinea pigs but duration of action is uncertain. Can be considered for oestrogen-induced mammary gland tumours in rats. The use of the implant in birds has been reported for a range of behavioural and reproductive (e.g. excessive egg laying) disorders but results appear to be variable.

Safety and handling: Pregnant women should not administer the product. If used in poultry, must be lifetime egg withhold.

Contraindications: Do not use in bitches.

Adverse reactions: Moderate swelling at the implant site may be observed for 14 days. A significant decrease in testicle size will be seen during the treatment period. In very rare cases, a testicle may be able to ascend the inguinal ring.

Drug interactions: No information available.

DOSES

Dogs: 1 implant per male dog.

Cats: No information available.

Small mammals: Ferrets: 1 implant per animal for removal of reproductive behaviour and breeding, as well as treatment of adrenal gland hyperplasia. The 9.4 mg implant (authorized in males only) lasts approximately 3–4 years. The 4.7 mg implant is not authorized in either sex and last approximately 2 years. Females will come into oestrus for approximately 2 weeks after implantation; Others: Effects are variable and depend on the exact pathology, species and sex.

Birds: 1 implant per animal regardless of size.

Reptiles: No information available.

Desmopressin

(DDAVP*, Desmospray*, Desmotabs*) **POM**

Formulations: Intranasal: 100 μg/ml solution; 10 μg metered spray. Injectable: 4 μg/ml solution. Oral: 100 μg, 200 μg tablets.

Action: Binds to and stimulates ADH receptors in the collecting ducts of the kidney. Desmopressin, a vasopressin analogue, has a longer duration of action than vasopressin and, unlike vasopressin, has no vasoconstrictor activity. Also increases von Willebrand factor, factor VIII and plasminogen concentrations.

Use: Diagnosis and treatment of central diabetes insipidus, and used to boost plasma levels of factor VIII and von Willebrand factor in patients with mild to moderate haemophilia A or von Willebrand's disease. Severe forms of these diseases are not successfully treated with desmopressin. Further advice on the use of this drug in the modified water deprivation test should be obtained from relevant texts and specialist laboratories. Assess adrenocortical function before performing the test.

Safety and handling: Normal precautions should be observed.

Contraindications: Do not perform the modified water deprivation test in patients with renal disease, dehydration or hypercalcaemia.

Adverse reactions: No information available.

Drug interactions: No information available.

DOSES

Dogs:
- Coagulopathies: 1–4 μg (micrograms)/kg i.v. once; dilute in 20 ml saline and administer over 10 min.
- Diabetes insipidus diagnosis: (using modified water deprivation test): 1–4 μg (micrograms)/dog i.v. once.
- Diabetes insipidus treatment: 1–4 μg (micrograms)/dog i.v., i.m. or 5–20 μg/dog or 0.05–0.2 ml/dog intranasally or on to the

conjunctiva q8–24h, or 5 µg/kg p.o. q8–24h initially (maximum dose 400 µg p.o. q8h). The dose and frequency of dosing can be increased or decreased according to response.

Cats: 5 µg (micrograms)/cat or 0.05 ml (1–2 drops) intranasally or on to the conjunctiva q8–24h, or 5 µg/cat p.o. q8–24h initially. The dose and frequency of dosing can be increased or decreased according to response.

Small mammals, Birds, Reptiles: No information available.

Dexamethasone

(Aurizon, Dexadreson, Dexafort, Dexa-ject, Rapidexon, Voren, Dexamethasone*, Maxidex*, Maxitrol*) **POM-V**

Formulations: Ophthalmic: 0.1% solution (Maxidex, Maxitrol). Maxitrol also contains polymyxin B and neomycin. Injectable: 2 mg/ml solution; 1 mg/ml, 3 mg/ml suspension; 2.5 mg/ml suspension with 7.5 mg/ml prednisolone. Oral: 0.5 mg tablet. (1 mg of dexamethasone is equivalent to 1.1 mg of dexamethasone acetate, 1.3 mg of dexamethasone isonicotinate or dexamethasone sodium phosphate, or 1.4 mg of dexamethasone trioxa-undecanoate.)

Action: Alters the transcription of DNA, leading to alterations in cellular metabolism which cause reduction in inflammatory response.

Use: Anti-inflammatory drug and in the assessment of adrenal function in suspected hyperadrenocorticism (HAC). Also used to prevent and treat anaphylaxis associated with transfusion or chemotherapeutic agents. Anti-inflammatory potency is 7.5 times greater than prednisolone. On a dose basis 0.15 mg dexamethasone is equivalent to 1 mg prednisolone. Dexamethasone has a long duration of action and low mineralocorticoid activity and is particularly suitable for short-term high-dose therapy in conditions where water retention would be a disadvantage. Unsuitable for long-term daily or alternate-day use. Animals on chronic therapy should be tapered off steroids when discontinuing the drug. Consult specialist texts and laboratories for advice on the performance and interpretation of dexamethasone suppression tests. Use shorter-acting preparations wherever possible in birds. The use of long-acting steroids in most cases of shock and spinal injury is of no benefit and may be detrimental. Use glucocorticoids with care in rabbits as they are sensitive to these drugs.

Safety and handling: Normal precautions should be observed.

Contraindications: Do not use in pregnant animals. Systemic corticosteroids are generally contraindicated in patients with renal disease and diabetes mellitus. Impaired wound healing and delayed recovery from infections may be seen. Topical corticosteroids are contraindicated in ulcerative keratitis.

Adverse reactions: A single dose of dexamethasone or dexamethasone sodium phosphate suppresses adrenal gland function for up to 32 hours. Prolonged use of glucocorticoids suppresses the hypothalamic-pituitary axis (HPA), causing adrenal atrophy, elevated liver enzymes, cutaneous atrophy, weight loss, PU/PD, vomiting and diarrhoea. GI ulceration may develop. Hyperglycaemia and decreased serum T4 values may be seen in patients receiving dexamethasone. Corticosteroids should be used with care in birds as there is a high risk of immunosuppression and side effects, such as hepatopathy and a diabetes mellitus-like syndrome. Even small single doses, or the use of topical, ocular and aural preparations, can cause severe adverse effects in rabbits.

Drug interactions: There is an increased risk of GI ulceration if used concurrently with NSAIDs. The risk of developing hypokalaemia is increased if corticosteroids are administered concomitantly with amphotericin B or potassium-depleting diuretics (furosemide, thiazides). Dexamethasone antagonizes the effect of insulin. The metabolism of corticosteroids may be enhanced by phenytoin or phenobarbital and decreased by antifungals such as itraconazole.

DOSES
See Appendix for immunosuppression protocols.
Dogs:
- Ophthalmic: Apply small amount of ointment to affected eye(s) q6–24h or 1 drop of solution in affected eye(s) q6–12h.
- Cerebral oedema: 2–3 mg/kg i.v., then 1 mg/kg s.c. q6–8h, taper off.
- Inflammation: 0.01–0.16 mg/kg i.m., s.c., p.o. q24h for 3–5 days maximum.
- Prevention and treatment of anaphylaxis: 0.5 mg/kg i.v. once.
- Immunosuppression: 0.3–0.64 mg/kg i.m., s.c., p.o. q24h for up to 5 days.
- Assessment of adrenal function: low dose dexamethasone suppression test (0.015 mg/kg i.v.).

Cats:
- Ophthalmic, Cerebral oedema, Inflammation, Anaphylaxis, Immunosuppression: doses as for dogs.
- Assessment of adrenal function: dexamethasone suppression test (0.15 mg/kg i.v.). NB: note difference to dogs.

Small mammals: Ferrets: 0.5–2.0 mg/kg s.c., i.m., i.v. q24h; Rabbits: 0.2–0.6 mg/kg s.c., i.m., i.v. q24h; Others: anti-inflammatory: 0.05–0.2 mg/kg i.m., s.c. q12–24h tapering dose over 3–14 days.
Birds: 2–6 mg/kg i.v., i.m. q12–24h.
Reptiles: Inflammatory, non-infectious respiratory disease: 2–4 mg/kg i.m., i.v. q24h for 3 days.

Dexmedetomidine
(Dexdomitor) **POM-V**

Formulations: Injectable: 0.1 mg/ml, 0.5 mg/ml solution.

Action: Agonist at peripheral and central alpha-2 adrenoreceptors producing dose-dependent sedation, muscle relaxation and analgesia.

Use: To provide sedation and premedication when used alone or in combination with opioid analgesics. Dexmedetomidine combined with ketamine is used to provide a short duration (20-30 min) of surgical anaesthesia in cats. Dexmedetomidine is also being increasingly used in very low doses to manage emergence excitation in dogs and cats during recovery from anaesthesia and for the provision of analgesia when administered by constant rate infusion. Dexmedetomidine is the pure dextroenantiomer of medetomidine. As the levomedetomidine enantiomer is largely inactive, dexmedetomidine is twice as potent as the racemic mixture (medetomidine). Administration of dexmedetomidine reduces the biological load presented to the animal, resulting in quicker metabolism of concurrently administered anaesthetic drugs and a potentially faster recovery from anaesthesia. Dexmedetomidine is a potent drug that causes marked changes in the cardiovascular system, including an initial peripheral vasoconstriction that results in an increase in blood pressure and a compensatory bradycardia. After 20–30 min vasoconstriction wanes, while blood pressure returns to normal values. Heart rate remains low due to the central sympatholytic effect of alpha-2 agonists. These cardiovascular changes result in a fall in cardiac output; central organ perfusion is well maintained at the expense of redistribution of blood flow away from the peripheral tissues. Respiratory system function in well maintained; respiration rate may fall but is accompanied by an increased depth of respiration. Oxygen supplementation is advisable in all animals that have received dexmedetomidine for sedation. The duration of analgesia from a 5 μg/kg dose of dexmedetomidine is approximately 1 hour. Combining dexmedetomidine with an opioid provides improved analgesia and sedation. Lower doses of dexmedetomidine should be used in combination with other drugs. Reversal of dexmedetomidine sedation or premedication with atipamezole at the end of the procedure shortens the recovery period, which is advantageous. Analgesia should be provided with other classes of drugs before atipamezole. The authorized dose range of dexmedetomidine for dogs and cats is very broad. High doses (>10 μg/kg) are associated with greater physiological disturbances than doses of 1–10 μg/kg. Using dexmedetomidine in combination with opioids in the lower dose range can provide good sedation and analgesia with minimal side effects. The lower concentration of dexmedetomidine is designed to increase the accuracy of dosing in dogs <20 kg body weight and cats.

Safety and handling: Normal precautions should be observed.

Contraindications: Do not use in animals with cardiovascular or other systemic disease. Use of dexmedetomidine in geriatric patients is not advisable. It should not be used in pregnant animals, nor in animals likely to require or receiving sympathomimetic amines.

Adverse reactions: Causes diuresis by suppressing ADH secretion, a transient increase in blood glucose by decreasing endogenous insulin secretion, mydriasis and decreased intraocular pressure. Vomiting after i.m. administration is common, so dexmedetomidine should be avoided when vomiting is contraindicated (e.g. foreign body, raised intraocular pressure). Due to effects on blood glucose, use in diabetic animals is not recommended. Spontaneous arousal from deep sedation following stimulation can occur with all alpha-2 agonists, aggressive animals sedated with dexmedetomidine must still be managed with caution.

Drug interactions: No information available.

DOSES

When used for sedation is generally given as part of a combination. See Appendix for sedation protocols in all species.
Dogs, Cats:
- Premedication: 3–5 µg (micrograms)/kg i.v., i.m, s.c. in combination with an opioid (use lower end of dose range i.v.).
- Emergence excitation: 1 µg (microgram)/kg i.v. can be given to manage emergence excitation during recovery from anaesthesia, although administration around the time of extubation will prolong the recovery period from anaesthesia and treated animals should be monitored carefully.
- Perioperative analgesia and rousable sedation: 1–2 µg (micrograms)/kg/h constant rate infusion is indicated, although the efficacy of analgesia will be improved in most animals if dexmedetomidine is used as an adjunt to opioid analgesia.

Small mammals: See Appendix.
Birds, Reptiles: No information available.

Dextrose see Glucose

Diazepam `CIL`
(Dialar*, Diazemuls*, Diazepam Rectubes*, Rimapam*, Stesolid*, Tensium*, Valclair*, Valium*) **POM**

Formulations: Injectable: 5 mg/ml emulsion (2 ml ampoules, Diazemuls). Oral: 2 mg, 5 mg, 10 mg tablets; 2 mg/5 ml solution. Rectal: 2 mg/ml (1.25, 2.5 ml tubes), 4 mg/ml (2.5 ml tubes) solutions; 10 mg suppositories.

Action: Enhances activity of the major inhibitory central nervous system neurotransmitter, gamma-aminobutyric acid (GABA), through binding to the benzodiazepine site of the $GABA_A$ receptor.

Use: Anticonvulsant, anxiolytic and skeletal muscle relaxant (e.g. urethral muscle spasm and tetanus). Diazepam is the drug of choice for the short-term emergency control of severe epileptic seizures and status epilepticus in dogs and cats. The anti-seizure effect in the dog is only maintained for around 20 minutes and should always be used as part of a balanced emergency seizure protocol; not effective as maintenance anti-seizure medication in the dog. In cats is effective as a maintenance medication. Diazepam is indicated in dogs with marked spinal pain due to muscle spasm, in combination with conventional pain relief. It may also be used in combination with ketamine to offset muscle hypertonicity associated with ketamine, and with opioids and/or acepromazine for pre-anaesthetic medication in the critically ill. It provides very poor sedation or even excitation when used alone in healthy animals. Diazepam is used in behavioural medicine for anxiety and fear-related disorders in dogs and cats, especially where there are signs of panic. In addition, its amnesic properties mean it can be used during or immediately following an aversive experience to minimize the impact of such exposure. Best if used approximately 30 minutes before a fear-inducing event. Higher range doses are required for amnesic activity. Although it has been used for the management of urine spraying in cats, a high relapse rate upon withdrawal should be expected. Used in birds for the short-term management of feather plucking. It is used in cats as an appetite stimulant. Diazepam has a high lipid solubility, which facilitates its oral absorption and rapid central effects. Liver disease will prolong duration of action. In the short term repeated doses of diazepam or a constant rate infusion will lead to drug accumulation and prolonged recovery. Flumazenil (a benzodiazepine antagonist) will reverse the effects of diazepam. The development of dependence to benzodiazepams may occur after regular use, even with therapy of only a few weeks, and the dose should be gradually reduced in these cases if the benzodiazepine is being withdrawn.

Safety and handling: Substantial adsorption of diazepam may occur on to some plastics and this may cause a problem when administering diazepam by continuous i.v. infusion. The use of diazepam in PVC infusion bags should be avoided; giving sets should be kept as short as possible and should not contain a cellulose propionate volume-control chamber. If diazepam is given by continuous i.v. infusion the compatible materials include glass, polyolefin, polypropylene and polyethylene.

Contraindications: Benzodiazepines should be avoided in patients with CNS depression, respiratory depression, severe muscle weakness or hepatic impairment (as may worsen hepatic encephalopathy). They are also contraindicated in the long-term treatment of canine and feline behavioural disorders due to the risks of disinhibition and interference with memory and learning.

Adverse reactions: Sedation, muscle weakness and ataxia are common. Rapid i.v. injection or oral overdose may cause marked paradoxical excitation (including aggression) and elicit signs of pain in normal dogs; i.v. injections should be made slowly (over at least 1 minute for each 5 mg). Intramuscular injection is painful and results in erratic drug absorption. Rectal administration is effective for emergency control of seizures if i.v. access is not possible, but the time to onset is delayed to 5–10 min. The duration of action may be prolonged after repeated doses in rapid succession, in older animals, those with liver dysfunction, and those receiving beta-1 antagonists. Fulminant hepatic necrosis in cats has been associated with repeated oral administration. Chronic dosing leads to a shortened half-life due to activation of the hepatic microsomal enzyme system and tolerance to the drug may develop in dogs. The propylene glycol formulation of injectable diazepam can cause thrombophlebitis, therefore the emulsion formulation is preferred for i.v. injection.

Drug interactions: Do not dilute or mix with other agents. Due to extensive metabolism by the hepatic microsomal enzyme system, interactions with other drugs metabolized in this way are common. Cimetidine and omeprazole inhibit metabolism of diazepam and may prolong clearance. Concurrent use of phenobarbital may lead to a decrease in the half-life of diazepam. An enhanced sedative effect may be seen if antihistamines or opioid analgesics are administered with diazepam, and diazepam will reduce the dose requirement of other anaesthetic agents. When given with diazepam the effects of digoxin may be increased. Diazepam may be used in combination with tricyclic antidepressant therapy for the management of more severe behavioural responses.

DOSES
When used for sedation is generally given as part of a combination. See Appendix for sedation protocols in all species.
Dogs:
- Anxiolytic: 0.5–2.0 mg/kg p.o as required.
- Sedation and premedication: 0.2–0.5 mg/kg i.v., i.m.
- Skeletal muscle relaxation: 2–10 mg/dog p.o. q8–12h.
- Emergency management of seizures, including status epilepticus: bolus dose of 0.5–1 mg/kg i.v. or intrarectally (if venous access is not available). Time to onset of clinical effect is 2–3 min for i.v. use; therefore repeat every 10 min if no clinical effect, up to three times. Additional doses may be administered if appropriate supportive care facilities are available (for support of respiration). Constant rate i.v. infusion for control of status epilepticus or cluster seizures: initial rate 1 mg/kg/h, may be titrated upwards to effect.

Cats:
- Anxiolytic: 0.2–0.4 mg/kg p.o. q8h.
- Appetite stimulant: 0.1–0.2 mg/kg i.v. once.
- Behavioural modification of urine spraying and muscle relaxation: 1.25–5 mg/cat p.o. q8h. The dose should be gradually increased to achieve the desired effect without concurrent sedation.
- Emergency management of seizures including status epilepticus: bolus dose of 0.5–1 mg/kg i.v. or intrarectally if venous access is not available. Time to onset of clinical effect is 2–3 min for i.v. use, therefore repeat every 10 min if there is no clinical effect, up to maximum of three times. Constant rate i.v. infusion for the control of status epilepticus or cluster seizures: initial rate of 0.5 mg/kg/h. Care should be taken in cats to avoid overdosing: if cats demonstrate excessive sedation then diazepam should be discontinued.

Small mammals: Ferrets: seizures: 2–5 mg/kg i.m. once; Rabbits: epileptic seizures: 1 mg/kg i.v.; Guinea pigs: 0.5–5.0 mg/kg i.m. once; Chinchillas, Hamsters, Gerbils, Rats, Mice: 2.5–5 mg/kg i.m., i.p. once.
Birds:
- Epileptic seizures: 0.1–1 mg/kg i.v., i.m. once.
- Appetite stimulant in raptors: 0.2 mg/kg p.o. q24h.
Reptiles: Epileptic seizures: 2.5 mg/kg i.m., i.v.

Diazoxide

(Eudemine*) **POM**

Formulations: Injectable: 15 mg/ml solution. Oral: 50 mg tablet.

Action: A diuretic that causes vasodilation and inhibits insulin secretion by blocking calcium mobilization.

Use: Used to manage hypoglycaemia caused by hyperinsulinism in dogs and ferrets. In humans it is also used in the short-term management of acute hypertension.

Safety and handling: Normal precautions should be observed.

Contraindications: No information available.

Adverse reactions: The commonest adverse effects are anorexia, vomiting and diarrhoea. Hypotension, tachycardia, bone marrow suppression, pancreatitis, cataracts and electrolyte and fluid retention may occur. Drug efficacy may diminish over a period of months.

Drug interactions: Phenothiazines and thiazide diuretics may increase the hyperglycaemic activity of diazoxide, whilst alpha-adrenergic blocking agents (e.g. phenoxybenzamine) may antagonize the effects of diazoxide.

DOSES
Dogs:
- Hypoglycaemia: 3.3 mg/kg p.o. q8h initially, increasing gradually to 20 mg/kg p.o. q8h.
- Hypertension: 1–3 mg/kg rapid i.v. injection (<30 seconds); maximum single dose of 150 mg.

Cats: No information available.
Small mammals: Ferrets: 5–30 mg/kg p.o. q12h.
Birds, Reptiles: No information available.

Dibotermin alfa (Recombinant human Bone Morphogenetic Protein-2, rhBMP-2)
(TruScient) **POM-V**

Formulations: 0.66 mg vial which when reconstituted produces 0.2 mg/ml of dibotermin alfa. Kit includes two sponges of bovine type I collagen.

Action: Dibotermin alfa is a human osteoinductive protein derived from a recombinant mammalian cell line, which causes induction of new bone tissue at the site of implantation by binding to receptors on the surface of mesenchymal cells and causing differentiation into bone-forming cells.

Use: Authorized for the treatment of diaphyseal fractures as an adjunct to standard surgical care using open fracture reduction in dogs. It has also been successfully applied for the stimulation of healing of feline diaphyseal fractures, canine and feline arthrodeses and delayed or non-union fracture revision surgery. Before using the product, definitive fracture reduction, fixation and haemostasis should be achieved. The sponge is prepared by saturating it with the solution a minimum of 15 minutes before it is inserted (the saturated sponges must be used within 2 hours). When preparing the solution it is important to follow the instructions on reconstitution carefully. Once reconstituted, 1.6 ml of the solution is uniformly distributed on to each sponge. Any pooled fluid should be removed from the fracture site. The prepared sponges should be cut into strips as needed prior to placement. The amount of prepared sponge required is determined by the fracture anatomy and the ability to close the wound with minimal compression of the sponge. The prepared sponge should be placed so that it bridges the fracture and makes good contact with the major proximal and distal fracture fragments. During placement, forceps should be used to handle the prepared sponge to avoid excessive fluid loss. The prepared sponge may be wrapped around the bone or placed up to the edges of a bone plate as the geometry of the fracture and fixation requires. The periosteal soft tissues should not be unnecessarily disturbed in order to place the sponges. Dibotermin alfa will not provide mechanical stability and should not be used to fill spaces in the presence of compressive forces.

Safety and handling: Intended for single-use only. It must not be re-sterilized.

Contraindications: Do not use in dogs that are skeletally immature, have an active infection at the surgical site, pathological fracture or any active malignancy. Bone plates should not be covered with the prepared sponge in order to facilitate plate removal if required following fracture healing. Do not irrigate the wound once the prepared sponge is placed across the fracture.

Adverse reactions: Local proliferation of mesenchymal tissue maturing to new bone occurs and so a firm swelling is often palpable within the first 3 weeks postoperatively, which gradually recedes over several months. A soft swelling which recedes within 3 weeks may also occur. Uncommonly, exuberant bony callus associated with a persistent (>10 weeks), moderate soft tissue swelling may occur. Normal complications of fracture repair (seroma, excessive licking of incision area, joint stiffness, local swelling, skin ulcer, incisional discharge, incisional dehiscence) can occur.

Drug interactions: None reported.

DOSES
Dogs, Cats: Use only the amount of prepared sponge needed to achieve coverage of accessible fracture lines and defects (maximum of two sponges).
Small mammals, Birds, Reptiles: No information available.

Dichlorophen

(Dichlorophen Tablets BP) **AVM-GSL**

Formulations: Oral: 500 mg tablet.

Action: Cestocide which acts by interfering with oxidative phosphorylation.

Use: Control of tapeworm infections in dogs and cats >6 months old. Effective against *Taenia* and *Dipylidium* but not *Echinococcus*. Affected worms are dislodged and disintegrate during their passage along the alimentary tract so they are not easily recognizable when passed 6–8h after dosing. Administer tablets whole or crushed in food.

Safety and handling: Normal precautions should be observed.

Contraindications: Do not repeat the treatment if vomiting occurs shortly after dosing. Do not administer to animals weighing <1.25 kg or under 6 months of age. Do not repeat the treatment in <10 days.

Adverse reactions: Vomiting may be seen. Rarely salivation, hyperaesthesia and loss of coordination.

Drug interactions: No information available.

DOSES

Dogs, Cats: 250 mg total dose (dogs, cats <2.5 kg), 500 mg/2.5 kg (larger animals) p.o. Give maximum 6 tablets at one time, and give the rest 3 hours later if there is no vomiting. The tablets are best administered immediately before the main feed of the day and may be given whole or crushed and given in food. Animals should be treated every 4–6 months.

Small mammals: No information available.

Birds: Pigeons: 10 mg/pigeon p.o. twice, 10 days apart.

Reptiles: No information available.

Diclofenac

(Voltarol Ophtha*, Voltarol Ophtha Multidose*) **POM**

Formulations: Ophthalmic: 0.1% solution in 5 ml bottle and in single-use vial.

Action: COX inhibitor that produces local anti-inflammatory effects.

Use: Used in cataract surgery to prevent intraoperative miosis and reflex (axonal) miosis caused by ulcerative keratitis. Used to control pain and inflammation associated with corneal surgery and in ulcerative keratitis when topical corticosteroid use is contraindicated.

Safety and handling: Normal precautions should be observed.

Contraindications: No information available.

Adverse reactions: As with other topical NSAIDs, diclofenac may cause local irritation. Topical NSAIDs should be used with caution in ulcerative keratitis as they can delay epithelial healing. Topical NSAIDs, and most specifically diclofenac, have been associated with an increased risk of corneal 'melting' (keratomalacia) in humans, although this has not been reported in the veterinary literature. Topical NSAIDs have the potential to increase intraocular pressure and should be used with caution in dogs predisposed to glaucoma. Regular monitoring is advised. Use of systemic formulations has been associated with death in some species of bird.

Drug interactions: Ophthalmic NSAIDs may be used safely with other ophthalmic pharmaceuticals, although concurrent use of drugs which adversely affect the corneal epithelium (e.g. gentamicin) may lead to increased corneal penetration of the NSAID. The concurrent use of topical NSAIDs with topical corticosteroids has been identified as a risk factor in humans for precipitating corneal problems.

DOSES
Dogs, Cats: 1 drop q30min for 2 h prior to cataract surgery (there is a wide variation in protocols for cataract surgery).
Small mammals: No information available.
Birds: See note above on adverse reaction.
Reptiles: No information available.

Difloxacin
(Dicural) **POM-V**

Formulations: Oral: 15 mg, 50 mg, 100 mg and 150 mg tablets. Injectable: 50 mg/ml solution.

Action: Bactericidal antimicrobial which works by inhibiting the bacterial DNA gyrase enzyme, causing damage to the bacterial DNA. The fluoroquinolones work in a concentration-dependent manner.

Use: Ideally fluoroquinolone use should be reserved for infections where culture and sensitivity testing predicts a clinical response and where first- and second-line antimicrobials would not be effective. Active against a wide range of Gram-negative organisms and also good to intermediate activity against Gram-positives (e.g. *Escherichia coli*, *Klebsiella*, *Pasteurella*, *Staphylococcus*, *Pseudomonas aeruginosa*). Activity against *Streptococcus* and *Proteus* is intermediate. Activity against anaerobes is limited. Main indications include infections associated with the skin and soft tissues, and bacterial cystitis. Capable of achieving exceptionally high concentrations in the urinary tract.

Safety and handling: Normal precautions should be observed.

Contraindications: Due to concerns about the development of arthropathy in young animals, do not use in dogs <8 months old or <18 months in large and giant breeds. Do not use in dogs with epilepsy.

Adverse reactions: Mild self-limiting GI disturbance has been reported. Fluoroquinolones have been associated with cartilage lesions in young animals. Neurotoxicity is associated with drug overdose.

Drug interactions: Substances containing divalent and trivalent cations, including sucralfate, antacids, multivitamins and compounds containing iron, magnesium, calcium and zinc, may interfere with the absorption of the drug from the GI tract.

DOSES
See Appendix for guidelines on responsible antibacterial use.
Dogs: 5 mg/kg p.o., s.c. q24h.
Cats, Small mammals, Birds, Reptiles: No information available.

Digoxin
(Digoxin*, Lanoxin*, Lanoxin PG*) **POM**

CIL

Formulations: Oral: 62.5 µg, 125 µg, 250 µg tablets; 50 µg/ml elixir. Injectable: 100 µg/ml, 250 µg/ml.

Action: Inhibits Na^+-K^+ ATPase, leading to an increase in intracellular sodium. Sodium is exchanged for calcium, resulting in an increase in intracellular calcium and hence a mild positive inotropic effect. Digoxin slows the heart rate by decreasing the rate of sinoatrial node firing and inhibiting AV nodal conduction. These effects result primarily from parasympathetic activation and sympathetic inhibition, although it may also have a modest direct depression of nodal tissue. The combination of a slower heart rate and increased force of contraction increases cardiac output in patients with supraventricular tachyarrhythmias. Digoxin improves baroreceptor reflexes that are impaired in heart failure.

Use: Management of heart failure and supraventricular tachyarrhythmias. It is primarily used to control the ventricular rate in cases of heart failure with concurrent atrial fibrillation. Effective to decrease the ventricular rate in dogs with atrial fibrillation either as monotherapy or in combination with diltiazem. Digoxin/diltiazem combination therapy results in more effective rate control than monotherapy. In ferrets and rabbits it is used in the treatment of dilated cardiomyopathy. Serum levels should be checked after 5–7 days, with a sample taken at least 8 hours post-pill. The bioavailability of digoxin varies between the different formulations: i.v. = 100%; tablets = 60%; and elixir = 75%. If toxic effects are seen or the drug is ineffective, serum levels of digoxin should be assessed; the ideal therapeutic level is a trough serum concentration in the region of 1 ng/ml to optimize beneficial effects and minimize toxic side effects, with a suggested range 0.6–1.2 ng/ml. The dose shown below achieves a therapeutic serum digoxin concentration (1.0–2.0 ng/ml) whilst minimizing adverse effects in dogs. Decreased dosages or an increase in dosing intervals may be required in geriatric patients, obese animals or those with significant renal dysfunction. The intravenous route is rarely indicated and, if used, should be done very slowly and with extreme care.

Safety and handling: Normal precautions should be observed.

Contraindications: Frequent ventricular arrhythmias or atrioventricular block.

Adverse reactions: Cats are more sensitive to the toxic effects of digoxin than dogs. Hypokalaemia predisposes to toxicity in all species. Signs of toxicity include anorexia, vomiting, diarrhoea, depression or arrhythmias (e.g. AV block, bigeminy, paroxysmal ventricular or atrial tachycardias with block, and multiform ventricular premature contractions). Lidocaine and phenytoin may be used to control digoxin-associated arrhythmias. Intravenous administration may cause vasoconstriction.

Drug interactions: Antacids, chemotherapy agents (e.g. cyclophosphamide, cytarabine, doxorubicin, vincristine), cimetidine and metoclopramide may decrease digoxin absorption from the GI tract. The following may increase the serum level, decrease the elimination rate or enhance the toxic effects of digoxin: amiodarone, antimuscarinics, diazepam, erythromycin, loop and thiazide diuretics (hypokalaemia), oxytetracycline, quinidine and verapamil. Spironolactone may enhance or decrease the toxic effects of digoxin.

DOSES
Dogs: 2.2–4.4 µg (micrograms)/kg i.v. q12h. Tablets: 3–7 µg/kg p.o. q12h based on lean body weight (decrease dose by 10% for elixir). Maximum dose 0.25 mg/dog p.o. q12h.
Cats: 1–1.6 µg (micrograms)/kg i.v. q12h, 10 µg/kg p.o. q24–48h, ¼ of a 125 µg tablet q24–48h.
Small mammals: Ferrets: 5–10 µg (micrograms)/kg p.o. q12–24h; Rabbits: 3–30 µg/kg p.o. q24–48h; Hamsters: 0.05–0.1 mg/kg p.o. q12–24h.
Birds: Raptors: 0.02–0.05 mg/kg p.o. q12h for 2–3 days then reduce to 0.01 mg/kg q12–24h; Pigeons, Parrots: 0.02 mg/kg p.o. q24h.
Reptiles: No information available.

Diltiazem
(Hypercard, Dilcardia SR*) **POM-V, POM**

Formulations: Oral: 10 mg (Hypercard), 60 mg (generic) tablets. Long-acting preparations authorized for humans, such as Dilcardia SR (60 mg, 90 mg, 120 mg capsules), are available but their pharmacokinetics have been little studied in animals to date.

Action: Inhibits inward movement of calcium ions through slow (L-type) calcium channels in myocardial cells, cardiac conduction tissue and vascular smooth muscle; vascular smooth muscle is more sensitive to diltiazem than myocardial tissues (relative activity of 7:1). Diltiazem causes a reduction in myocardial contractility (negative inotrope, although less effective than verapamil), depressed electrical activity (retarded atrioventricular conduction) and decreases vascular resistance (vasodilation of cardiac vessels and peripheral arteries and arterioles).

Use: Primarily used to control supraventricular tachyarrhythmias in dogs and cats. It is authorized for use in cats with hypertrophic cardiomyopathy. Effective to decrease the ventricular rate in dogs with atrial fibrillation either as monotherapy or in combination with digoxin. Digoxin/diltiazem combination therapy results in more effective rate control than monotherapy. Diltiazem is preferred to verapamil by many because it has effective antiarrhythmic properties with minimal negative inotropy. Diltiazem is less effective than amlodipine in the management of hypertension. In cats with hypertrophic cardiomyopathy beta-adrenergic blockers are now more commonly used than diltiazem. Reduce the dose in patients with hepatic or renal impairment.

Safety and handling: Normal precautions should be observed.

Contraindications: Diltiazem is contraindicated in patients with second or third degree AV block, marked hypotension or sick sinus syndrome, and should be used cautiously in patients with systolic dysfunction or acute or decompensated congestive heart failure.

Adverse reactions: In dogs, bradycardia is the commonest adverse effect, whilst in cats it is vomiting. Lethargy can be seen in both species.

Drug interactions: If diltiazem is administered concurrently with beta-adrenergic blockers (e.g. propranolol), there may be additive negative inotropic and chronotropic effects. The co-administration of diltiazem and beta-blockers is not recommended. The activity of diltiazem may be adversely affected by calcium salts or vitamin D. There are conflicting data regarding the effect of diltiazem on serum digoxin levels and monitoring of these levels is recommended if the drugs are used concurrently. Cimetidine inhibits the metabolism of diltiazem, thereby increasing plasma concentrations. Diltiazem enhances the effect of theophylline, which may lead to toxicity. It may affect quinidine and ciclosporin concentrations. Diltiazem may displace highly protein-bound agents from plasma proteins. Diltiazem may increase intracellular vincristine levels by inhibiting outflow of the drug from the cell.

DOSES
Dogs: 0.05–0.25 mg/kg i.v. over 1–2 minutes, 0.5–2.0 mg/kg p.o. q8h or up to 3.0 mg/kg p.o. q12h for sustained/extended release preparations. Lower doses are preferred in the presence of heart failure. Long-acting preparations have been used at a dose of 10 mg/kg p.o. q24h but there is little experience with such formulations in animals.
Cats: 0.05–0.25 mg/kg i.v. over 1–2 minutes, 0.5–2.5 mg/kg p.o. q8h, or one 10 mg tablet for cats of 3–6.25 kg p.o. q8h.
Small mammals: Ferrets: 1.5–7.5 mg/kg p.o. q12h.
Birds, Reptiles: No information available.

Dimercaprol (British anti-lewisite)
(Dimercaprol*) **POM**

Formulations: Injectable: 50 mg/ml solution in peanut oil.

Action: Chelates heavy metals.

Use: Treatment of acute toxicity caused by arsenic, gold, bismuth and mercury, and used as an adjunct (with edetate calcium disodium) in lead poisoning.

Safety and handling: Normal precautions should be observed.

Contraindications: Severe hepatic failure.

Adverse reactions: Intramuscular injections are painful. Dimercaprol-metal complexes are nephrotoxic. This is particularly so with iron, selenium or cadmium; do not use for these metals. Alkalinization of urine during therapy may have protective effects for the kidney.

Drug interactions: Iron salts should not be administered during therapy.

DOSES
Dogs, Cats: 2.5–5 mg/kg i.m. q4h for 2 days, then q8h for 10 days or until recovery. (Note: the 5 mg/kg dose should only be used on the first day when severe acute intoxication occurs.) Arsenic poisoning when gastroenteritis is present: 6–7 mg/kg i.m. q8h or 3–4 mg/kg i.m. q6h. Increase intervals between doses on 3rd day and q12h dosing at the lower dosage levels may begin on day 4; continue to day 10. Aggressive supportive therapy should be maintained throughout the treatment period.
Small mammals: No information available.
Birds: 2.5 mg/kg i.m. q4h for 2 days then q12h until signs resolve.
Reptiles: No information available.

Dimethylsulfoxide (DMSO)
(Rimso-50*) **POM**

Formulations: Injectable: 50%, 90% liquid; medical grade only available as a 50% solution, other formulations are available as an industrial solvent. Topical: 70%, 90% gel; 70% cream.

Action: The mechanism of action is not well understood. Antioxidant activity has been demonstrated in certain biological settings and is thought to account for the anti-inflammatory activity.

Use: Management of otitis externa and haemorrhagic cystitis induced by cyclophosphamide. Although efficacy is unproven it has been used in the treatment of renal amyloidosis. In humans, DMSO is authorized for the treatment of interstitial cystitis. DMSO is very rapidly absorbed through the skin following administration by all routes and is distributed throughout the body. Metabolites of DMSO are excreted in the urine and faeces. DMSO is also excreted through the lungs and skin, producing a characteristic sulphuric odour. Humans given DMSO experience a garlic-like taste sensation after administration.

Safety and handling: Should be kept in a tightly closed container because it is very hygroscopic. Gloves should be worn during topical application and the product should be handled with care.

Contraindications: No information available.

Adverse reactions: Changes in refractive index and lens opacities have been seen in dogs given high doses of DMSO chronically, these are slowly reversible upon discontinuation of the drug. Other adverse effects include local irritation and erythema caused by local histamine release. Administration i.v. of solutions with concentrations >20% may cause haemolysis and diuresis.

Drug interactions: DMSO should not be mixed with other potentially toxic ingredients when applied to the skin because of profound enhancement of systemic absorption.

DOSES
Dogs:
- Otic: 4–6 drops of a 60% solution in affected ear q12h for up to 14 days.
- Renal amyloidosis: 80 mg/kg s.c. 3 times/week; 125–300 mg/kg p.o. q24h.
- Topical: Apply 90% solution to affected areas q8–12h. Total daily dose should not exceed 20 ml. Do not apply for longer than 14 days.

Cats, Small mammals: No information available.
Birds: May be applied topically to lesions, e.g. bumblefoot, as an anti-inflammatory presurgery. May be combined with other drugs as a carrying agent.
Reptiles: No information available.

Dinoprost tromethamine
(Prostaglandin F2)
(Enzaprost, Lutalyse) **POM-V**

Formulations: Injectable: 5 mg/ml solution.

Action: Stimulates uterine contraction, causes cervical relaxation and inhibits progesterone production by the corpus luteum.

Use: Used in the termination of pregnancy at any stage of gestation and to stimulate uterine contractions in the treatment of open pyometra.

Safety and handling: Pregnant woman and asthmatics should avoid handling this agent.

Contraindications: Do not use for the treatment of closed pyometra as there is a risk of uterine rupture.

Adverse reactions: Hypersalivation, panting, tachycardia, vomiting, urination, defecation, transient hyperthermia, locomotor incoordination and mild CNS signs have been reported. Such effects usually diminish within 30 min of drug administration. There is no adverse effect on future fertility. Severe adverse effects are reported in birds.

Drug interactions: The effect of oxytocin would be potentiated by prostaglandins and inhibited by progestogens.

DOSES
Dogs:
- Abortifacient: First half of gestation: 0.05–0.25 mg/kg s.c. q12h for 4 days starting at least 5 days after the onset of cytological dioestrus. Second half of gestation: 0.05–0.25 mg/kg s.c. q12h until abortion is complete; monitor radiographically or ultrasonographically. Use low doses initially (0.05–0.1 mg/kg s.c. q12h) to assess the severity of any adverse effects. Assess serum progesterone concentration at the end of treatment to ensure that complete luteolysis has occurred.
- Open pyometra: 0.1–0.25 mg/kg s.c. q12h until the uterus is empty; usually 3–5 days treatment required.

Cats: Abortifacient: 0.025 mg/kg s.c. q24h for up to 5 days, after day 40 of pregnancy.

Small mammals: Rabbits: 0.2 mg/kg single i.m. injection following 3 days of oral liquid paraffin to assist in emptying impacted caecal contents.

Birds: Do not use.

Reptiles: No information available.

Dinoprostone (Prostaglandin E2)
(Prostin E2*) **POM**

Formulations: Topical: 0.4 mg/ml gel.

Action: Stimulates uterine contraction, causes cervical relaxation and inhibits progesterone production by the corpus luteum.

Use: Used to relax the vagina and induce uterine contractions in egg-bound birds.

Safety and handling: Pregnant woman and asthmatics should avoid handling this agent.

Contraindications: No information available.

Adverse reactions: Uterine rupture may occur.

Drug interactions: No information available.

DOSES
Birds: Apply a thin layer of gel to the cloacal mucosa once.
Dogs, Cats, Small mammals, Reptiles: No information available.

Dioctyl sodium sulfosuccinate see **Docusate sodium**

Diphenhydramine
(Dreemon*, Nytol*) **P**

Formulations: Oral: 25 mg tablet; 2 mg/ml solution. Other products are available of various concentrations and most contain other active ingredients.

Action: The antihistaminergic (H1) effects are used to reduce pruritus and prevent motion sickness. It is also a mild anxiolytic and sedative.

Use: Control of mild anxiety conditions in dogs and cats, including anxiety related to car travel. Management of night-time activity in cats and compulsive scratching. In birds it is used in the management of allergic rhinitis and hypersensitivity reactions. In ferrets it is used before vaccination if a previous vaccine reaction has been encountered. Liquid is very distasteful.

Safety and handling: Normal precautions should be observed.

Contraindications: Urine retention, glaucoma and hyperthyroidism.

Adverse reactions: Paradoxical excitement may be seen in cats.

Drug interactions: An increased sedative effect may occur if used with benzodiazepines or other anxiolytics/hypnotics. Avoid the concomitant use of other sedative agents. Diphenhydramine may enhance the effect of adrenaline and partially counteract anticoagulant effects of heparin.

DOSES
Dogs:
- Antiemesis: 2–4 mg/kg p.o. q6–8h.
- Suppression of pruritus: 1–2 mg/kg p.o. q8–12h.

Cats: 2–4 mg/kg p.o. q6-8h, 1 mg/kg i.v., i.m. q8h.

Small mammals: Ferrets: 0.5–2 mg/kg p.o. q8–12h; Guinea pigs: 5 mg/kg s.c. prn; Chinchillas, Hamsters, Rats, Mice: 1–2 mg/kg p.o., s.c. q12h.

Birds: 2–4 mg/kg p.o. q12h.

Reptiles: No information available.

Diphenoxylate (Co-phenotrope)   **CIL**
(Lomotil* (with atropine)) **POM**

Formulations: Oral: 2.5 mg diphenoxylate + 0.025 mg atropine tablet.

Action: Increases intestinal segmental smooth muscle tone, decreases the propulsive activity of smooth muscle, and decreases electrolyte and water secretion into the intestinal lumen. Atropine is added in a sub-therapeutic dose to discourage abuse by diphenoxylate overdose.

Use: Management of acute diarrhoea and irritable bowel syndrome in dogs. Concurrent correction of water and electrolyte imbalance is indicated whilst investigations into the cause of the diarrhoea are undertaken. Little is known about the safety and efficacy of Lomotil in cats.

Safety and handling: Normal precautions should be observed.

Contraindications: Intestinal obstruction.

Adverse reactions: Sedation, constipation and ileus. Do not use in animals with liver disease, intestinal obstruction, neoplastic or toxic bowel disease.

Drug interactions: Diphenoxylate may potentiate the sedative effects of barbiturates and other tranquillizers.

DOSES
Dogs: 0.05–0.1 mg/kg diphenoxylate p.o. q6–8h.
Cats, Small mammals, Birds, Reptiles: No information available.

Dipyrone see **Metamizole**

Dirlotapide
(Slentrol) **POM-V**

Formulations: Oral: 5 mg/ml solution.

Action: Causes a reduced uptake of dietary lipids, dose-dependent decrease in serum cholesterol and triglyceride, and an increased presence of triglyceride-containing droplets in enterocytes. Also has an appetite-decreasing effect.

Use: Aid to the management of overweight and obese adult dogs. Should be used as part of an overall weight management programme. In clinical trials, treated animals rapidly regained weight following cessation of treatment when diet was not restricted. Treatment should be given with food. Duration of treatment must not exceed 12 months.

Safety and handling: Light-sensitive. Store in the original container.

Contraindications: Do not use in dogs that are pregnant, lactating, <18 months of age or have impaired liver function. Do not use in dogs in which overweight or obesity is caused by a concomitant systemic disease (e.g. hypothyroidism, hyperadrenocorticism). Do not use in cats.

Adverse reactions: Vomiting, diarrhoea or softened stools may occur during treatment. Reversible decreases in serum albumin, globulin, total protein, calcium and alkaline phosphatase and increases in ALT, AST and potassium may occur. Risk of hepatic lipidosis in cats.

Drug interactions: Unknown at this time but could be considerable with fat-soluble drugs, therefore do not mix with other drugs.

DOSES
Dogs: 0.05 mg/kg initial body weight per day (0.01 ml/kg/day). After 2 weeks of therapy, the initial dose should be increased by 100% for a further 2 weeks. Following these initial 4 weeks of therapy, dogs should be weighed monthly during treatment with the product and dose adjustments made according to effect. The aim is to achieve a 3% weight loss per month. If this is not achieved then the dose can be increased by 50%, up to a maximum dose of 0.2 ml/kg. If weight loss is excessive then the dose should be reduced by 25%. A mean weight loss of about 18–20% after 6 months of therapy can be anticipated.
Cats, Small mammals: Do not use.
Birds, Reptiles: No information available.

Dobutamine
(Dobutamine*, Dobutrex*, Posiject*) **POM**

Formulations: Injectable: 12.5 mg/ml, 50 mg/ml solution.

Action: Dobutamine is a direct-acting synthetic catecholamine and derivative of isoprenaline with direct beta-1 adrenergic agonist effects and mild beta-2 and alpha-1 adrenergic effects at standard doses. Positive inotropy results primarily from stimulation of the beta-1 adrenoreceptors of the heart, while producing less marked chronotropic, arrhythmogenic and vasodilatory effects. Dobutamine does not cause the release of endogenous noradrenaline.

Use: Short-term inotropic support of patients with heart failure due to systolic dysfunction (e.g. dilated cardiomyopathy), septic and cardiogenic shock. It is used to support myocardial function during anaesthesia in animals that are hypotensive when reduced myocardial contractility is suspected as the primary cause. Dobutamine is a potent and short-acting drug, therefore it should be given in low doses by continuous rate infusion; accurate dosing is important. The dose of dobutamine should be adjusted according to clinical effect, therefore monitoring of arterial blood pressure during administration is advisable. All sympathomimetic drugs have pro-arrhythmic properties, therefore the ECG should be monitored during drug infusion. The dose should be titrated upwards until improvement in blood pressure, perfusion or clinical status is seen, or adverse effects (usually tachyarrhythmias) develop. The beneficial effects of dobutamine diminish over 48 hours due to down regulation of beta receptors.

Safety and handling: Dilute to a 25 μg/ml solution in dextrose or normal saline and store solution in the fridge when not in use. Degradation of dobutamine solution causes a pink discoloration. The reconstituted solution is stable for at least 24h, after this discoloured solutions should be discarded.

Contraindications: Avoid in patients with a cardiac outflow obstruction (e.g. aortic stenosis).

Adverse reactions: Dobutamine is short-acting, therefore adverse reactions such as tachycardia, pro-arrhythmia and hypertension can usually be managed by stopping the drug infusion. Hypokalaemia can develop with prolonged use; this can predispose to tachyarrhythmias. Complex ventricular arrhythmias may also be treated with lidocaine. Use cautiously in cases of atrial fibrillation as may increase ventricular rate. Prior and concurrent treatment with digoxin is recommended. Nausea, vomiting and seizures (particularly in cats) are also possible.

Drug interactions: Diabetic patients treated with dobutamine may experience increased insulin requirements. Increased systemic vascular resistance may develop if dobutamine is administered with beta-blocking drugs such as propranolol, doxapram or monoamine oxidase inhibitors (e.g. selegiline). Concomitant use with halothane may result in an increased incidence of arrhythmias.

DOSES
Dogs: 2.5–20 µg (micrograms)/kg/min i.v. by constant rate infusion. Start at the bottom end of the dose range and increase slowly until the desired effect is achieved. Adverse effects are more commonly seen at doses >10 µg/kg/min. Administer with an i.v. infusion pump or other i.v. flow controlling device.
Cats: 1–5 µg (micrograms)/kg/min i.v. by constant rate infusion. Start at the bottom end of the dose range and increase slowly until the desired effect is achieved. Adverse effects are more commonly seen at doses >2.5 µg/kg/min. Administer with an i.v. infusion pump or other i.v. flow controlling device.
Small mammals, Birds, Reptiles: No information available.

Docusate sodium (Dioctyl sodium sulfosuccinate, DSS)
(Co-danthrusate*, Docusol*, Norgalax*, Waxsol*) **P, GSL**

Formulations: Oral: 100 mg capsule (Dioctyl); 2.5 mg/ml liquid (Docusol Paediatric Solution), 10 mg/ml liquid (Docusol), 50 mg dantron plus 60 mg docusate/5 ml (Co-danthrusate). Rectal: 120 mg enema (Norgalax). Topical: 0.5% docusate in water-miscible base (Waxsol). Docusate is also a component of many other mixed topical preparations.

Action: Anionic surfactant acting as emulsifying, wetting and dispersing agent.

Use: Constipation and ceruminous otitis.

Safety and handling: Normal precautions should be observed.

Contraindications: Intestinal obstruction.

Adverse reactions: Avoid the concurrent use of docusate and mineral oil.

Drug interactions: No information available.

DOSES

Dogs:
- Constipation: 50–100 mg p.o. q12–24h or 10–15 ml of 5% solution mixed with 100 ml of water instilled per rectum prn.
- Otitis: A few drops in the affected ear q8–12h or 5–15 min prior to flushing.

Cats:
- Constipation: 50 mg p.o. q12–24h or 2 ml of a 5% solution mixed with 50 ml of water instilled per rectum prn.
- Otitis: dose as for dogs.

Small mammals, Birds, Reptiles: No information available.

Dog appeasing pheromone (Adaptil, Appeasines)
(D.A.P.) **GSL**

Formulations: Plug-in diffuser, topical environmental spray, collar.

Action: The mixture is based on derivatives of the dermal secretions produced by the bitch after whelping, which help to keep pups within the safety of the den. The signal causes an innate emotional bias in the perception of the environment and does not require learning. A similar signal appears to form part of the social signal controlling groups of adult dogs. Associated limbic activity helps to antagonize the effect of certain forms of aversion in the environment, but does not cause sedation or reduce the startle response.

Use: Helps control signs of stress associated with separation, noise sensitivity, travel, introduction to a new home, visits to a novel environment (e.g. veterinary clinic) and other anxiogenic circumstances. The diffuser should be placed in the room most frequently occupied by the dog and, in the management of behavioural disorders, where the inappropriate behaviour most frequently occurs. For behavioural problems involving hyperattachment to the owner, a treatment period of 3 months is recommended. The spray can be used inside and outside the home environment. It can be used in cars, hospitalization cages, kennels, indoor pens or refuge areas, and applied directly on to bedding. It can be sprayed with the bottle in an upside down position. The collar formulation is particularly useful to help control reactions which occur outside the home. If multiple dogs are affected by a problem, each dog should wear a collar and possibly a diffuser considered for problems based around the home. Do not spray directly on to animals or near an animal's face. The collar formulation should not be used for animals with a known reactivity to collars. Avoid contact with water when the collar is in use as this may wash out the active ingredients.

Safety and handling: Normal precautions should be observed.

Contraindications: No information available.

Adverse reactions: No information available.

Drug interactions: None known, although anecdotally an apparently synergistic action with benzodiazepines has been reported in some instances.

APPLICATION

Dogs: The diffuser is active over an area of approximately 50–70 m². If the total target area exceeds this, a second diffuser should be used. One vial will last for approximately 4 weeks of continuous use. It should not be repeatedly switched on and off. Follow manufacturer's instructions for each formulation. In the house, DAP spray can complement the use of the diffuser device where a more local application is needed. Spray 8–10 pumps of DAP on to the required surface 15 min before the effect is required, and before the dog is introduced into the environment, to allow the alcohol carrier to evaporate. The effect should last for 1–2 h, although each animal will respond individually. The application can be renewed after 1–2 h or when the effects appear to be reducing.

Cats, Small mammals, Birds, Reptiles: Not applicable.

Domperidone

(Domperidone*, Motilium*) **POM**

Formulations: Oral: 10 mg tablet, 1 mg/ml suspension.

Action: A potent antiemetic with a similar mechanism of action to metoclopramide, but with fewer adverse CNS effects as it cannot penetrate the blood-brain barrier. It is gastrokinetic in humans but may not be a prokinetic in dogs.

Use: Treatment of vomiting. However, maropitant is authorized for veterinary use and there is more clinical experience with metoclopramide and ondansetron.

Safety and handling: Normal precautions should be observed.

Contraindications: Intestinal obstruction or perforation.

Adverse reactions: There is little information on the use of this drug in veterinary medicine, but it may cause gastroparesis in dogs.

Drug interactions: No information available.

DOSES

Dogs, Cats: 2–5 mg per animal q8h.
Small mammals: Rabbits: 0.5 mg/kg p.o. q12h. Contraindicated in GI obstruction.
Birds, Reptiles: No information available.

Dopamine
(Dopamine*) **POM**

Formulations: Injectable: 200 mg in 5 ml vial (40 mg/ml solution), 800 mg in a 5 ml vial (160 mg/ml solution).

Action: Dopamine is an endogenous catecholamine and precursor of noradrenaline, with direct and indirect (via release of noradrenaline) agonist effects on dopaminergic and beta-1 and alpha-1 adrenergic receptors.

Use: Improvement of haemodynamic status. Main indications are treatment of shock following correction of fluid deficiencies, acute heart failure, and support of blood pressure during anaesthesia. Dobutamine is preferred for support of systolic function in patients with heart failure. Dopamine is a potent and short-acting drug, therefore it should be given in low doses by continuous rate infusion, and accurate dosing is important. Dopamine should be diluted in normal saline to an appropriate concentration. At low doses (<10 µg/kg/min) dopamine acts on dopaminergic and beta-1 adrenergic receptors, causing vasodilation, increased force of contraction and heart rate, and resulting in an increase in cardiac output and organ perfusion; systemic vascular resistance remains largely unchanged. At higher doses (>10 µg/kg/min) dopaminergic effects are overridden by the alpha effects, resulting in an increase in systemic vascular resistance and reduced peripheral blood flow. Dopamine has been shown to vasodilate mesenteric blood vessels via DA1 receptors. There may be an improvement in urine output but this may be entirely due to inhibition of proximal tubule sodium ion reabsorption and an improved cardiac output and blood pressure rather than directly improving renal blood flow. The dose of dopamine should be adjusted according to clinical effect, therefore monitoring of arterial blood pressure during administration is advisable. All sympathomimetic drugs have pro-arrhythmic properties, therefore ECG monitoring is advised.

Safety and handling: Solution should be discarded if it becomes discoloured.

Contraindications: Discontinue or reduce the dose of dopamine should cardiac arrhythmias arise.

Adverse reactions: Extravasation of dopamine causes necrosis and sloughing of surrounding tissue due to tissue ischaemia. Should extravasation occur, infiltrate the site with a solution of 5–10 mg phentolamine in 10–15 ml of normal saline using a syringe with a fine needle. Nausea, vomiting, tachyarrhythmias and changes in blood pressure are the most common adverse effects. Hypotension may develop with low doses, and hypertension may occur with high doses. Sudden increases in blood pressure may cause a severe bradycardia. All dopamine-induced arrhythmias are most effectively treated by stopping the infusion.

Drug interactions: Risk of severe hypertension when monoamine oxidase inhibitors, doxapram and oxytocin are used with dopamine. Halothane may increase myocardial sensitivity to catecholamines. The effects of beta-blockers and dopamine are antagonistic.

DOSES
Dogs: 2–10 μg (micrograms)/kg/min i.v. as a constant rate infusion.
Cats: 1-5 μg (micrograms)/kg/min i.v. as a constant rate infusion.
Small mammals: Guinea pigs: 0.08 mg/kg i.v. once.
Birds, Reptiles: No information available.

Dorzolamide
(CoSopt*, Dorzolamide*, Dorzolamide with Timolol*, Trusopt*) **POM**

Formulations: Ophthalmic drops: 20 mg/ml (2%) (Dorzolamide, Trusopt), 2% dorzolamide + 0.5% timolol (CoSopt, Dorzolamide with Timolol); 5 ml bottle, single-use vials (CoSopt, Trusopt).

Action: Reduces intraocular pressure by reducing the rate of aqueous humour production by inhibiting the formation of bicarbonate ions within the ciliary body epithelium.

Use: In the control of all types of glaucoma in dogs and cats, either alone or in combination with other topicals. Dorzolamide/timolol combination may be more effective in dogs than either drug alone. It may be less tolerated than brinzolamide because of its less physiological pH of 5.6. The concurrent use of a topical and a systemic carbonic anhydrase inhibitor is not beneficial as there is no additional decrease in intraocular pressure compared with either route alone.

Safety and handling: Normal precautions should be observed.

Contraindications: Severe hepatic or renal impairment. Dorzolamide/timolol is not the drug of choice in uveitis or anterior lens luxation.

Adverse reactions: Local irritation and blepharitis. Dorzolamide may cause more local irritation than brinzolamide. Dorzolamide/timolol causes miosis. Rarely, dorzolamide has been reported to cause hypokalaemia in cats as a result of systemic absorption.

Drug interactions: No information available.

DOSES
Dogs, Cats: 1 drop/eye q8–12h.
Small mammals: Rabbits: 1 drop/eye q8–12h; Rats: 1 drop 1% solution (dilute standard formulation with sterile water) q12h.
Birds: 1 drop/eye q12h.
Reptiles: No information available.

Doxapram

(Dopram-V) **POM-VPS, POM-V**

Formulations: Injectable: 20 mg/ml solution. Oral: 20 mg/ml drops.

Action: Stimulates respiration by increasing the sensitivity of aortic and carotid body chemoreceptors to arterial gas tensions.

Use: Stimulates respiration during and after general anaesthesia. In neonatal puppies and kittens, used to stimulate or initiate respiration after birth, particularly in animals delivered by caesarean section. The dose should be adjusted according to the requirements of the situation; adequate but not excessive doses should be used. A patent airway is essential. Must not be used indiscriminately to support respiratory function. Severe respiratory depression should be controlled by tracheal intubation, followed by IPPV and then resolution of the initiating cause. Duration of effect in mammals is 15–20 minutes. Has also been used to aid assessment of laryngeal function under light anaesthesia. Not effective at stimulating respiration in the face of hypoxaemia (pre-oxygenation of hypoventilating neonates is recommended, along with removal of obstructive secretions).

Safety and handling: Protect from light.

Contraindications: Do not use in animals without a patent airway.

Adverse reactions: Overdose can cause excessive hyperventilation, which may be followed by reduced carbon dioxide tension in the blood leading to cerebral vasoconstriction. This could result in cerebral hypoxia in some animals. Doxapram is irritant and may cause a thrombophlebitis, avoid extravasation or repeated i.v. injection into the same vein. Use doxapram injection with caution in neonates because it contains benzyl alcohol which is toxic. Overdosage symptoms include hypertension, skeletal muscle hyperactivity, tachycardia and generalized CNS excitation including seizures; treatment is supportive using short-acting i.v. barbiturates or propofol and oxygen. Effects in pregnant/lactating animals are not known.

Drug interactions: Hypertension may occur with sympathomimetics. The use of theophylline concurrently with doxapram may cause increased CNS stimulation. As doxapram may stimulate the release of adrenaline, its use within 10 min of the administration of anaesthetic agents that sensitize the myocardium to catecholamines (e.g. halothane) should be avoided. Doxapram is compatible with 5% dextrose or normal saline but is incompatible with sodium bicarbonate or thiopental. High doses administered during or after anaesthesia with halogenated hydrocarbon anaesthetics, such as halothane, may precipitate cardiac arrhythmias. Doxapram injection should be used with extreme caution in dogs that have been sedated with morphine. Administration of doxapram at 10 mg/kg to such animals may be followed by convulsions.

DOSES

Dogs, Cats: 2–5 mg/kg i.v., repeat according to need. Neonates: 1–2 drops under the tongue (oral solution) or 0.1 ml i.v. into the umbilical vein; this should be used once only. For assessment of laryngeal function: 1–2 mg/kg i.v.

Small mammals: Ferrets, Rabbits, Chinchillas, Hamsters, Gerbils, Rats, Mice: 5–10 mg/kg i.v., i.m., i.p., sublingual once; Guinea pigs: 2–5 mg/kg i.v., s.c., i.p. once.

Birds: 5–20 mg/kg i.m., i.v., intratracheal, intraosseous once.

Reptiles: 4–12 mg/kg i.m., i.v., p.o. once.

Doxepin

(Sinepin*, Sinequan*, Zonalon*) **POM**

Formulations: Oral: 25 mg, 50 mg capsules.

Action: Doxepin blocks noradrenaline and serotonin re-uptake in the brain, resulting in antidepressive activity, while the H1 and H2 blockage result in antipruritic effects. Its metabolite, desmethyldoxepin, is also psychoactive.

Use: Management of pruritus and psychogenic dermatoses where there is a component of anxiety, including canine acral lick dermatitis and compulsive disorders. Data are lacking as to its efficacy at the suggested doses. The atypical tricyclic antidepressant clomipramine is an authorized preparation for use in dogs. Also used in birds for organophosphate toxicity. When used in birds it is important to monitor for cardiac arrhythmias.

Safety and handling: Normal precautions should be observed.

Contraindications: Hypersensitivity to tricyclic antidepressants, glaucoma, history of seizure or urinary retention and severe liver disease.

Adverse reactions: Sedation, dry mouth, diarrhoea, vomiting, excitability, arrhythmias, hypotension, syncope, increased appetite, weight gain and, less commonly, seizures and bone marrow disorders have been reported in humans.

Drug interactions: Should not be used with monoamine oxidase inhibitors or drugs which are metabolized by cytochrome P450 2D6, e.g. chlorphenamine and cimetidine.

DOSES

Dogs: 3–5 mg/kg p.o. q12h, maximum dose 150 mg q12h.

Cats: 0.5–1.0 mg/kg p.o. q12–24h.

Small mammals: No information available.

Birds: Feather plucking: 1–2 mg/kg p.o. q12h; organophosphate toxicity: 0.2 mg/kg i.m. q4h.

Reptiles: No information available.

A
B
C
D
E
F
G
H
I
J
K
L
M
N
O
P
Q
R
S
T
U
V
W
X
Y
Z

Doxorubicin (Adriamycin)
(Doxorubicin*) **POM**

Formulations: Injectable: 10 mg, 50 mg powders for reconstitution; 10 mg, 50 mg/vial solutions.

Action: Inhibits DNA synthesis and function.

Use: Treatment of lymphoma, soft tissue sarcomas, osteosarcoma and haemangiosarcoma, and may have a role in the management of carcinomas in the dog and soft tissue sarcomas in the cat. It may be used alone or in combination with other antineoplastic therapies. Premedication with i.v. chlorphenamine or dexamethasone is recommended. Doxorubicin is highly irritant and must be administered via a preplaced i.v. catheter. The reconstituted drug should be administered over a minimum period of 10 min into the side port of a freely running i.v. infusion of 0.9% NaCl. Do not use heparin flush. Use with care in breeds predisposed to cardiomyopathy. May need to reduce dose in patients with liver disease. Use with caution in patients previously treated with radiation as can cause radiation recall. See specialist texts for protocols and further advice.

Safety and handling: **Potent cytotoxic drug that should only be prepared and administered by trained personnel. See Appendix and specialist texts for further advice on chemotherapeutic agents.** After reconstitution the drug is stable for at least 48h at 4°C. A 1.5% loss of potency may occur after 1 month at 4°C but there is no loss of potency when frozen at −20°C. Filtering through a 0.22 µm filter will ensure adequate sterility of the thawed solution. Store unopened vials under refrigeration.

Contraindications: Do not use in patients with existing cardiac disease. Do not use in cats with renal disease/dysfunction.

Adverse reactions: Allergic reactions have been reported; acute anaphylactic reactions should be treated with adrenaline, steroids and fluids. Doxorubicin causes a dose-dependent cumulative cardiotoxicity in dogs (leading to cardiomyopathy and congestive heart failure). The risk of cardiotoxicity is greatly increased when the cumulative dose is >240 mg/m^2. It may also cause tachycardia and arrhythmias on administration; monitor with ECG and/or echocardiograms. Anorexia, vomiting, severe leucopenia, thrombocytopenia, haemorrhagic gastroenteritis and nephrotoxicity (in cats if dosages >100 mg/m^2) are the major adverse effects. A CBC and platelet count should be monitored whenever therapy is given. If neutrophil count drops below 3 x 10^9/l or platelet count drops below 50 x 10^9/l, treatment should be suspended. Once counts have stabilized, doxorubicin can be restarted at the same dose. If haematological toxicity occurs again, or if GI toxicity is recurrent, the dose should be reduced by 10–25%. Extravasation injuries secondary to perivascular administration may be serious, with severe tissue ulceration and necrosis possible. Dexrazoxane can be used to treat extravasation if it occurs. Ice compresses may also be beneficial (applied for 15 min q6h).

Drug interactions: Barbiturates increase plasma clearance of doxorubicin. Concurrent administration with cyclophosphamide increases the risk of nephrotoxicity in cats. The agent causes a reduction in serum digoxin levels. Do not mix doxorubicin with other drugs. Doxorubicin is incompatible with dexamethasone, 5-fluorouracil and heparin; concurrent use will lead to precipitate formation.

DOSES
See Appendix for chemotherapy protocols and conversion of body weight to body surface area.
Dogs: 30 mg/m² i.v. q3w, or 10 mg/m² on days 1, 2 and 3 every 4 weeks. Maximum total dose not to exceed 240 mg/m².
Cats: 20–25 mg/m² i.v. q3–5w for a maximum of 5 doses.
Small mammals: Ferrets: 20 mg/m² or 1–2 mg/kg i.v. every 3 weeks for a maximum of 5 doses. Also used for 2 doses as part of specific multi-drug protocols for lymphoma in ferrets. See relevant specialist texts.
Birds, Reptiles: No information available.

Doxycycline
(Doxyseptin 300, Ornicure, Pulmodox, Ronaxan, Vibramycin*, Vibravenos*) **POM-V**

Formulations: Oral: 20 mg, 100 mg tablets (Ronaxan), 300 mg tablets (Doxyseptin); 260 mg/sachet powder (Ornicure). Injectable: 20 mg/ml long-acting injection (Vibravenos; import on an STC).

Action: Bacteriostatic agent inhibiting protein synthesis at the initiation step by interacting with the 30S ribosomal subunit.

Use: Antibacterial (including spirochaetes such as *Helicobacter* and *Campylobacter*), antirickettsial, antimycoplasmal (e.g. *Mycoplasma haemofelis*) and antichlamydial activity. It is the drug of choice to treat feline and avian chlamydophilosis; treatment may be required for 3–4 weeks in cats. It is not affected by, and does not affect, renal function as it is excreted in faeces, and is therefore recommended when tetracyclines are indicated in animals with renal impairment. It is preferred by some authors to oxytetracycline for use in birds. Being extremely lipid-soluble, it penetrates well into prostatic fluid and bronchial secretions. Administer with food. Injection is very irritant in birds: must alternate injection sites or divide dose if large volume to inject.

Safety and handling: Normal precautions should be observed.

Contraindications: Do not administer Doxyseptin to dogs <15 kg. Do not administer to pregnant animals. Do not administer if there is evidence of oesophagitis or dysphagia.

Adverse reactions: Nausea, vomiting and diarrhoea. Oesophagitis and oesophageal ulceration may develop; administer with food or a water bolus to reduce this risk. Administration during tooth development may lead to discoloration of the teeth, although the risk is less than with other tetracyclines.

Drug interactions: Absorption of doxycycline is reduced by antacids, calcium, magnesium and iron salts, although the effect is less marked than seen with water-soluble tetracyclines. Phenobarbital and phenytoin may increase its metabolism, thus decreasing plasma levels. Do not use in combination with bactericidal antimicrobials.

DOSES
See Appendix for guidelines on responsible antibacterial use.
Dogs, Cats: 10 mg/kg p.o. q24h with food.
Small mammals: Rabbits: 2.5–4 mg/kg p.o. q24h; Rats, Mice: 5 mg/kg p.o. q12h; Other rodents: 2.5 mg/kg p.o. q12h.
Birds: Parrots: 15–50 mg/kg p.o. q24h, 1000 mg/kg in soft food/dehulled seed, 75–100 mg/kg i.m. q7d (Vibravenos; lowest dose rate for macaws); course of treatment with doxycycline for chlamydophilosis = 45 days; Raptors: 50 mg/kg p.o. q12h, 100 mg/kg i.m. q7d (Vibravenos); Passerines/Pigeons: 40 mg/kg p.o. 12–24h, 200–500 mg/l in water (soft or deionized water only).
Reptiles: 50 mg/kg i.m. once, then 25 mg/kg i.m. q72h.

Edetate calcium disodium (CaEDTA)
(Ledclair*) **POM**

Formulations: Injectable: 200 mg/ml solution.

Action: Heavy metal chelating agent.

Use: Lead and zinc poisoning. Dilute strong solution to a concentration of 10 mg/ml in 5% dextrose before use. Blood lead levels may be confusing, therefore monitor clinical signs during therapy. Measure blood lead levels 2–3 weeks after completion of treatment in order to determine whether a second course is required or if the animal is still being exposed to lead. Ensure there is no lead in the GI tract before administering (e.g. use laxatives).

Safety and handling: Normal precautions should be observed.

Contraindications: Use with caution in patients with impaired renal function.

Adverse reactions: Reversible nephrotoxicity is usually preceded by other clinical signs of toxicity (e.g. depression, vomiting, diarrhoea). Dogs showing GI effects may benefit from zinc supplementation. Injections are painful.

Drug interactions: No information available.

DOSES
Dogs, Cats: 25 mg/kg s.c. q6h for 2–5 days. The total daily dose should not exceed 2 g. Dogs that respond slowly or have an initial (pre-treatment) blood lead level of >4.5 μmol/l may need another 5–day course of treatment after a rest period of 5 days.
Small mammals: Ferrets: 20–30 mg/kg s.c. q12h; Rabbits: 27.5 mg/kg s.c. q6h for 5 days; Rodents: 25–30 mg/kg s.c. q6–12h.
Birds: 35–50 mg/kg i.m., s.c. q12h for 5 days followed by 2 days of no treatment, then repeat until metal particles are no longer visible on radiographs. 100 mg/kg i.m. weekly has been proposed in zinc toxicosis.
Reptiles: 10–40 mg/kg i.m. q12h.

Edrophonium
(Edrophonium Injection BP) **POM**

Formulations: Injectable: 10 mg/ml solution.

Action: Edrophonium is a reversible and short-acting competitive inhibitor of acetylcholinesterase with a very rapid onset of action. It blocks the breakdown of acetylcholine at the neuromuscular junction, thereby prolonging its action.

Use: To differentiate myasthenia gravis from other causes of exercise intolerance (previously known as the Tensilon test). Also used to treat atrial tachycardia (vagal effects) and to antagonize non-depolarizing neuromuscular blockade. Also used to distinguish between under- and over-treatment of myasthenia gravis with other anticholinesterases by giving doses at the lower end of the range for diagnostic tests. If treatment has been inadequate, edrophonium will improve muscle weakness; in over-treatment, edrophonium will temporarily exacerbate muscle weakness. Use with caution in patients with bronchial disease (especially feline asthma), bradycardia (and other arrhythmias), hypotension, renal impairment or epilepsy.

Safety and handling: Normal precautions should be observed.

Contraindications: Do not use in patients with mechanical GI or urinary tract obstructions or peritonitis.

Adverse reactions: Include nausea, vomiting, increased salivation and diarrhoea. Overdosage may lead to muscle fasciculations and paralysis. Severe bradyarrhythmias, even asystole, may occur if edrophonium is used to antagonize neuromuscular block without the co-injection of atropine. In overdose, respiration should be supported and atropine administered i.v. to counteract muscarinic effects.

Drug interactions: Do not use at higher doses in conjunction with depolarizing neuromuscular relaxants (e.g. suxamethonium) as this may potentiate neuromuscular blockade.

DOSES
Dogs:
- Diagnosis of myasthenia gravis: 0.1 mg/kg i.v. (maximum 5 mg). Improvement should be noted within 30 seconds, with the effects dissipating within 5 min, for a positive test. Atropine should be available (0.05 mg/kg) to control cholinergic side effects (e.g. salivation, urination). If there is no response, repeat test after 10–20 min using 0.2 mg/kg.
- Atrial tachycardia after failure of vagal manoeuvres: 1.5 mg i.v. once (Note: This procedure is not advised in cases of heart failure).
- Antagonism of non-depolarizing neuromuscular blockade: edrophonium (0.5–1.0 mg/kg) is mixed with atropine (0.04 mg/kg) and injected i.v. over 2 min once signs of spontaneous recovery from block, e.g. diaphragmatic 'twitching' are present. Continued ventilatory support should be provided until full respiratory muscle activity is restored.

Cats:
- Diagnosis of myasthenia gravis: 0.25–0.5 mg total dose/cat i.v. Doses >6 mg/kg have been experimentally reported in cats but will result in bradycardia and are not required for confirmation of myasthenia gravis. Improvement should be noted within 30 seconds, with the effects dissipating within 5 min, for a positive test. Atropine should be available (0.04 mg/kg) to control cholinergic side effects (e.g. salivation, urination).
- Atrial tachycardia after failure of vagal manoeuvres: doses as for dogs.

Small mammals, Birds, Reptiles: No information available.

Emodepside
(Profender) **POM-V**

Formulations: Topical: 21.4 mg/ml emodepside with praziquantel solution in spot-on pipettes. An oral formulation for dogs is available in several European countries.

Action: Stimulates presynaptic secretin receptors resulting in paralysis and death of the parasite.

Use: Treatment of roundworms (adult and immature) and tapeworms (adult) including *Toxocara cati*, *Toxascaris leonina*, *Ancylostoma tubaeforme*, *Aelurostrongylus abstrusus*, *Dipylidium caninum*, *Taenia taeniaeformis*, *Echinococcus multilocularis*. Do not shampoo until substance has dried.

Safety and handling: Women of child-bearing age should avoid contact with this drug or wear disposable gloves when using it.

Contraindications: Do not use in cats <8 weeks or <0.5 kg. Do not use in rabbits.

Adverse reactions: Ingestion may result in salivation or vomiting. Harmful to aquatic animals.

Drug interactions: Possible interaction with P-glycoprotein substrates/inhibitors.

DOSES
Dogs: No information available.
Cats: Minimum dose 0.14 ml/kg applied topically once per treatment cycle. Do not use in cats <8 weeks or <0.5 kg.
Small mammals: Rabbits: Do not use.
Birds, Reptiles: No information available.

Enalapril
(Enacard) **POM-V**

Formulations: Oral: 1 mg, 2.5 mg, 5 mg, 10 mg, 20 mg tablets.

Action: Angiotensin converting enzyme (ACE) inhibitor. It inhibits conversion of angiotensin I to angiotensin II and inhibits the breakdown of bradykinin. Overall effect is a reduction in preload and afterload via venodilation and arteriodilation, decreased salt and water retention via reduced aldosterone production and inhibition of the angiotensin-aldosterone-mediated cardiac and vascular remodelling. Efferent arteriolar dilation in the kidney can reduce intraglomerular pressure and therefore glomerular filtration. This may decrease proteinuria.

Use: Treatment of congestive heart failure caused by mitral regurgitation or dilated cardiomyopathy in dogs and cats. Often used in conjunction with diuretics when heart failure is present as most effective when used in these cases. Can be used in combination with other drugs to treat heart failure (e.g. pimobendan, spironolactone, digoxin). May be beneficial in cases of chronic renal insufficiency, particularly protein-losing nephropathies. May reduce blood pressure in hypertension. ACE inhibitors are more likely to cause or exacerbate prerenal azotaemia in hypotensive animals and those with poor renal perfusion (e.g. acute, oliguric renal failure). Use cautiously if hypotension, hyponatraemia or outflow tract obstruction are present. Regular monitoring of blood pressure, serum creatinine, urea and electrolytes is strongly recommended with ACE inhibitor treatment. Hypotension, azotaemia and hyperkalaemia are all indications to stop or reduce ACE inhibitor treatment in rabbits. The use of ACE inhibitors in cats with cardiac disease stems from extrapolation from theoretical benefits and studies showing a benefit in other species with heart failure and different cardiac diseases (mainly dogs and humans).

Safety and handling: Normal precautions should be observed.

Contraindications: Do not use in cases of cardiac output failure.

Adverse reactions: Potential adverse effects include hypotension, hyperkalaemia and azotaemia. Monitor blood pressure, serum creatinine and electrolytes when used in cases of heart failure. Dosage should be reduced if there are signs of hypotension (weakness, disorientation). Anorexia, vomiting and diarrhoea are rare. No adverse effects were seen in normal dogs given 15 mg/kg/day for up to 1 year. It is not recommended for breeding, pregnant or lactating bitches, as safety has not been established. In rabbits, treatment with ACE inhibitors can be associated with an increase in azotaemia.

Drug interactions: Concomitant treatment with potassium-sparing diuretics (e.g. spironolactone) or potassium supplements could result in hyperkalaemia. However, in practice, spironolactone and ACE inhibitors appear safe to use concurrently. There may be an increased risk of nephrotoxicity and decreased clinical efficacy when used with NSAIDs. There is a risk of hypotension with concomitant administration of diuretics, vasodilators (e.g. anaesthetic agents, antihypertensive agents) or negative inotropes (e.g. beta-blockers).

DOSES
Dogs:
- Cardiac disease: 0.5 mg/kg p.o. q24h increasing to 0.5 mg/kg p.o. q12h after 2 weeks in the absence of a clinical response.
- Protein-losing nephropathy: 0.25–1 mg/kg p.o. q12–24h.
- Hypertension: Doses up to 3 mg/kg have been used.

Cats: Cardiac disease, protein-losing nephropathy: 0.25–0.5 mg/kg p.o. q12–24h.

Small mammals: Ferrets: 0.25–0.5 mg/kg p.o. q24–48h; Rabbits: 0.25–0.5 mg/kg p.o. q24–48h.

Birds: 1.25 mg/kg p.o. q12h.

Reptiles: No information available.

Enilconazole
(Imaverol) **POM-VPS**

Formulations: Topical: 100 mg/ml (10%) liquid.

Action: Inhibition of cytochrome P450-dependent synthesis of ergosterol in fungal cells, causing increased cell wall permeability and allowing leakage of cellular contents.

Use: Fungal infections of the skin and nasal aspergillosis.

Safety and handling: Normal precautions should be observed.

Contraindications: No information available.

Adverse reactions: Hepatotoxic if swallowed. Avoid contact with eyes. Hypersalivation, gastrointestinal signs and muscle signs reported in cats.

Drug interactions: No information available.

DOSES
Dogs:
- Dermatological indications: Dilute 1 volume enilconazole in 50 volumes of water to produce a 0.2 mg/ml (0.2%) solution. Apply every 3 days for 3–4 applications.
- Nasal aspergillosis: 10 mg/kg q12h instilled into the nasal cavities and sinuses through indwelling tubes for 7–10 days. Dilute the solution of enilconazole (100 mg/ml) 50:50 with water. The instilled volume should be kept low (<10 ml) to reduce the risk of inhalation and the tubes flushed with an equivalent volume of air. Make up a fresh solution as required.

Cats: Dermatological indications: doses as for dogs.

Small mammals: Rabbits: Dilute (1:50 volume enilconazole to 50 volumes water) and apply topically to lesions every 3 days for 3–4 applications and then check success of therapy with fungal culture; Hamsters: 0.2% rinse topically q14d until fungal cultures negative.

Birds: Dilute 1 volume of 10% solution with 10 volumes of water and give 0.5 ml/kg/day intratracheally for 7–14 days.

Reptiles: Apply topically to lesions correctly diluted (1:50 volume enilconazole to 50 volumes water) q48–72h.

Enrofloxacin
(Baytril, Enrocare, Enrotab, Enrotron, Enrox, Enroxil, Floxabactin, Floxibac, Powerflox, Quinoflox, Xeden, Zobuxa) **POM-V**

Formulations: Injectable: 25 mg/ml, 50 mg/ml, 100 mg/ml solutions. Oral: 15 mg, 50 mg, 150 mg, 250 mg tablets; 25 mg/ml solution.

Action: Enrofloxacin is a bactericidal antimicrobial which inhibits bacterial DNA gyrase. The bactericidal action is concentration-dependent, meaning that 'pulse' dosing regimens may be effective, particularly against Gram-negative bacteria.

Use: Ideally fluoroquinolone use should be reserved for infections where culture and sensitivity testing predicts a clinical response and where first- and second-line antimicrobials would not be effective. Active against *Mycoplasma* and many Gram-positive and Gram-negative organisms, including *Pasteurella*, *Staphylococcus*, *Pseudomonas aeruginosa*, *Klebsiella*, *Escherichia coli*, *Mycobacterium*, *Proteus* and *Salmonella*. Relatively ineffective against obligate anaerobes. Fluoroquinolones are highly lipophilic drugs that attain high concentrations within cells in many tissues and are particularly effective in the management of soft tissue, urogenital (including prostatic) and skin infections. For the treatment of non-tubercular mycobacterial disease, enrofloxacin can be combined with clarithromycin and rifampin. Administration by i.v. route is not authorized but has been used in cases of severe sepsis. If this route is used, administer slowly as the carrier contains potassium. Careful dosing in cats is facilitated by accurate body weight and use of a 1 ml syringe. Dilute solution for injection 1 in 4 with water if dosing small mammals orally. Switch to oral medications in birds as soon as possible.

Safety and handling: Normal precautions should be observed.

Contraindications: Fluoroquinolones are relatively contraindicated in growing dogs and rabbits, as cartilage abnormalities have been reported in young dogs and rabbits (but not cats). Enrofloxacin is not authorized in cats <8 weeks of age; dogs <1 year of age; large-breed dogs <18 months of age.

Adverse reactions: In birds, joint lesions have been induced in nestling pigeons with high doses of enrofloxacin, and muscle necrosis may be seen following i.m. administration. Enrofloxacin should be used with caution in epileptics until further information is available, as in humans they potentiate CNS adverse effects when administered concurrently with NSAIDs. In cats, irreversible retinal blindness has occurred at dosing rates higher than those currently recommended, although at least one case reported in the literature was being dosed within the 5 mg/kg q24h rate.

Drug interactions: Adsorbents and antacids containing cations (Mg^{2+}, Al^{3+}) may bind to fluoroquinolones and prevent their absorption from the GI tract. The absorption of fluoroquinolones may also be inhibited by sucralfate and zinc salts; separate doses of these drugs by at least 2 hours. Fluoroquinolones increase plasma theophylline concentrations. Cimetidine may reduce the clearance of fluoroquinolones and so should be used with caution in combination with these drugs.

DOSES
See Appendix for guidelines on responsible antibacterial use.
Dogs, Cats: 5 mg/kg s.c., i.v. q24h; 2.5 mg/kg p.o. q12h or 5 mg/kg p.o. q24h. Some isolates of *Pseudomonas aeruginosa* may require higher doses, contact the manufacturer to discuss individual cases.

Small mammals: Ferrets: 5–10 mg/kg p.o., s.c., i.m. q12h or 10–20 mg/kg p.o., s.c., i.m. q24h; Rabbits: 10–30 mg/kg p.o., s.c., i.v. q24h; Rodents: 5–10 mg/kg s.c., p.o. q12–24h; Others: 5–10 mg/kg s.c., p.o. q12h or 20 mg/kg s.c., p.o. q24h.
Birds: 10–15 mg/kg i.m. (but see note above), p.o. q12h (sensitive infections can be treated q24h) or 100–200 mg/l drinking water.
Reptiles: 5–10 mg/kg i.m., p.o. q24–48h.

Ephedrine
(Enurace, Ephedrine hydrochloride*) **POM-V, POM**

Formulations: 10 mg, 15 mg, 30 mg, 50 mg tablets; 3 mg/ml, 30 mg/ml solutions for injection; 0.5% and 1% nasal drops.

Action: Non-catecholamine sympathomimetic stimulates alpha- and beta-adrenergic receptors directly, and indirectly through endogenous release of noradrenaline. Also causes contraction of internal urethral sphincter muscles and relaxation of bladder muscles. Compared to more powerful sympathomimetics, e.g. oxymetazoline and xylometazoline, there is less of a rebound effect.

Use: Treatment of hypotension during anaesthesia. As well as constricting peripheral vessels, accelerates heart rate and can therefore assist in bradycardia. Also used orally in the treatment of urinary incontinence and nasal congestion (and may be of some benefit in cat 'flu). Can be used in conjunction with phenylpropanolamine. Polyuria should be excluded before treatment is given for urinary incontinence, as many conditions that cause polyuria would be exacerbated by ephedrine. Use with caution in dogs and cats with cardiovascular disease, partial urethral obstruction, hypertension, diabetes mellitus, hyperadrenocorticism, hyperthyroidism or other metabolic disorders.

Safety and handling: Pregnant women should take particular care to wear gloves for administration.

Contraindications: Do not use in pregnant or lactating patients or those with glaucoma.

Adverse reactions: Even at recommended therapeutic doses may cause more generalized sympathetic stimulation (panting, mydriasis, CNS stimulation) and cardiovascular effects (tachycardia, atrial fibrillation and vasoconstriction). May also cause reduction of the motility and tone of the intestinal wall.

Drug interactions: Synergistic with other sympathomimetics. Volatile anaesthetics will enhance the sensitivity of the myocardium to the effects of ephedrine. Concomitant use with cardiac glycosides (digoxin) and tricyclic antidepressants (amitriptyline) can cause arrhythmias. Will enhance effects of theophylline and may cause hypertension when given with MAO inhibitors (e.g. selegeline).

DOSES
Dogs:
- Urinary incontinence: 1 mg/kg p.o. q12h. Dose should be adjusted according to effect but there is a maximum dose of 2.5 mg/kg p.o. q12h.
- Nasal congestion: No dose determined. Suggest start at 1 drop of 0.5% solution intranasally q12h. If giving orally, suggest 0.5 mg/kg p.o. q12h.
- Hypotension: 0.05–0.2 mg/kg i.v.; repeat as necessary; duration of effect is short (5–15 minutes).

Cats:
- Nasal congestion: 1 drop of 0.5% solution intranasally q12h. Oral formulations not convenient for administration to most cats.
- Hypotension: 0.05–0.1 mg/kg i.v.; repeat as necessary; duration of effect is short (5–15 minutes).

Small mammals, Birds, Reptiles: No information available.

Epinephrine see Adrenaline

Epirubicin (4'-Epi-doxorubicin)
(Epirubicin*, Pharmorubicin*) **POM**

Formulations: Injectable: 10 mg, 20 mg, 50 mg powder for reconstitution; 2 mg/ml solution.

Action: Intracellularly its metabolism results in production of cytotoxic free radicals. It also binds irreversibly to DNA, thereby preventing replication. It also alters membrane functions.

Use: Cytotoxic anthracycline glycoside antibiotic that has demonstrated efficacy against several human neoplasms. In the dog the drug has been assessed against lymphoma (similar efficacy to doxorubicin) and also as an adjunct in the management of splenic haemangiosarcoma. It may be used alone or in combination with other antineoplastic therapies. The drug must be given i.v. Premedication with i.v. chlorphenamine or dexamethasone is recommended. As extravasation of the drug is likely to result in severe tissue necrosis, use of an indwelling catheter taped in place is recommended for administration. The reconstituted drug should be administered over a minimum period of 10 min into the side port of a freely running i.v. infusion of 0.9% NaCl. Reported to be less cardiotoxic than doxorubicin, epirubicin should still be used with caution in patients with or predisposed to cardiac disease.

Safety and handling: Potent cytotoxic drug that should only be prepared and administered by trained personnel. See Appendix and specialist texts for further advice on chemotherapeutic agents. After reconstitution the drug is stable for 24h at room temperature (protect from light). Store under refrigeration.

Contraindications: No information available.

Adverse reactions: Acute anaphylactic reactions should be treated with adrenaline, steroids and fluids. Epirubicin causes a dose-dependent cumulative cardiotoxicity in dogs (leading to cardiomyopathy and congestive heart failure) but possibly at a lower incidence than that of doxorubicin. This rarely develops in dogs given a total dose of <240 mg/m^2. It may also cause tachycardia and arrhythmias on administration. Dogs with pre-existing cardiac disease should be routinely monitored with ECGs and/or echocardiograms. Anorexia, vomiting, pancreatitis, severe leucopenia, thrombocytopenia, haemorrhagic gastroenteritis and nephrotoxicity are major adverse effects. A complete CBC and platelet count should be monitored whenever therapy is given. If the neutrophil count drops below 3 x 10^9 or if the platelet count drops below 50 x 10^9, treatment should be suspended. Once the counts have stabilized, epirubicin can then be restarted at the same dose. If haematological toxicity occurs again, or if GI toxicity is recurrent the dose should be reduced by 10–25%.

Drug interactions: Epirubicin is incompatible with heparin; a precipitate will form. Increased risk of myelosuppression when used in combination with cyclophosphamide. In humans cimetidine increased the area under the dose curve of epirubicin by 50% and should not be used concurrently.

DOSES
See Appendix for chemotherapy protocols and conversion of body weight to body surface area.
Dogs: 30 mg/m^2 i.v. q3wk; maximum total dose not to exceed 240 mg/m^2.
Cats, Small mammals, Birds, Reptiles: No information available.

Epoetin alfa, Epoetin beta see **Erythropoietin**
Equine chorionic gonadotrophin see **Serum gonadotrophin**

Erythromycin `CIL`
(Erythrocin, Erythromycin*, Erythroped*) **POM-V, POM**

Formulations: Injectable: 200 mg/ml solution; 1 g/vial powder for reconstitution. Oral: 250 mg, 500 mg tablets/capsules; 25 mg/ml suspension; powder authorized for chickens.

Action: May be bactericidal (time-dependent) or bacteriostatic, depending upon drug concentration and bacterial susceptibility. It binds to the 50S ribosome, inhibiting peptide bond formation.

Use: Has a similar antibacterial spectrum to penicillins. It is active against Gram-positive cocci (some *Staphylococcus* species are resistant), Gram-positive bacilli and some Gram-negative bacilli (*Pasteurella*). Some strains of *Actinomyces*, *Nocardia*, *Chlamydophila* and *Rickettsia* are also inhibited by erythromycin. Most of the

Enterobacteriaceae (*Pseudomonas*, *Escherichia coli*, *Klebsiella*) are resistant. It is used in hamsters to treat proliferative ileitis (*Lawsonia intracellularis*) and in ferrets to control *Campylobacter* infection, although it may not eliminate intestinal carriage of this organism. Being a lipophilic weak base, it is concentrated in fluids that are more acidic than plasma, including milk, prostatic fluid and intracellular fluid. Resistance to erythromycin can be quite high, particularly in staphylococcal organisms. Erythromycin acts as a GI prokinetic by stimulating motilin receptors. Different esters of erythromycin are available. It is likely that the kinetics and possibly the toxicity will differ, depending on the ester used. Erythromycin's activity is enhanced in an alkaline pH. As the base is acid-labile it should be administered on an empty stomach.

Safety and handling: Normal precautions should be observed.

Contraindications: In humans the erythromycin estolate salt has been implicated in causing cholestatic hepatitis. Although not demonstrated in veterinary medicine, this salt should be avoided in animals with hepatic dysfunction.

Adverse reactions: The commonest adverse effect is GI upset. Care should be taken in cases of hepatic or renal impairment. Erythromycin can cause enterotoxaemia in rodents and rabbits.

Drug interactions: Erythromycin may enhance the absorption of digoxin from the GI tract and increase serum levels of cisapride, methylprednisolone, theophylline and terfenadine. The interactions with terfenadine and cisapride proved particularly significant in human medicine, leading to fatal or near-fatal arrhythmias in some patients receiving both drugs. Erythromycin should not be used in combination with other macrolide, lincosamide or chloramphenicol antimicrobials as antagonism may occur.

DOSES
See Appendix for guidelines on responsible antibacterial use.
Dogs, Cats: 10–20 mg/kg p.o. q8–12h. GI prokinetic: 0.5–1 mg/kg p.o. q8h.
Small mammals: Ferrets: 10 mg/kg p.o. q6h; Hamsters: 20 mg/kg p.o. q12h or 0.13 mg/ml drinking water.
Birds: 20 mg/kg i.m., s.c. q8h; 60 mg/kg p.o. q12h or 125 mg/l of drinking water; 200 mg/kg soft feed.
Reptiles: No information available.

Erythropoietin (Epoetin alfa, Epoetin beta)
(Eprex*, Neorecormon*) **POM**

CIL

Formulations: Injectable: 1000 IU, 2000 IU, 5000 IU powders for reconstitution; 2000 IU/ml, 4000 IU/ml, 10,000 IU/ml, 40,000 IU/ml solutions. Eprex is epoetin alfa. Neorecormon is epoetin beta.

Action: Stimulates division and differentiation of red blood cells.

Use: Recombinant human erythropoietin (r-HuEPO) is predominantly used to treat anaemia associated with chronic renal failure, although it is also used to treat anaemic human patients with cancer and rheumatoid arthritis, and cats with FeLV-associated anaemia. Erythropoietin is not indicated in conditions where high serum concentrations of the hormone already exist (e.g. haemolytic anaemia, anaemia due to blood loss), where the anaemia is due to iron deficiency or where systemic hypertension is present. Monitoring and/or supplementation of iron may be necessary, especially if response to treatment is poor. Darbepoetin may be a better choice in many cases.

Safety and handling: Normal precautions should be observed.

Contraindications: Conditions where high serum concentrations of erythropoietin already exist.

Adverse reactions: Local and systemic allergic reactions may rarely develop (skin rash at the injection site, pyrexia, arthralgia and mucocutaneous ulcers). The production of cross-reacting antibodies to r-HuEPO occurs in 20% of treated dogs and 30% of treated cats 4 weeks or more after treatment. These antibodies reduce the efficacy of the drug and can cause pure red cell aplasia. The drug should be discontinued if this develops.

Drug interactions: No information available.

DOSES

Dogs, Cats: Epoetin alfa/beta: 50 IU/kg i.v., s.c. 3 times/week until PCV is normal, then gradually reduce frequency of dosing to maintain PCV at lower end of normal. If response is inadequate then increasingly higher doses (up to 100 IU/kg) can be given. Dose changes should only be made at 3-weekly intervals.
Small mammals: Ferrets, Rabbits: epoetin alfa: 50–150 IU/kg i.m., s.c. q48h. Once desired PCV reached, administer q7d for maintenance.
Birds, Reptiles: No information available.

Esmolol
(Brevibloc*) **POM**

Formulations: Injectable: 10 mg/ml solution.

Action: An ultra-short-acting beta-blocker. It is relatively cardioselective and blocks beta-1 adrenergic receptors in the heart. It has a negative inotropic and chronotropic action which can lead to a decreased myocardial oxygen demand. Blood pressure is reduced. It has an antiarrhythmic effect through its blockade of adrenergic stimulation of the heart.

Use: Therapy of, or as an assessment of the efficacy of beta-adrenergic blockers in the treatment of, supraventricular tachycardias (including atrial fibrillation, atrial flutter and atrial tachycardia). Its effect is brief, persisting only 10–20 min after i.v. infusion. Other beta-blockers must be used for chronic or maintenance therapy.

Safety and handling: Normal precautions should be observed.

Contraindications: Patients with bradyarrhythmias, acute or decompensated congestive heart failure. Relatively contraindicated in animals with medically controlled congestive heart failure as is poorly tolerated. Do not administer concurrently with alpha-adrenergic agonists.

Adverse reactions: Most frequently seen in geriatric patients with chronic heart disease or in patients with acute or decompensated heart failure. Include bradycardia, AV block, myocardial depression, heart failure, syncope, hypotension, hypoglycaemia, bronchospasm and diarrhoea. Depression and lethargy are occasionally seen and are a result of esmolol's high lipid solubility and penetration into the CNS. Esmolol may reduce the glomerular filtration rate and therefore exacerbate any pre-existing renal impairment.

Drug interactions: The hypotensive effect of esmolol is enhanced by many agents that depress myocardial activity including anaesthetics, phenothiazines, antihypertensives, diuretics and diazepam. There is an increased risk of bradycardia, severe hypotension, heart failure and AV block if esmolol is used concurrently with calcium-channel blockers. Concurrent digoxin administration potentiates bradycardia. Esmolol may increase serum digoxin levels by up to 20%. Morphine may increase esmolol serum concentration by up to 50%. Esmolol may enhance the effects of muscle relaxants. The bronchodilatory effects of theophylline may be blocked by esmolol.

DOSES
Dogs, Cats: 0.05–0.5 mg/kg i.v. bolus over 5 min; 25–200 µg (micrograms)/kg/min constant rate infusion.
Small mammals, Birds, Reptiles: No information available.

Estriol (Oestriol)
(Incurin) **POM-V**

Formulations: Oral: 1 mg tablet.

Action: Synthetic, short-acting oestrogen with a high affinity for oestrogen receptors in the lower urogenital tract. It increases muscle tone, improving urodynamic function.

Use: Management of urethral sphincter mechanism incompetence that develops in spayed bitches.

Safety and handling: Normal precautions should be observed.

Contraindications: Do not use in intact bitches. Do not use if PU/PD present. Manufacturer states that this drug should not be used in animals <1 year old.

Adverse reactions: Oestrogenic effects are seen in 5–9% of bitches receiving 2 mg q24h.

Drug interactions: No information available.

DOSES
Dogs: The dose has to be determined for each animal individually. Start at a dose of 1 mg/dog p.o. q24h. If treatment is successful reduce the dose to 0.5 mg/dog p.o. q24h. If treatment is unsuccessful increase to 2 mg/dog p.o. q24h. Alternate-day dosing can be considered once a response has been seen. The minimum effective dose is 0.5 mg/dog p.o. q24–48h. The maximum dose is 2 mg/dog p.o. q24h.
Cats: Do not use.
Small mammals, Birds, Reptiles: No information available.

Etamiphylline
(Millophylline V) **POM-V**

Formulations: Oral: 100 mg, 200 mg, 300 mg tablets. Injectable: 140 mg/ml solution.

Action: Phosphodiesterase inhibitor.

Use: Bronchial constriction and pulmonary oedema. It has a mild diuretic action and is a mild cardiac and respiratory stimulant. It is recommended that the drug should not be used in animals <3 kg.

Safety and handling: Normal precautions should be observed.

Contraindications: No information available.

Adverse reactions: Occasional CNS stimulation may develop; treat with a sedative (e.g. diazepam).

Drug interactions: No information available.

DOSES
Dogs, Cats: 10 mg/kg p.o. q8h or 14 mg/kg i.m., s.c. q8h; may also be given slowly i.v. after 1:1 dilution in water for injection.
Small mammals, Birds, Reptiles: No information available.

Ethanol
(Alcohol*) **POM**

Formulations: Injectable: Medical grade alcohol is a 95% solution. To prepare a solution for i.v. use, dilute to 20% in sterile water and administer through a 22 μm filter. Other commercially available forms of alcohol are less safe as they usually contain other substances which make i.v. administration hazardous (vodka is likely to be the least dangerous).

Action: Competitive inhibition of alcohol dehydrogenase.

Use: Prevents metabolization of ethylene glycol (antifreeze) or methanol to toxic metabolites. Also used to cleanse and de-grease skin. When treating ethylene glycol toxicity, adjust dose to maintain blood ethanol levels above 35 mg/dl in dogs. Monitor fluid and electrolyte balance during ethanol therapy. Unlikely to be effective if administered >8 hours after toxin ingestion. Fomepizole, if available, is safer than ethanol.

Safety and handling: Normal precautions should be observed.

Contraindications: No information available.

Adverse reactions: Ethanol will cause diuresis and may cause additive depression that will mask CNS signs of ethylene glycol toxicity. Adverse events occur frequently with intravenous ethanol infusions.

Drug interactions: Avoid concurrent fomepizole administration (increases risk of alcohol toxicity).

DOSES

Dogs: 5.5 ml of 20% ethanol solution/kg given i.v. q4h for 5 treatments, then i.v. q6h for 4 additional treatments. Alternatively, give an i.v. loading dose of 1.3 ml/kg of 30% solution then begin a constant rate infusion of 0.42 mg/kg/h for 48h. For clinically mild cases (minimal CNS signs), particularly if using vodka, oral administration is also possible.
Cats: 5 ml of 20% ethanol solution/kg i.v. q6h for 5 treatments, then q8h for 4 additional treatments.
Small mammals, Birds, Reptiles: No information available.

Etherified starch
(eloHAES*, HAES-steril*, Hemohes*, Tetraspan*, Venofundin*, Volulyte*, Voluven*) **POM**

Formulations: Injectable: 6%, 10% solutions.

Action: Promotes retention of the fluid in the vascular system through the exertion of oncotic pressure.

Use: Expansion and maintenance of blood volume in various forms of shock including hypovolaemic, haemorrhagic and septic shock. The duration of plasma expansion is dependent on various factors including molecular weight and molar substitution ratio. Plasma persistence of colloidal molecules may be prolonged (up to 24 h). Hetastarch administration increases plasma volume, generally by at least the volume administered but it can be up to 172%. Initial plasma expansion may be greater with pentastarch but the duration of action is shorter. In hypoalbuminaemic dogs the administration of hetastarch is associated with an increase in colloid osmotic pressure and a decrease in peripheral oedema. In humans the half-life of hetastarch varies with time after administration and dose, and administration of consecutive doses increases the half-life

hypersecretory conditions secondary to gastrinoma, mast cell neoplasia or short bowel syndrome. Reduction of vomiting due to gastric ulceration is typically achieved in about 2 weeks. However, animals should be treated for at least 2 weeks after the remission of clinical signs, so a minimum treatment duration of 28 days is recommended. Currently cimetidine is the only antiulcer drug with a veterinary market authorization. There is little information on the use of famotidine in dogs compared with cimetidine or ranitidine. Famotidine has little effect on GI motility in humans. There is one study in healthy Beagles showing that famotidine somewhat increases gastric pH.

Safety and handling: Normal precautions should be observed.

Contraindications: No information available.

Adverse reactions: In humans famotidine has fewer side effects than cimetidine.

Drug interactions: Famotidine is devoid of many of the interactions of the H2 related antagonist cimetidine.

DOSES
Dogs, Cats: 0.5–1.0 mg/kg p.o. q12–24h.
Small mammals: Ferrets: 0.25–0.5 mg/kg p.o., i.v., s.c. q24h; Chinchillas: 0.5 mg/kg s.c. q24h; Guinea pigs: 0.4 mg/kg p.o., s.c. q24h.
Birds, Reptiles: No information available.

Febantel see Pyrantel

Feline facial fraction F3 (Feline facial pheromone F3, Familiarization pheromone)
(Feliway) **GSL**

Formulations: Plug-in diffuser, topical environmental spray.

Action: A synthetic analogue of the F3 fraction of the 'feline facial pheromones' that are used in facial marking of the physical environment by cats. Believed to provide a feeling of security for cats in unfamiliar or stressful situations. F3 is believed to stimulate receptors in the vomeronasal organ, resulting in anxiolytic activity within the limbic system in response to particular classes of stimuli, especially those associated with threats to physical resources.

Use: Management of indoor urine marking, inappropriate scratching and changes to the animal's physical environment at home or outside (e.g. during transport, within the cattery or the veterinary clinic). Additional indications include management of situational anxiety-related disorders. It can aid handling for anaesthesia induction and during other medical examinations when the spray may be applied to the consultation or preparation table. The diffuser should be placed in the room most frequently occupied by the cat and, in the case of management of behavioural disorders, where the inappropriate behaviour most frequently occurs. The pump spray should not mark or stain but it is sensible to patch-test fabrics and polished surfaces before using extensively.

Safety and handling: Humans with known sensitivity to the ingredients should avoid using the product in their homes.

Contraindications: No information available.

Adverse reactions: No information available.

Drug interactions: None.

APPLICATION

Cats: Follow manufacturer's instructions. Pump spray: F3 is applied to the environment in locations where the inappropriate behaviour is occurring and in locations that are of behavioural significance. When being used as a familiarization signal for cats in potentially stressful situations, or in new environments, the spray should be applied 30 min before the cat has access to the area. In the case of management of existing urine marking, one dose (one depression of the nozzle) should be applied daily from about 10 cm from the soiled site at a height of about 20 cm from the floor. In multicat households the spray should be applied 2–3 times/day on previously marked sites and once a day on other locations which are of behavioural significance. When using to prevent urine marking, spray once per day in locations of behavioural significance. For best results allow the spray to come to room temperature before it is applied and adjust cleaning regimes for indoor marking. Rinse well and allow areas to dry after cleaning, with biological washing powder followed by surgical spirit, before applying the F3 spray. The diffuser is active over an area of approximately 50–70 m^2. If the total target area exceeds this, a second diffuser should be used. One vial will last for approximately 4 weeks if the device is left switched on 24h per day. Do not repeatedly switch the diffuser on and off; it is designed to be left on at all times.
Dogs, Small mammals, Birds, Reptiles: Not applicable.

Feline facial fraction F4 (Feline facial pheromone F4)

(Felifriend) **GSL**

Formulations: Topical environmental spray; hand gel.

Action: A synthetic analogue of the F4 fraction of the 'feline facial pheromones' that are used in facial marking of the social environment by cats. F4 is believed to stimulate receptors in the vomeronasal organ, resulting in anxiolytic activity within the limbic system especially in response to social stimuli. Effect is greatest when there are no learned associations with these stimuli. Do not spray close to the animal's head, specifically in the region of the eyes.

Use: Used to familiarize cats to unfamiliar humans or those to whom they show apprehensive or fearful behaviour. The primary use is to improve tolerance of handling during veterinary examination and grooming. It may also be used to increase tolerance between cats but caution is warranted as it is not authorized for direct application to cats.

Safety and handling: Normal precautions should be observed.

Contraindications: No information available.

Adverse reactions: In some cases a paradoxical increase in agitation and aggression is witnessed due to contradictory chemical and visual signals. If cats exhibit vocalization and threatening behaviour after the application, terminate the contact and attempt reintroduction slowly later. Stop if aggression continues.

Drug interactions: None.

APPLICATION

Cats: Follow manufacturer's instructions. To aid familiarization to humans, apply 2 sprays of the solution to the palm of each hand and rub the hands and wrists together as required. Place the hands 20 cm in front of the cat's nose and wait for one minute before attempting to initiate contact. For familiarization to cats, apply 2 sprays of the solution on to a compress and apply to the flank and neck regions of each cat. It is best to avoid using the pump spray in front of the cat since this can lead to fear responses. Wait for at least one minute after application before introducing the cats to each other and ensure that they are supervised.

Dogs, Small mammals, Birds, Reptiles: Not applicable.

Fenbendazole

(Bob Martin Easy to Use Wormer, Granofen, Lapizole, Panacur, Zerofen) **NFA-VPS**

Formulations: Oral: 222 mg/g granules (22%); 20 mg/ml oral suspension (2%); 25 mg/ml oral suspension (2.5%); 100 mg/ml oral suspension (10%); 187.5 mg/g oral paste (18.75%).

Action: Inhibits fumarate reductase system of parasites thereby blocking the citric acid cycle and also reduces glucose absorption by the parasite.

Use: Treatment of ascarids (including larval stages), hookworms, whipworms, tapeworms (*Taenia*), *Oslerus osleri*, *Aelurostrongylus abstrusus*, *Angiostrongylus vasorum*, *Capillaria aerophila*, *Ollulanus tricuspis*, *Physaloptera rara* and *Paragonimus kellicotti* infections. There is 60–70% efficacy against *Dipylidium caninum*. Fenbendazole has 100% efficacy in clearing *Giardia* cysts. It is used in rabbits for the treatment of *Encephalitozoon cuniculi*. Unlike some other benzimidazoles, fenbendazole is safe to use in pregnant animals.

Safety and handling: Normal precautions should be observed.

Contraindications: No information available.

Adverse reactions: Bone marrow hypoplasia has been reported in a dog. Birds, especially vultures and storks, and some raptors, are more sensitive to adverse reactions affecting bone marrow, intestinal and liver functions. In pigeons and doves, mortality of 50% has occurred at doses of 20 mg/kg p.o. given on 3 consecutive days. Vomiting, depression and death within 96 h are recorded in some raptors. Feather damage also reported in pigeons. Potential toxicity in some reptiles, e.g. ball pythons.

Drug interactions: No information available.

DOSES
Dogs:
- Roundworms, tapeworms: dogs <6 months old: 50 mg/kg p.o. q24h for 3 consecutive days; >6 months old: 100 mg/kg as a single dose p.o. Treatment of *Capillaria* may need to be extended to 10 days. Repeat q3months. For pregnant bitches 25 mg/kg p.o. q24h from day 40 until 2 days post-whelping (approximately 25 days).
- *Angiostrongylus vasorum*: 50 mg/kg p.o. for a minimum of 10 days, although the duration of treatment has yet to be defined.
- *Oslerus osleri*: 50 mg/kg p.o. q24h for 7 days, although a repeat course of treatment may be required in some cases.
- *Aelurostrongylus abstrusus*: 20 mg/kg p.o. q24h for 3 days.
- Giardiasis: 50 mg/kg p.o. q24h for 5 days.

Cats:
- Roundworms, tapeworms: cats <6 months old: 20 mg/kg p.o. q24h for 5 days; >6 months old: 100 mg/kg as a single dose p.o.
- *Aelurostrongylus abstrusus*: 20 mg/kg p.o. q24h for 5 days.
- Giardiasis: 20 mg/kg p.o. for 5 days.

Small mammals: Rabbits: *E. cuniculi*: 20 mg/kg p.o. q24h for 28 days; Other small mammals: 20-50 mg/kg p.o. q24h for 5 consecutive days; the higher end of the range is suggested for giardiasis only.

Birds:
- Nematodes: 20–100 mg/kg p.o., administer 2 doses separated by 10 days; capillariasis: 25 mg/kg p.o. q24h for 5 consecutive days; Pigeons: 16 mg/kg p.o. once, repeat after 10 days if necessary or 10–20 mg/kg p.o. q24h for 3 days, repeat after 2 weeks; Passerines: 20 mg/kg p.o. q24h for 3 doses. Not advisable to give more than 50 mg/kg in unfamiliar species.
- Giardiasis: 50 mg/kg p.o. q24h for 3 doses.

Reptiles:
- Nematodes: 50–100 mg/kg once p.o., per cloaca; repeat after 2 and 4 weeks.
- Giardiasis and flagellates: 50 mg/kg p.o. q24h for 3–5 days. In species with potential toxicity, e.g. ball pythons (*Python regius*): 25 mg/kg p.o.

Fentanyl

CIL

(Fentadon, Recuvyra, Durogesic*, Fentanyl*, Fentora*, Sublimaze*) **POM-V CD SCHEDULE 2, POM CD SCHEDULE 2**

Formulations: Oral: 100 µg, 200 µg, 400 µg, 600 µg, 800 µg tablets. Injectable: 50 µg/ml solution. Transdermal: 50 mg/ml solution; 12.5 µg/h, 25 µg/h, 50 µg/h, 75 µg/h, 100 µg/h patches.

Action: Synthetic pure mu (OP3) receptor agonist.

Use: Very potent opioid analgesic (50 times more potent than morphine) used to provide profound intraoperative analgesia in dogs and cats. Can also be used at low dose rates for postoperative analgesia. Use of potent opioids during anaesthesia contributes to a balanced anaesthesia technique, therefore the dose of other concurrently administered anaesthetic agents should be reduced. Fentanyl has a rapid onset of action after i.v. administration and short duration of action (10–20 min depending on dose). After prolonged administration (>4 hours) or high doses its duration of action is significantly prolonged as the tissues become saturated. It can be used intraoperatively to provide analgesia by intermittent bolus doses or by a continuous rate infusion. Postoperatively fentanyl can be given by continuous rate infusion to provide analgesia, doses at the low end of the dose range should be used and respiratory function monitored. Its clearance is similar to morphine whilst its elimination half-life is longer, reflecting its higher lipid solubility and volume of distribution. A very concentrated (50 mg/ml) solution of fentanyl for transdermal administration to dogs is authorized for the control of postoperative pain associated with major orthopaedic and soft tissue surgery. The solution is applied to the skin on the dorsal neck area 2–4 hours before the start of surgery and plasma concentrations within the therapeutic range for analgesia are maintained for 4 days after application, providing medium term opioid analgesia for dogs that are discharged from hospital after surgery. The solution should only be applied to intact skin. The solution is licensed for use as the sole opioid analgesic to be applied during the perioperative period; however, additional top-up opioid analgesia can be given if transdermal fentanyl is insufficient. It is advisable to monitor body temperature in dogs that have received transdermal fentanyl for at least 40 hours after application and support body temperature if hypothermia is identified. Dogs >20 kg must be hospitalized for at least 48 hours after application before discharge to owners. The transdermal preparation has significant human health considerations associated with use (see below) and an application system designed to minimize the risk of human exposure to fentanyl has been developed. Transdermal fentanyl patches can be used to provide analgesia for up to 72 hours after surgery or for the management of chronic pain. However, in dogs, licensing of a transdermal solution makes use of patches redundant. Following patch application, it takes approximately 7 hours in cats and 24 hours in dogs to attain adequate plasma concentrations to provide analgesia. Alternative forms of analgesia must be provided during this period, or patches must be placed before surgery. Systemic plasma concentrations of fentanyl can be very variable after transdermal absorption from patches and some animals may not develop adequate plasma concentrations to achieve analgesia. Therefore, it is preferable to use transdermal fentanyl as an adjunctive analgesic in combination with other drugs. Direct application of heat sources to transdermal fentanyl patches (e.g. during anaesthesia) will significantly increase the uptake of fentanyl and may result in higher than expected plasma concentrations.

Safety and handling: Veterinary surgeons must undergo training in order to become authorized to prescribe transdermal fentanyl and receive the drug from veterinary wholesalers. The transdermal solution of fentanyl is very concentrated with the potential to cause opioid overdose (associated with respiratory depression) if absorbed systemically by humans (e.g. through contact with the skin or mucosal surfaces such as the eyes and mouth). Personal protective clothing consisting of latex or nitrile gloves, eye protection and suitable protective clothing must be worn when handling the product. Following application to the skin, the site must not be touched for at least 5 min until the solution is dry. It is advisable to wear gloves when handling dogs to which transdermal fentanyl has been applied for up to 72 hours following application or to wash hands immediately after handling the dog in this time window. Dog owners should be advised that children <15 kg body weight should not be allowed to come into contact with dogs treated with transdermal fentanyl until 72 hours after application. The manufacturer provides information to give to the dog owner at the time of discharge, detailing the effects of the drug and the risks of human exposure. Other dogs and cats should not be allowed to come into contact with the site of application on treated dogs for 72 hours following application. If animals are sent home with transdermal fentanyl patches the owners must be warned about the dangers of patch ingestion by humans or other animals.

Contraindications: Do not use transdermal fentanyl solution in cats.

Adverse reactions: Intraoperative administration is likely to cause respiratory depression, therefore, respiration should be monitored and facilities must be available to provide positive pressure ventilation. Rapid i.v. injection can cause severe bradycardia, even asystole, therefore the drug should be given slowly. A reduction in heart rate is likely whenever fentanyl is given, atropine can be administered to counter bradycardia if necessary. Apart from the effects on heart rate, fentanyl has limited other effects on cardiovascular function when used at clinical dose rates.

Drug interactions: Fentanyl can be used to reduce the dose requirement for other anaesthetic drugs in patients with cardiovascular instability or systemic disease.

DOSES
Dogs:
- Intraoperative analgesia: 1–5 μg (micrograms)/kg i.v. q20min.

- Anaesthesia: 2.5–10 µg (micrograms)/kg/h by continuous rate infusion during anaesthesia, reduced to 1–5 µg/kg/h during the postoperative period. Continuous rate infusions should be preceded by a loading dose (5–10 µg/kg).
- Transdermal solution: 2.6 mg/kg (0.052 ml/kg); the total volume should be divided so that a maximum of 0.5 ml transdermal solution is applied at any one site; a distance of 2.5 cm should be allowed between application sites.
- Transdermal patch: 4 µg (micrograms)/kg/h patch (e.g. 100 µg/h patch for a 25 kg dog).

Cats:
- Intraoperative analgesia: 5 µg (micrograms)/kg bolus, repeated injections may be required q20min.
- Anaesthesia: Continuous rate infusions as for dogs.
- Transdermal patch: 25 µg (micrograms)/h patch for cats 3–5 kg; in smaller cats and kittens the 12.5 µg/h patch can be applied.

Small mammals, Birds, Reptiles: No information available.

Fentanyl/Fluanisone
(Hypnorm) POM-V CD SCHEDULE 2

Formulations: Injectable: 0.2 mg/ml fentanyl with 10 mg/ml fluanisone.

Action: Fentanyl is a pure mu opioid agonist and fluanisone is a butyrophenone; the combination produces neuroleptanalgesia.

Use: Sedation and analgesia for restraint and to allow minor procedures to be carried out in mice, rats, rabbits and guinea pigs. Combined with a benzodiazepine it can be used to produce anaesthesia with muscle relaxation for surgery. It can be used for premedication prior to induction of anaesthesia with propofol in rabbits. Fentanyl/fluanisone produces a long duration of sedation and analgesia in small mammals (30–60 min), the duration of action is dependent on dose and varies between species. When used in combination with a benzodiazepine to produce anaesthesia, the lowest end of the dose range of fentanyl/fluanisone should be used. Hypnorm is miscible with midazolam at appropriate dilutions, enabling a single injection to produce anaesthesia. Duration of anaesthesia is approximately 20–40 min, although recovery can be very prolonged. Various dose regimens for different species have been published. Prolonged respiratory depression in the recovery period can be avoided by the administration of a partial mu agonist (buprenorphine) at the end of the procedure. This will reverse respiratory depression induced by fentanyl and provide continued analgesia. Small mammals should be weighed before drug administration, accurate dosing is imperative to prevent overdose. Oxygen supplementation via a face mask is recommended during sedation and anaesthesia of all animals.

Safety and handling: Normal precautions should be observed.

Contraindications: Animals with pre-existing respiratory compromise.

Adverse reactions: Respiratory depression can occur when given in high doses, particularly during the recovery period. Administration of buprenorphine in the recovery period can ameliorate respiratory depression and sedation, and provide ongoing analgesia. Measures should be taken to maintain normothermia during the sedation/anaesthesia and recovery period.

Drug interactions: No information available.

DOSES
When used for sedation is generally given as part of a combination. See Appendix for sedation protocols in all species.
Dogs, Cats: Not recommended.
Small mammals: Rabbits: 0.1–0.5 ml/kg i.m.; Guinea pigs: 0.5–1 ml/kg i.m.; Rats: 0.2–0.5 ml/kg i.m., i.p.; Mice: 0.1–0.5 ml/kg i.p.
Birds, Reptiles: No information available.

Filgrastim (Granulocyte colony stimulating factor, G-CSF)
(Neupogen*) **POM**

Formulations: Injectable: 30 million IU (300 μg)/ml solution.

Action: Filgrastim is recombinant human granulocyte colony stimulating factor (rhG-CSF). It activates proliferation and differentiation of granulocyte progenitor cells, enhances granulopoiesis.

Use: In humans it is indicated in the management of neutropenia, especially in patients receiving high-dose chemotherapy. Neutrophil counts rise within 24 hours. Following discontinuation of therapy, neutrophil counts drop to normal after 5 days. There are few reports on the use of G-CSF in dogs or cats. It is most likely to be used in the management of febrile patients, particularly those receiving cytotoxic drugs with neutrophil counts <1x10^9/l. It may also be used as an adjunct in the treatment of infections, e.g. canine erlichiosis, parvovirus, FeLV or FIV, in the treatment of bone marrow neoplasia and for cyclic haemopoiesis in dogs.

Safety and handling: Normal precautions should be observed.

Contraindications: Dogs or cats that have developed antibodies to G-CSF (with resultant neutropenia) should probably not receive it in the future.

Adverse reactions: Normal dogs produce neutralizing antibodies to rhG-CSF. This limits repeated use and may result in neutropenia. This does not appear to be the case in canine chemotherapy patients. A variety of adverse effects have been reported in humans, including musculoskeletal pain, transient hypotension, dysuria, allergic reactions, proteinuria, haematuria, splenomegaly and increased liver enzymes. Reported adverse effects are bone pain at high doses and irritation at the injection site.

Drug interactions: Steroids and lithium may potentiate the release of neutrophils during G-CSF therapy. Concurrent administration with chemotherapy may increase incidence of adverse effects. G-CSF should be given at least 24 hours after the last dose of chemotherapy, as the stimulatory effects of G-CSF on haemopoietic precursors renders them more susceptible to the effects of chemotherapy.

DOSES
Dogs, Cats: 100,000–500,000 IU (1–5 micrograms)/kg/day s.c. for 3–5 days.
Small mammals, Birds, Reptiles: No information available.

Finasteride
(Proscar*) **POM**

Formulations: Oral: 5 mg tablet.

Action: Competitively inhibits dihydrotestosterone (DHT) production within the prostate. DHT is the main hormonal stimulus for the development of benign prostatic hyperplasia.

Use: Treatment of benign prostatic hyperplasia as an alternative to castration. Not authorized for veterinary use and therefore should only be used when delmadinone or osaterone are not appropriate.

Safety and handling: Women of child-bearing age should avoid handling crushed or broken tablets as finasteride is potentially teratogenic.

Contraindications: Do not use in breeding dogs.

Adverse reactions: Secreted into semen and causes fetal anomalies.

Drug interactions: No information available.

DOSES
Dogs: 5 mg per dog p.o. q24h.
Cats, Small mammals, Birds, Reptiles: No information available.

Fipronil
(Certifect, Effipro, Eliminall, Felevox, Fipronil, Fiprospot, Frontline) **NFA-VPS, POM-V**

Formulations: Topical: 10% w/v fipronil spot-on pipettes in a wide range of sizes (Effipro, Frontline); with *S*-methoprene (Frontline Combo); with *S*-methoprene and amitraz (Certifect). Also 0.25% w/v fipronil spray in alcohol base (Effipro and Frontline sprays) in a range of sizes.

Action: Fipronil interacts with ligand-gated (GABA) chloride channels, blocking pre- and post-synaptic transfer of chloride ions, resulting in death of parasites on contact.

Use: Treatment and prevention of flea infestations and tick prevention in dogs and cats >8 weeks of age and >2 kg (dogs) or >1 kg (cats). Elimination of canine and feline biting lice (*Trichodectes canis*, *Felicola subrostratus*). For treatment of flea infestations the additional use of an approved IGR is recommended and the product should be applied every 4 weeks to all in contact cats and dogs. Minimum treatment interval 4 weeks. Frontline spray may be used in treating very young puppies with sarcoptic acariasis. Bathing between 48 hours before and 24 hours after application is not recommended. Can be used in pregnant and lactating females. Beware of use in juvenile reptiles and immediately after skin slough due to increased permeability of skin and associated toxicity. Treatment of the environment is also recommended.

Safety and handling: Normal precautions should be observed.

Contraindications: Do not use in rabbits. May be harmful to aquatic organisms.

Adverse reactions: Local pruritus or alopecia may occur at the site of application.

Drug interactions: A low dose of amitraz has been shown to have a synergistic effect on the speed of tick kill, thus reducing the risk of transmission for tick-borne pathogens.

DOSES
Dogs:
- Flea infestations: spray 3–6 ml/kg (6–12 pumps/kg 100 ml application, 2–4 pumps/kg 250 ml or 500 ml application) or apply 1 pipette per dog according to body weight. Treatment should be repeated not more frequently than every 4 weeks.
- Cheyletiellosis, Otocariasis (*Otodectes cyanotis*): same dose but for two applications.

Cats: Spray 3–6 ml/kg (6–12 pumps/kg 100 ml application) or apply 1 pipette per cat. Treatment should be repeated not more frequently than every 4 weeks.

Small mammals: Ferrets: spray 3–6 ml/kg q30–60d; Rodents: 7.5 mg/kg topically q30–60d. Do not use in rabbits.

Birds: Use spray form q30–60d. Apply to cotton wool and dab behind head, under wings and at base of tail (raptors/parrots) or lightly under each wing (pigeon/passerine).

Reptiles: Spray on to cloth first then wipe over surface of reptile q7–14d until negative for ectoparasites. Beware of use in reptiles which have recently shed their skin and in small species where overdosage and toxicity may occur.

Firocoxib
(Previcox) **POM-V**

Formulations: Oral: 57 mg, 227 mg tablets.

Action: NSAID that selectively inhibits the COX-2 enzyme thereby limiting the production of prostaglandins involved in inflammation. It has also has analgesic and antipyretic effects.

Use: Relief of pain and inflammation associated with osteoarthritis and with soft tissue and orthopaedic surgery in dogs. When used for perioperative pain, it is recommended to give the first dose 2 hours before surgery. Studies investigating the safety of firocoxib in dogs were only carried out for 90 days, therefore animals receiving firocoxib for more prolonged periods should be monitored carefully for NSAID-induced side effects. Administration of firocoxib to animals with renal disease must be carefully evaluated. Firocoxib may have a synergistic role with platinum-based chemotherapeutic agents in the treatment of transitional cell carcinomas of the urinary bladder and may have some antitumour effects on its own.

Safety and handling: Normal precautions should be observed.

Contraindications: All NSAIDs should be administered cautiously in the perioperative period as they may adversely affect renal perfusion during periods of hypotension. If hypotension during anaesthesia is anticipated, delay firocoxib administration until the animal is fully recovered and normotensive. Do not give to dehydrated, hypovolaemic or hypotensive patients or those with GI disease or blood clotting problems. Do not give to pregnant animals, animals <10 weeks old or <3 kg. Do not use in cats.

Adverse reactions: GI signs may occur in all animals after NSAID administration. Stop therapy if this persists beyond 1–2 days. Some animals develop signs with one NSAID and not another. A 1–2-week wash-out period should be allowed before starting another NSAID after cessation of therapy. Stop therapy immediately if GI bleeding is suspected. There is a small risk that NSAIDs may precipitate cardiac failure in animals with cardiovascular disease. Liver disease will prolong the metabolism of firocoxib, leading to the potential for drug overdose with repeated dosing.

Drug interactions: Do not administer concurrently or within 24 hours of other NSAIDs and glucocorticoids. Do not administer with other potentially nephrotoxic agents, e.g. aminoglycosides.

DOSES
Dogs: 5 mg/kg p.o. q24h, with or without food.
Cats: Do not use.
Small mammals, Birds, Reptiles: No information available.

Flucloxacillin
(Floxapen*, Flucloxacillin*) **POM**

Formulations: Injectable: Flucloxacillin sodium: 250 mg, 500 mg, 1 g powders for reconstitution. Oral: Flucloxacillin sodium: 250 mg or 500 mg capsules; powder for reconstitution with water giving a final concentration of 125 mg/5 ml, 250 mg/5 ml. Formulations of flucloxacillin with ampicillin are available (Co-fluampicil, Magnapen).

Action: Beta-lactamase-resistant, narrow-spectrum beta-lactam antibiotic. It binds to penicillin-binding proteins, decreasing bacterial cell wall strength and rigidity, and affecting cell division, growth and septum formation. Flucloxacillin is bactericidal and works in a time-dependent fashion.

Use: Stable in gastric acid so can be given orally but food significantly reduces its bioavailability. It is less active than penicillin G or V against *Streptococcus* and obligate anaerobic bacteria, and is indicated for the treatment of infections caused by beta-lactamase-producing *Staphylococcus*. Patients with significant renal or hepatic dysfunction may need dosage adjustment. The amount of sodium in flucloxacillin sodium may be clinically important for patients on restricted sodium intakes. Although flucloxacillin is absorbed from the GI tract, food has a significant inhibitory effect on its bioavailability; doses must be given on an empty stomach. As flucloxacillin kills in a time-dependent fashion, dosing regimens should be designed to maintain tissue concentrations above the MIC throughout the interdosing interval. Use with care in hepatic disease or hepatic impairment.

Safety and handling: Normal precautions should be observed.

Contraindications: Do not administer to hamsters, gerbils, guinea pigs, chinchillas or rabbits. Do not administer to animals with a history of sensitivity to beta-lactam antimicrobials.

Adverse reactions: Nausea, diarrhoea and skin rashes are the commonest adverse effects. Cholestatic hepatitis has been reported in humans.

Drug interactions: Avoid the concomitant use of bacteriostatic antibiotics. The aminoglycosides (e.g. gentamicin) may inactivate penicillins when mixed together in parenteral solutions. A synergistic effect is seen when beta-lactam and aminoglycoside antimicrobials are used concurrently.

DOSES
See Appendix for guidelines on responsible antibacterial use.
Dogs, Cats: Flucloxacillin sodium: 15 mg/kg i.v., i.m., p.o. q6h.
Small mammals: Rats: 200 mg/kg s.c. q8h.
Birds, Reptiles: No information available.

Fluconazole
(Diflucan*, Fluconazole*) **POM**

Formulations: Oral: 50 mg, 150 mg, 200 mg capsules; 40 mg/ml suspension. Injectable: 2 mg/ml solution.

Action: Inhibition of the synthesis of ergosterol in fungal cell membranes, thus causing increased cell wall permeability and allowing leakage of cellular contents.

Use: Effective against *Blastomyces*, *Candida*, *Cryptococcus*, *Coccidioides*, *Histoplasma* and *Microsporum canis* infections and variably effective against *Aspergillus* and *Penicillium* infections. It attains therapeutic concentrations in the CNS and respiratory tract. It is excreted by the kidney, producing high concentrations in urine. Reduce dose in animals with renal impairment and liver disease. This drug should be used until clinical signs have resolved and the organism is no longer present; this may take up to 2 months in some cases.

Safety and handling: Normal precautions should be observed.

Contraindications: Do not use in pregnant/lactating animals.

Adverse reactions: Adverse effects may include nausea and diarrhoea. May be hepatotoxic. May cause vomiting in birds.

Drug interactions: Fluconazole (due to inhibition of cytochrome P450-dependent liver enzymes) may increase plasma theophylline concentrations. In humans, fluconazole has led to terfenadine toxicity when the two drugs were administered together. Fluconazole increases ciclosporin blood levels.

DOSES
Dogs: 2.5–5 mg/kg p.o. q12h.
Cats:
- Ocular/CNS cryptococcosis: 50 mg/cat i.v. infusion, p.o. q24h. Systemic infections: give double the calculated dose on day 1. Doses up to 100 mg/cat q12h are sometimes used for systemic/CNS *Cryptococcus* infection.
- Dermatophytosis, nasal cryptococcosis: 5 mg/kg p.o. q24h. For dermatophytosis administer for three periods of 7 days, with 7 days without treatment in between.

Dogs, Cats: Urinary candidiasis: 5–10 mg/kg q24h.
Small mammals: Rabbits: 25–43 mg/kg i.v. infusion (slow) q12h.
Birds: 2–5 mg/kg p.o. q24h.
Reptiles: 5 mg/kg p.o. q24h (iguanas with dermatophytosis).

Flucytosine
(Ancotil*) **POM**

Formulations: Injectable: 10 mg/ml solution. Flucytosine tablets are available from special order manufacturers or specialist importing companies.

Action: Fungal cells convert flucytosine (5-FC) into 5-fluorouracil (5-FU), which inhibits DNA and RNA synthesis in the cell. Mammalian cells are spared. Penetrates well into cerebrospinal fluid.

Use: Cryptococcosis (often in conjunction with amphotericin B or itraconazole) particularly if involving meninges, systemic and urinary yeast infections (e.g. candidiasis). Little used in veterinary medicine compared with other antifungals. Use flucytosine with caution in patients with hepatic or renal impairment; reduce the dose and monitor haematological, renal and hepatic parameters. Resistance can develop quickly when used as a sole agent.

Safety and handling: Normal precautions should be observed.

Contraindications: No information available.

Adverse reactions: Drug eruptions, including toxic epidermal necrolysis. Vomiting and diarrhoea may develop as well as myelosuppression, renal and hepatic toxicity; alleviate by dosing over 15 min. Flucytosine may be teratogenic.

Drug interactions: Synergy with amphotericin B has been demonstrated, although there is an increased risk of nephrotoxicity.

DOSES
Dogs: 25–35 mg/kg i.v. q8h or 50–65 mg/kg p.o. q8h.
Cats: 25–50 mg/kg i.v. q6h or 50–65 mg/kg p.o. q8h.
Small mammals, Birds, Reptiles: No information available.

Fludrocortisone   CIL
(Florinef*) **POM**

Formulations: Oral: 0.1 mg tablets.

Action: Aldosterone analogue that increases potassium excretion and sodium retention but which also has some glucocorticoid properties.

Use: Treatment of adrenocortical insufficiency (Addison's disease). Fludrocortisone is about 125 times more potent as a mineralocorticoid than is hydrocortisone but it is also about 12 times more potent as a glucocorticoid (and therefore about 3 times more potent than prednisolone). Monitor sodium and potassium concentrations separately (not just the ratio) 4–6 hours post-pill. Some dogs only require q24h dosing but if using this dose then check sodium and potassium concentrations pre-pill as well as 4–6 hours post-pill. Supplemental doses of prednisolone may be required at times of metabolic or physical stress.

Safety and handling: Normal precautions should be observed.

Contraindications: No information available.

Adverse reactions: Hypertension, oedema (including cerebral oedema) and hypokalaemia with overdosages. Long-term overdose may result in clinical signs of hypercortisolism.

Drug interactions: Hypokalaemia may develop if fludrocortisone is administered concomitantly with amphotericin B or potassium-depleting diuretics (furosemide, thiazides).

DOSES
Dogs: Start at 0.01 mg/kg p.o. q12h. Most patients when stable require <0.05 mg/kg p.o. q12h.
Cats: Doses as for dogs (very few reports).
Small mammals: Ferrets: post-adrenalectomy: 0.01 mg/kg p.o. q24h.
Birds, Reptiles: No information available.

Fluorometholone
(FML*) **POM**

Formulations: Ophthalmic: 0.1% drops in 5 ml, 10 ml bottles.

Action: Phospholipase A2 inhibition (COX and lipoxygenase inhibition).

Use: Superficial ocular inflammation or anterior uveitis. However, it is now rarely used in veterinary ophthalmology.

Safety and handling: Normal precautions should be observed.

Contraindications: Corneal ulceration and infectious keratitis.

Adverse reactions: Topical corticosteroids can cause cataracts and glaucoma in humans. Although raised intraocular pressure associated with topical corticosteroids has been reported in dogs and cats, it is rarely important in the clinical setting. Steroid-induced cataracts have not been reported in small animals, although they have been documented in experimental cats. Systemic effects may be apparent with prolonged use.

Drug interactions: Concurrent use of topical NSAIDs with topical corticosteroids has been identified as a risk factor in humans for precipitating corneal problems.

DOSES
Dogs, Cats: 1 drop per eye q6–12h, although dose frequency is dependent on the severity of inflammation and response to therapy.
Small mammals, Birds, Reptiles: No information available.

Fluorouracil (5-FU)
(Efudix*, Fluorouracil*) **POM**

Formulations: Injectable: 250 mg/vial, 500 mg/vial, 2500 mg/vial solutions. Topical: 5% cream (Efudix).

Action: Metabolites of fluorouracil inhibit pyrimidine synthesis, resulting in inhibition of DNA synthesis and function.

Use: Treatment of basal cell and squamous cell carcinoma (topically), intestinal carcinoma, transitional cell carcinoma of the bladder and mammary carcinoma. Consult relevant texts for specific protocols prior to use.

Safety and handling: Cytotoxic drug; see Appendix and specialist texts for further advice on chemotherapeutic agents.

Contraindications: Do not use in cats in any form (including topical) as it can cause a potentially fatal neurotoxicity.

Adverse reactions: Anorexia, vomiting, stomatitis, diarrhoea, leucopenia with a nadir between 7 and 14 days, thrombocytopenia, anaemia, alopecia, hyperpigmentation, dermatitis, cerebellar ataxia and seizures.

Drug interactions: Cimetidine inhibits the metabolism of 5-FU. In human oncology there is synergism between 5-FU and carboplatin but this combination has not been widely used in small animals and may be more toxic. Methotrexate is synergistic if administered before 5-FU but is antagonistic if administered afterwards. Vincristine increases the cytotoxicity of 5-FU.

DOSES
See Appendix for chemotherapy protocols and conversion of body weight to body surface area.
Dogs: 150–200 mg/m^2 i.v. once weekly for 6 weeks. In patients that have liver, renal or bone marrow impairment, reduce dose by half. Topical use: Apply to affected area q24h.
Cats: Do not use.
Small mammals, Birds, Reptiles: No information available.

Fluoxetine
(Reconcile, Prozac*) **POM-V, POM**

Formulations: Oral: 8 mg, 16 mg, 20 mg, 32 mg, 64 mg tablets; 4 mg/ml liquid. Liquid formulation and some tablet sizes are available in the UK but not under veterinary authorization. Veterinary formulation (Reconcile) only available in certain European regions (not the UK).

Action: Fluoxetine and its primary metabolite norfluoxetine block serotonin re-uptake in the brain, resulting in antidepressive activity and a raising in motor activity thresholds. It also has minor noradrenaline re-uptake inhibition properties.

Use: Authorized in other countries for the management of canine separation anxiety in association with a behaviour modification plan. Also used for the management of compulsive disorders and some forms of aggression in dogs. Use in the latter indication should be with a specifically constructed behaviour modification plan and with caution. Fluoxetine may also be used in the cat to control urine spraying and other anxiety-related behaviour problems, such as psychogenic alopecia and certain forms of aggression, especially if not responsive to anxiolytic intervention. Similar precautions are warranted when used for aggression in cats as apply to its use in dogs. Has also been used to control feather-picking and other compulsive type behaviours in psittacines but relapse following the discontinuation of therapy is common.

Safety and handling: Normal precautions should be observed.

Contraindications: Known sensitivity to fluoxetine or other SSRIs, history of seizures.

Adverse reactions: Common reactions include lethargy, decreased appetite and vomiting, which may result in minor weight loss. Trembling, restlessness and other GI disturbances may also occur and must be distinguished from a paradoxical increase in anxiety which has been reported in some cases. Owners should be warned of a potential increase in aggression in response to medication.

Drug interactions: Fluoxetine should not be used within 2 weeks of treatment with an MAOI (e.g. selegiline) and an MAOI should not be used within 6 weeks of treatment with fluoxetine. Fluoxetine, like other SSRIs, antagonizes the effects of anticonvulsants and so is not recommended for use with epileptic patients or in association with other agents which lower seizure threshold, e.g. phenothiazines. Caution is warranted if fluoxetine is used concomitantly with aspirin or other anticoagulants since the risk of increased bleeding in the case of tissue trauma may be increased.

DOSES
Dogs: 1–2 mg/kg p.o. q24h.
Cats: 0.5–1.0 mg/kg p.o. q24h.
Small mammals: Rats:1–1.5 mg/kg p.o. q24h.
Birds: 1–4 mg/kg p.o. q24h.
Reptiles: No information available.

Flurbiprofen
(Ocufen*) **POM**

Formulations: Ophthalmic: 0.03% solution in single-use vials.

Action: Inhibits prostaglandin synthesis producing an anti-inflammatory and analgesic action. Prostaglandins also play a role in the miosis produced during intraocular surgery by constricting the iris sphincter independently of cholinergic mechanisms.

Use: Before cataract surgery. It is also useful for anterior uveitis and ulcerative keratitis when topical corticosteroids are contraindicated. Topical NSAIDs have the potential to increase intraocular pressure and should be used with caution in dogs predisposed to glaucoma.

Safety and handling: Normal precautions should be observed.

Contraindications: No information available.

Adverse reactions: As with other topical NSAIDs, flurbiprofen may cause local irritation. Topical NSAIDs can be used in ulcerative keratitis but with caution as they can delay epithelial healing. Topical NSAIDs have been associated with an increased risk of corneal 'melting' (keratomalacia) in humans, although this has not been reported in the veterinary literature. Regular monitoring is advised.

Drug interactions: Ophthalmic NSAIDs may be used safely with other ophthalmic pharmaceuticals, although concurrent use of drugs which adversely affect the corneal epithelium (e.g. gentamicin) may lead to increased corneal penetration of the NSAID. The concurrent use of topical NSAIDs with topical corticosteroids has been identified as a risk factor in humans for precipitating corneal problems.

DOSES
Dogs, Cats, Small mammals, Birds, Reptiles: 1 drop per eye q6–12h depending on severity of inflammation. 1 drop q30min for 4 doses preoperatively (presurgery protocols vary widely).

Fluticasone

CIL

(Flixotide*) **POM**

Formulations: Inhalational: 50 μg, 125 μg, 250 μg metered inhalations (Evohaler).

Action: Binds to specific nuclear receptors and affects gene transcription such that many aspects of inflammation are suppressed.

Use: Used as an inhaled corticosteroid in the management of inflammatory airway disease in dogs and cats. Administer via commercially available chambers and masks specifically designed for veterinary use. Not useful for acute bronchospasm (and cases of fluticasone-induced bronchospasm reported in humans).

Safety and handling: Normal precautions should be observed.

Contraindications: No information available.

Adverse reactions: Inhaled steroids are known to suppress the hypothalamic-pituitary-adrenal axis, although they are considered generally safer than systemic steroids.

Drug interactions: No information available.

DOSES

Dogs: 125–500 μg (micrograms)/dog q12–24h.
Cats: 50–250 μg (micrograms)/cat q12–24h.
Small mammals: Rabbits: 50–250 μg (micrograms)/rabbit q12–24h via spacer chamber administration (anecdotal).
Birds, Reptiles: No information available.

Fluvoxamine

(Faverin*, Fluvoxamine*) **POM**

Formulations: Oral: 50 mg, 100 mg tablets.

Action: Serotonin uptake inhibitor that causes increased serotonin concentrations at the brain synapses with resultant anxiolytic, antidepressant and compulsive effects.

Use: Treatment of canine compulsive disorders, anxieties, phobias and panic attacks, especially when involving signs of impulsiveness and aggression. May be of use for the management of maternal aggression. In cats it has been suggested for use in a range of fears and anxieties and in the treatment of wool-eating. Plasma levels appear to increase in an exponential way with increased dosage. Only anecdotal reports of efficacy in the veterinary literature.

Safety and handling: Normal precautions should be observed.

Contraindications: Known sensitivity to other selective serotonin re-uptake inhibitors (SSRIs) such as fluoxetine. Do not use in pregnant and lactating animals or those with epilepsy, cardiovascular disease, diabetes mellitus, a history of bleeding disorder, or renal or hepatic compromise.

Adverse reactions: GI upset, inappetence, lethargy and vomiting may occur, resulting in minor weight loss. Occasional paradoxical signs of increased anxiety may be apparent. Tachycardia or bradycardia may develop.

Drug interactions: Fluvoxamine may be an inhibitor of cytochrome P450 3A4 and so should not be given in association with drugs metabolized by this cytochrome, such as alprazolam, cisapride and erythromycin. Do not give fluvoxamine in combination with, or within 2 weeks of therapy with, monoamine oxidase inhibitors, e.g. selegiline.

DOSES
Dogs: 1–2 mg/kg p.o. q24h.
Cats: 0.25–0.5 mg/kg p.o. q24h.
Small mammals, Birds, Reptiles: No information available.

Fomepizole (4-Methylpyrazole)
(Antizol*) **POM**

Formulations: Injectable: 1.5 g/1.5 ml vial; dilute 1:19 (i.e. 1.5 ml vial added to 28.5 ml of 0.9% saline, giving a 50 mg/ml solution) solution. Discard after 72 hours. Available from special order manufacturers or specialist importing companies.

Action: Competitive inhibition of alcohol dehydrogenase.

Use: Treatment of ethylene glycol (antifreeze) toxicity in dogs. Available for import on a named-patient basis.

Safety and handling: Normal precautions should be observed.

Contraindications: No information available.

Adverse reactions: No information available.

Drug interactions: Increases risk of ethanol toxicity if co-administered.

DOSES
Dogs: 20 mg/kg i.v. infusion of 30 min initially, then 15 mg/kg i.v. slowly over 15–30 min 12 h and 24 h later, then 5 mg/kg i.v. q12h until ethylene glycol concentration is negligible or the dog has recovered. Most effective if started within 8 hours of intoxication.
Cats: (Not approved in cats) 125 mg/kg slow i.v. then 31.25 mg/kg i.v. q12h for 3 additional doses. Efficacy has been shown if treated with 3 hours of ingestion.
Small mammals, Birds, Reptiles: No information available.

Framycetin
(Canaural) **POM-V**

Formulations: Topical: 5 mg/g suspension (Canaural also contains fusidic acid, nystatin and prednisolone).

Action: Aminoglycosides inhibit bacterial protein synthesis and require an oxygen-rich environment to be effective, thus they are ineffective in low-oxygen sites (abscesses, exudates), making all obligate anaerobic bacteria resistant. They are bactericidal and their mechanism of killing is concentration-dependent, leading to a marked post-antibiotic effect, allowing pulse-dosing regimens which may limit toxicity.

Use: Treatment of aural infections. Framycetin is particularly effective against Gram-negative bacteria, although the combination preparation Canaural has a broad spectrum of activity.

Safety and handling: Normal precautions should be observed.

Contraindications: Do not use in animals with a perforated tympanum. Do not use in conjunction with other products known to be ototoxic.

Adverse reactions: Aminoglycosides are potentially ototoxic, and ataxia, deafness and nystagmus may be observed in cats where drops have been administered with a perforated tympanum. Local irritation.

Drug interactions: No information available.

DOSES
See Appendix for guidelines on responsible antibacterial use.
Dogs, Cats: 2–10 drops per ear q12h.
Small mammals: Widely used anecdotally for the treatment of otitis externa in several species and for parasitic otitis (*Otodectes*) in the ferret at a dose of 2–10 drops per ear q12h.
Birds, Reptiles: No information available.

Furosemide (Frusemide)
(Dimazon, Frusecare, Frusedale, Frusol*) **POM-V, POM**

Formulations: Injectable: 50 mg/ml solution. Oral: 20 mg, 40 mg, 1 g tablets; 40 mg/5 ml oral solution.

Action: Loop diuretic, inhibiting the $Na^+/K^+/Cl^-$ cotransporter in the thick ascending limb of the loop of Henle. The net effect is a loss of sodium, potassium, chloride and water in the urine. It also increases excretion of calcium, magnesium and hydrogen as well as renal blood flow and glomerular filtration rate. Transient venodilation may occur following i.v. administration and in some species, bronchodilation may occur; the exact mechanism for both is unclear.

Use: Management of congestive heart failure (acute and chronic), non-cardiogenic oedema, hypercalcuric nephropathy, acute renal failure, hyperkalaemia and hypertension. The use of diuretic monotherapy for the chronic management of heart failure due to mild regurgitation or dilated cardiomyopthy in dogs is not recommended, as patients receiving concomitant therapy with ACE inhibitors, pimobendan (and spironolactone in dogs with mitral regurgitation) have a better clinical outcome. Use with caution in patients with severe electrolyte depletion, hepatic failure and diabetes mellitus.

Safety and handling: Normal precautions should be observed.

Contraindications: Dehydration and anuria. Do not use in dehydrated or hyperuricaemic birds.

Adverse reactions: Hypokalaemia, hypochloraemia, hypocalcaemia, hypomagnesaemia and hyponatraemia; dehydration, polyuria/polydipsia and prerenal azotaemia occur readily. A marked reduction in cardiac output can occur in animals with severe pulmonary disease, low-output heart failure, hypertrophic cardiomyopathy, pericardial or myocardial disorders, cardiac tamponade and severe hypertension. Other adverse effects include ototoxicity (especially in cats), GI disturbances, leucopenia, anaemia, weakness and restlessness.

Drug interactions: Nephrotoxicity/ototoxicity associated with aminoglycosides may be potentiated when furosemide is also used. Furosemide may induce hypokalaemia, thereby increasing the risk of digoxin toxicity. Increased risk of hypokalaemia if furosemide given with acetazolamide, corticosteroids, thiazides and theophylline. Concurrent administration of NSAIDs with furosemide may decrease efficacy and may predispose to nephrotoxicity, particularly in patients with poor renal perfusion. Furosemide may inhibit the muscle relaxation qualities of tubocurarine, but increase the effects of suxamethonium.

DOSES
Dogs, Cats:
- Acute, life-threatening congestive heart failure: 1–4 mg/kg i.v., i.m. q1–4h as required, based on improvement in respiratory rate and effort. Once clinical signs improve, increase dosing interval to q8–12h, monitor urea, creatinine and electrolytes, and start oral therapy once tolerated.
- Chronic, congestive heart failure: 1–5 mg/kg p.o. q8–48h. Typical maintenance doses for mild to moderate CHF are 1–2 mg/kg p.o. q12–24h (dogs) and 1–2 mg/kg p.o. q12–48h (cats). The goal is to use the lowest dose of furosemide that effectively controls clinical signs. Doses in excess of 12 mg/kg/day are unlikely to be beneficial and warrant the addition of a different class of diuretic (e.g. thiazide) to control refractory failure. In patients with ascites, use of s.c. instead of p.o. furosemide can have a marked clinical benefit.
- Hypercalcuric nephropathy: hydrate before therapy. Give 5 mg/kg bolus i.v., then begin 5 mg/kg/h infusion, or give 2–5 mg/kg i.v., s.c., p.o. q8–24h. Maintain hydration status and electrolyte

balance with normal saline and added KCl. Furosemide generally reduces serum calcium levels by 0.5–1.5 mmol/l.
- Acute renal failure/uraemia: after replacing fluid deficit give furosemide at 2 mg/kg i.v. If no diuresis within 1 hour repeat dose at 4 mg/kg i.v. If no response within 1 hour give another dose at 6 mg/kg i.v. The use of low-dose dopamine as adjunctive therapy is often recommended.
- To promote diuresis in hyperkalaemic states: 2 mg/kg i.v. q6h.

Small mammals: Ferrets: 1–4 mg/kg i.v., i.m., p.o. q8–12h; Rabbits: 1–4 mg/kg i.v., i.m. q4–6h initially; maintenance doses are often 1–2 mg/kg p.o. q8–24h; Rodents: 1–4 mg/kg s.c., i.m. q4–6h or 5–10 mg/kg s.c., i.m. q12h.
Birds: 0.1–6.0 mg/kg i.m., s.c., i.v. q6–24h.
Reptiles: 5 mg/kg i.m. q12–24h.

Fusidic acid
(Canaural, Fuciderm, Fucithalmic Vet) **POM-V**

Formulations: Topical: 5 mg/g fusidate suspension (Canaural also contains framycetin, nystatin and prednisolone); 0.5% fusidic acid + 0.1% betamethasone cream (Fuciderm); 1% fusidic acid viscous solution (Fucithalmic Vet).

Action: Inhibits bacterial protein synthesis.

Use: Active against Gram-positive bacteria, particularly *Staphylococcus pseudintermedius*. It is used topically in the management of staphylococcal infections of the conjunctiva, skin or ear. Fusidic acid is able to penetrate skin and penetrate the cornea gaining access to the anterior chamber of the eye. The carbomer gel vehicle in the ocular preparation may also be efficacious as a surface lubricant.

Safety and handling: Avoid contamination of the container on application.

Contraindications: Do not use preparations containing corticosteroids in pregnant animals, birds and rabbits.

Adverse reactions: No information available.

Drug interactions: No information available.

DOSES
See Appendix for guidelines on responsible antibacterial use.
Dogs:
- Otic: 2–10 drops per affected ear q12h.
- Ophthalmic: 1 drop per eye q12–24h.
- Skin: Apply to affected area q12h for 5 days.

Cats: Otic, Ophthalmic: doses as for dogs.
Small mammals: Rabbits: Fucithalmic Vet: 1 drop per eye q12–24h.
Birds: Skin: apply a thin layer q24h; Ophthalmic: 1 drop per affected eye q12–24h.
Reptiles: No information available.

Gabapentin (Gabapentinum)

(Neurontin*) **POM**

CIL

Formulations: Oral: 100 mg, 300 mg, 400 mg capsules; 600 mg, 800 mg film-coated tablets; 50 mg/ml solution.

Action: Gabapentin is an analogue of the neurotransmitter gamma-aminobutyric acid (GABA). The precise mechanism of action of gabapentin is unknown; however, it has been suggested that it mediates its anticonvulsive effect by increasing synaptic levels of GABA in the CNS, most likely through increased synthesis of GABA. Gabapentin has also been demonstrated to decrease the influx of calcium ions into neurons via a specific subunit of voltage-dependent calcium channels. It is believed that some of the therapeutic effect of gabapentin is mediated through binding to these channels. Gabapentin does not interact with sodium-dependent channels and demonstrates no affinity for the common neurotransmitter receptors, including benzodiazepine, glutamate, glycine and dopamine. The mode of action of the analgesic effect of gabapentin is unknown.

Use: Adjunctive therapy in the treatment of seizures refractory to treatment with conventional therapy. Also treatment of neuropathic pain, particularly if insensitive to opioid analgesics. After multiple dosing, peak plasma concentrations of gabapentin are usually achieved within 2 hours of a dose and steady state achieved within 1–2 days. Gabapentin therapy should only be withdrawn slowly. Monitoring of serum levels in dogs and in human patients does not appear useful. Use with caution in patients with renal impairment, behavioural abnormalities or severe hepatic disease.

Safety and handling: Normal precautions should be observed.

Contraindications: No information available.

Adverse reactions: The most commonly reported adverse effect in dogs is mild sedation and ataxia. False-positive readings have been reported with some urinary protein tests in human patients taking gabapentin. Hepatic toxicity has been reported as a rare side effect in human patients.

Drug interactions: The absorption of gabapentin from the GI tract is reduced by antacids containing aluminium with magnesium; it is recommended that gabapentin is taken at least 2 hours after the administration of such an antacid. Cimetidine has been reported to reduce the renal clearance of gabapentin but the product information does not consider this to be of clinical importance.

DOSES

Dogs: 10–60 mg/kg p.o. daily, divided q8–12h. Incremental dosing is recommended.
Cats: 5–10 mg/kg p.o. q8–12h.

Small mammals: Ferrets: 3–5 mg/kg p.o. q8h; Rabbits: 2–5 mg/kg p.o. q8h; Rats: 30 mg/kg p.o. q8h; Hamsters: 50 mg/kg p.o. q24h.
Birds: 10 mg/kg p.o. q12–24h.
Reptiles: No information available.

Gelatine (Oxypolygelatine, Polygeline)
(Gelofusine, Haemaccel) **POM-V**

Formulations: Injectable: 4% solution of succinylated gelatine in 0.7% sodium chloride (Gelofusine); 35 g/dl degraded urea-linked gelatine with NaCl, KCl, CaCl$_2$ (Haemaccel).

Action: Promotes retention of fluid in the vascular system through the exertion of oncotic pressure.

Use: The expansion and maintenance of blood volume in various forms of shock including hypovolaemic and haemorrhagic shock. The main difference between gelatine-based solutions and other synthetic colloids is that they have lower molecular weights (and hence are excreted rapidly), appear to have few antigenic or anticoagulative effects. The plasma half-life of most gelatines is approximately 8 hours (oxypolygelatine 2–4 hours), so that the duration of plasma expansion is much shorter than with etherified starch. There appears to be little effect on coagulation or blood loss following gelatine administration. Use with caution in animals with congestive heart failure or renal insufficiency as will increase risk of circulatory overload.

Safety and handling: Normal precautions should be observed.

Contraindications: No information available.

Adverse reactions: Anaphylactoid reactions to gelatine solutions are rare; it is uncertain whether these reactions represent a specific immune response. In human medicine there are concerns over the safety of these solutions when used in patients with kidney disease.

Drug interactions: No information available.

DOSES
Dogs, Cats, Small mammals: Infuse a volume similar to the estimated blood loss. In normal circumstances do not exceed replacement of >25% of circulating blood volume with gelatines in a 24 h period.
Birds, Reptiles: No information available.

Gentamicin
(Clinagel Vet, Easotic, Genta, Otomax, Tiacil, Genticin*) **POM-V, POM**

Formulations: Injectable: 40 mg/ml solution for i.v., i.m., s.c. injection (human preparation), 100 mg/ml solution for i.v., i.m., s.c.

injection (Genta). Ophthalmic/aural solution: 0.5% solution (Tiacil); 0.3% ophthalmic gel (Clinagel). Gentamicin is a component of some topical ear preparations.

Action: Aminoglycosides inhibit bacterial protein synthesis and require an oxygen-rich environment to be effective, thus they are ineffective in low-oxygen sites (abscesses, exudates), making all obligate anaerobic bacteria resistant. They are bactericidal and their mechanism of killing is concentration-dependent, leading to a marked post-antibiotic effect, allowing pulse-dosing regimens which may limit toxicity.

Use: Active against Gram-negative bacteria, but some staphylococcal and streptococcal (*Streptococcus faecalis*) species are also sensitive. All obligate anaerobic bacteria and many haemolytic streptococci are resistant. Use in domestic animals is limited by nephrotoxicity and, more rarely, ototoxicity and neuromuscular blockade. Microbial resistance is a concern, although many bacteria resistant to gentamicin may be susceptible to amikacin. Monitoring serum gentamicin levels is recommended for all dogs receiving systemic therapy. Consider specific glomerular filtration rate measurements to assess risk prior to initiating therapy. The trough serum level should be allowed to fall below 2 μg/ml. When used for 'blind' therapy of undiagnosed serious infections, gentamicin is usually given in conjunction with a penicillin and/or metronidazole. Aminoglycosides are more active in an alkaline environment. Geriatric animals or those with reduced renal function should only be given this drug systemically when absolutely necessary, although the move to dosing q24h should reduce the likelihood of nephrotoxicity. Use with caution in rabbits, birds and reptiles. Fluid therapy is essential during treatment of reptiles; monitor uric acid levels in birds and reptiles.

Safety and handling: Normal precautions should be observed.

Contraindications: Do not use the aural preparation if the tympanum is perforated. Do not use in conjunction with other drugs considered to be nephrotoxic.

Adverse reactions: Gentamicin delays epithelial healing of corneal ulcers and may cause local irritation. Nephrotoxicity and ototoxicity are potential side effects. Cellular casts in urine sediment are an early sign of impending nephrotoxicity; however, urine must be examined immediately to detect their presence and their absence is not a guarantee of safety. Serum creatinine levels rise later and fatal acute renal failure may be inevitable when they do. Gentamicin should not be used during pregnancy. In rabbits oral administration (including beads) can cause fatal enteritis. Toxic to birds and reptiles.

Drug interactions: Avoid concurrent use of other nephrotoxic, ototoxic or neurotoxic agents (e.g. amphotericin B, furosemide). Increase monitoring and adjust dosages when these drugs must be used together. Aminoglycosides may be chemically inactivated by beta-lactam antibiotics (e.g. penicillins, cephalosporins) or heparin when mixed *in vitro*. The effect of non-depolarizing muscle relaxants (e.g. atracurium, pancuronium, vecuronium) may be enhanced by aminoglycosides. Synergism may occur when aminoglycosides are used with beta-lactam antimicrobials. Activity may be reduced if used in conjunction with bacteriostatic antimicrobials.

DOSES
See Appendix for guidelines on responsible antibacterial use.
Dogs, Cats:
- Otic: 2–8 drops (depending on weight of the animal) in affected ear or apply ointment to affected area q12h. Easotic preparation: apply 1 ml to each ear q24h using metered dose delivery.
- Ophthalmic: 1 drop per eye q6–8h. Severe ocular infections may require dosing q1–2h. A fortified topical solution (100 mg gentamicin in 5 ml of 0.3% solution, making 14.3 mg/ml) can be used.
- Systemic: 5–10 mg/kg slowly i.v. (over 30 min), i.m., s.c. q24h.

Small mammals: Ferrets: 2–4 mg/kg i.v. (over 30 min), i.m., s.c. q6–12h; topically q6–8h; Rabbits: 1.5–2.5 mg/kg s.c., i.m., i.v. q8h; can be incorporated into antibiotic-impregnated beads (1 g/20 g methylmethacrylate) in surgical sites (e.g. in rabbits following abscess debridement). Beads require surgical removal at a later date; Guinea pigs: 6 mg/kg s.c. q24h; Rats and Mice: 4–20 mg/kg i.m. q12h; Other rodents: 2–5 mg/kg s.c., i.m. q8–24h. Ensure adequate renal function and hydration status before use. All species: nebulize 50 mg in 10 ml saline for 15 min q8–12h; ophthalmic: 1 drop per eye q6–8h.
Birds: 2–5 mg/kg i.v., i.m. q6–12h; topically q6–8h; nebulize 50 mg in 10 ml saline for 15 min q8–12h.
Reptiles: Chelonians: 2–4 mg/kg i.m. q72h; may also be nebulized at dilution of 10–20 mg gentamicin/15 ml saline for 15–20 min q8–12h for respiratory tract infections in chelonians and lizards; Snakes: 2.5 mg/kg i.m. q72h.

Glipizide
(Glipizide*, Minodiab*) **POM**

Formulations: Oral: 2.5 mg, 5 mg tablets.

Action: Increases insulin secretion, thereby reducing blood glucose.

Use: Management of type II non-insulin-dependent diabetes mellitus, where there is some residual insulin production. May be effective alone or administered with insulin to reduce insulin requirements. It is ineffective when there is an absolute insulin deficiency or when insulin resistance is present. An effect on blood glucose may not be seen for 4–8 weeks. Administer with food. Preferred to metformin and glibenclamide, as better researched.

Safety and handling: Normal precautions should be observed.

Contraindications: Do not use if ketoacidosis present. Do not use if there is evidence of reduced hepatic or renal function.

Adverse reactions: Glipizide may cause GI disturbances (e.g. vomiting) and sensitivity reactions (e.g. jaundice, rashes, fever).

Drug interactions: The effects of glipizide may be enhanced by ACE inhibitors, NSAIDs, chloramphenicol, potentiated sulphonamides and fluoroquinolones.

DOSES
Dogs: Do not use.
Cats: 0.25–0.5 mg/kg p.o. q12h. Start at the lower end of the dose range, increasing the dose as required if no adverse effects are reported after 2 weeks.
Small mammals, Birds, Reptiles: No information available.

Glucagon
(Glucagen) **POM**

Formulations: Injectable: 1 mg vial for reconstitution.

Action: Binds to specific receptor and counteracts most of the effects of insulin.

Use: Insulin overdose. Use only when feeding and glucose administration has failed to maintain a response. Duration of activity is unknown in dogs but likely to be 1–2 hours. When using glucagon, blood glucose levels should be monitored hourly.

Safety and handling: Store at room temperature until reconstituted and then use immediately.

Contraindications: Normoglycaemia. Contraindicated in humans with insulinomas.

Adverse reactions: Vomiting is the main one reported in humans. Anaphylaxis may occur but is rare. Experience with dogs is too limited to provide clear guidance.

Drug interactions: No information available.

DOSES
Dogs, Cats: 50 ng (nanograms)/kg i.v. once followed by infusion of 10–15 ng/kg/min i.v.; may increase up to 40 ng/kg/min i.v. depending on blood glucose measurements.
Small mammals, Birds, Reptiles: No information available.

Glucose (Dextrose)
(Aqupharm, 50% Glucose for injection, Vetivex) **POM-V, POM-VPS, POM**

Formulations: Injectable: sodium chloride 0.9% w/v, glucose monohydrate 5.5% w/v (Aqupharm No. 3 and Vetivex 3), sodium chloride 0.18% w/v, glucose monohydrate 4.4% w/v (Aqupharm No.

18 and Vetivex 6), other electrolyte solutions with glucose for i.v. use: Glucose 40% and 50% w/v.

Action: Source of energy for cellular metabolism. Osmotic agent.

Use: Dilute glucose solutions are used for fluid replacement (primarily where intracellular and interstitial losses have occurred). Concentrated glucose solutions are used parenterally as an energy source or in the treatment of hypoglycaemia. Patients requiring parenteral nutritional support will require mixtures comprising combinations of amino acids, glucose solutions and fat. See also Amino acid solutions and Lipid emulsions for use in parenteral nutrition. Solutions containing >5% glucose are hypertonic and irritant if given other than i.v. The 50% solutions contain 1.7 kcal/ml (8.4 kJ/ml) glucose and are extremely hypertonic (2525 mOsm/l). Use with caution in patients with insulin resistance and diabetes mellitus.

Safety and handling: Multi-use vials of 5% glucose or higher rapidly support bacterial growth and strict aseptic technique is required, single patient use is advised.

Contraindications: No information available.

Adverse reactions: 10–50% solutions are irritant and hyperosmolar; administer through a jugular catheter or dilute appropriately. Glucose infusions may produce severe hypophosphataemia in some patients with prolonged starvation. If glucose loading produces signs of hyperglycaemia, insulin may be added to correct it. See comments under Amino acid solutions for use in parenteral nutrition solutions.

Drug interactions: No information available.

DOSES
Dogs:
- Fluid therapy: Fluid requirements depend upon the degree of dehydration and ongoing losses. **See Parenteral fluids table in Appendix.**
- Parenteral nutrition: The amount required will be governed by the animal's physiological status, the parenteral nutrition admixture and its ability to tolerate high blood glucose levels. Generally glucose is used to supply 40–60% of the energy requirement. Seek specialist advice before giving parenteral nutrition. See Amino acid solutions.
- Hypoglycaemia: 1–5 ml 50% dextrose i.v. slowly over 10 min. Note that to meet minimum needs for maintenance 1 ml/kg/h of 50% glucose is needed.

Cats: Doses as for dogs for fluid therapy and hypoglycaemia. Specific advise regarding nutrient admixtures and the use of concentrated glucose solutions for provision of energy in cats requiring nutritional support should be sought.

Small mammals: Doses as for dogs.

Birds: Hypoglycaemia: 50–100 mg/kg i.v. as slow bolus.

Reptiles: 50 mg/kg dextrose administered as a 5–10% solution by dilution in crystalloids given by i.v. slowly.

Glutamine
(Dipeptiven) **POM, GSL**

Formulations: Parenteral: N(2)-L-alanyl-L-glutamine (POM). Oral: 500 mg powder or tablet (GSL).

Action: Conditionally essential amino acid required for energy synthesis in the enterocytes. Supplementation in patients with stress starvation is believed to have beneficial effects on intestinal cell proliferation and for prevention of mucosal atrophy.

Use: GI protectant in stress starvation (i.e. when nutritional support by any route is indicated) and to enhance GI healing in patients with severe GI epithelium damage, such as that caused by parvovirus enteritis. Use with caution in cases with epilepsy or liver disease.

Safety and handling: Normal precautions should be observed.

Contraindications: Avoid in patients with acute hepatic encephalopathy as it is partially metabolized to ammonia and glutamate.

Adverse reactions: May have CNS effects at high doses.

Drug interactions: Glutamine may antagonize the effects of lactulose in patients with hepatic encephalopathy and could potentially affect the efficacy of antiseizure medications.

DOSES
Dogs, Cats: 0.3 g/kg i.v. in maintenance fluids; 0.5 g/kg p.o. q24h.
Small mammals: Ferrets: 0.5 g/kg p.o. in divided doses daily (anecdotal).
Birds, Reptiles: No information available.

Glyceryl trinitrate (Nitroglycerin(e))
(Glyceryl trinitrate*, Nitrocine*, Percutol*, Sustac*) **POM**

Formulations: Topical: 2% ointment to be applied to skin (Percutol). Oral: 2.6 mg, 6.4 mg modified-release tablets (Sustac). Injectable: 1 mg/ml, 5 mg/ml solutions (Glyceryl trinitrate, Nitrocine).

Action: Systemic vasodilator. Although a potent coronary vasodilator, its major benefit in small animals follows from a reduction in venous return as a consequence of venodilation. A decrease in venous return reduces left ventricular filling pressures.

Use: Short-term management of cardiogenic oedema (particularly acute pulmonary oedema) in animals with congestive heart failure. It is normally only used for 1–2 days. Its efficacy is debatable. Rotate application sites; suggested sites include the thorax, groin and inside the ears. Rub ointment well into the skin.

Safety and handling: Owners should be cautioned to avoid contact with areas where the ointment has been applied and to wear non-permeable gloves when applying.

Contraindications: Hypotension, hypovolaemia, cerebral haemorrhage, head trauma.

Adverse reactions: Hypotension (reduce dose), tachycardia and a rash at the site of application. Tachyphylaxis can occur. Headaches are common in humans and may be an adverse effect in animals also.

Drug interactions: Concurrent use of ACE inhibitors, anaesthetics, beta-blockers, calcium-channel blockers, corticosteroids and diuretics may enhance the hypotensive effect. NSAIDs may antagonize its hypotensive effects.

DOSES
Dogs: 6–50 mm applied topically to the skin q6–8h; 2.6–6.4 mg p.o. q8–12h (modified-release tablets). Where it is used chronically for the management of heart failure (e.g. nocturnal dyspnoea) use q24h to avoid tolerance.
Cats: 3–6 mm topically to the skin q6–8h; 2.6 mg p.o. q8–12h (modified-release tablets).
Small mammals: Ferrets: 1–3 mm topically to the skin q12–24h.
Birds, Reptiles: No information available.

Glycopyrronium (Glycopyrrolate)
(Robinul*) POM

Formulations: Injectable: 200 µg/ml solution.

Action: Blocks the action of acetylcholine at muscarinic receptors at the terminal ends of the parasympathetic nervous system, reversing parasympathetic effects. Its quaternary structure prevents it from crossing the blood-brain barrier and so it is devoid of central effects.

Use: Potent antisialagogue agent and has been used preoperatively to decrease oral and bronchial secretions. It is also used to inhibit vagal efferent activity and manage bradycardias caused by the administration of potent opioid drugs. Glycopyrronium is used with long-acting anticholinesterase drugs (e.g. neostigmine, pyridostigmine) during antagonism of neuromuscular block. Glycopyrronium is longer acting than atropine. Routine administration of glycopyrronium prior to anaesthesia as part of premedication is no longer recommended. It causes a reduction in oral and bronchial secretions by decreasing the water content, therefore secretions become more sticky. Administration of potent opioids in the perioperative period can promote bradyarrhythmias but it is better to monitor heart rate and give glycopyrronium to manage a low heart rate if necessary. Administration of very low doses of glycopyrronium i.v. can cause exacerbation of bradyarrhythmias due to a vagal stimulatory effect; giving another dose i.v. will usually cause an increase in heart rate. Glycopyrronium is devoid of central effects and therefore does not cause mydriasis. Glycopyrronium is preferred over atropine in rabbits due to the variable and unpredictable effects of atropine in this species.

Safety and handling: Normal precautions should be observed.

Contraindications: No information available.

Adverse reactions: Tachycardias following overdose of glycopyrronium are usually transient and do not require management. Ventricular arrhythmias may be treated with lidocaine if severe. The incidence of adverse effects is lower than that seen with atropine.

Drug interactions: When mixed with alkaline drugs (e.g. barbiturates) a precipitate may form. Antimuscarinics may enhance the actions of sympathomimetics and thiazide diuretics. The following may enhance the activity of glycopyrronium: antihistamines, quinidine, pethidine, benzodiazepines and phenothiazines. Combining glycopyrronium and alpha-2 adrenergic agonists is not recommended.

DOSES
Dogs, Cats:
- Premedication and management of vagally mediated bradyarrhythmias: 2–10 μg (micrograms)/kg i.v., i.m. 10–15 min prior to anaesthetic induction.
- Neuromuscular blockade antagonism: glycopyrronium (10 μg (micrograms)/kg i.v. once) with neostigmine (50 μg (micrograms)/kg i.v. once).

Small mammals: Rabbits: 11 μg (micrograms)/kg i.v., i.m. once; Rodents: 10–20 μg/kg i.v., i.m. once.
Birds: Premedication: 10–30 μg (micrograms)/kg i.m., i.v. once.
Reptiles: 10 μg (micrograms)/kg i.m., i.v.

Haemoglobin glutamer
(Oxyglobin) **POM-V**

Formulations: Injectable: 130 mg/ml solution in 60 ml and 125 ml oxygen-impermeable delivery bags.

Action: An ultrapurified, polymerized haemoglobin of bovine origin in modified Ringer's lactate solution which can carry oxygen.

Use: Provides oxygen-carrying capacity for anaemic dogs. It has an intravascular half-life of 30–40 h in healthy dogs. Because there is no red cell membrane, pre-treatment compatibility testing is not required. The effect of repeated dosing is unknown. It is isosmotic to blood and has a lower viscosity. The product is not authorized for use in cats but has been used, albeit given at a slower rate. Use with caution in animals with advanced heart disease or renal impairment (oliguria/anuria) as it can cause volume overload.

Safety and handling: It has a long shelf-life (>2 years) but once the overwrap is removed, the solution must be used within 24 hours, even if stored in a refrigerator, as it has no preservative and slow oxygenation results in methaemoglobin formation.

Contraindications: Not to be used in animals with fluid overload, overhydration or at risk of congestive heart failure. Should not be used in animals previously treated with oxyglobin.

Adverse reactions: Rapid administration to normovolaemic animals could result in hypervolaemia. The solution causes a discoloration of plasma (red, brown) and mucous membranes, sclera, urine and skin (yellow, brown or red). Vomiting, diarrhoea and fever have been reported. There is an increase in plasma total protein and haemoglobin that can artefactually change derived red cell indices on blood screens. Increased liver enzymes have been noted in toxicity trials in Beagles. Haemoglobinuria is expected and significant urine discoloration can interfere with other colorimetric changes on dipsticks. The package insert contains notes of known interferences with clinical chemistry analysers. Ideally obtain all diagnostic blood and urine samples before administration. The main complication of administration to cats is volume overload, leading to pulmonary oedema and pleural effusions; partly due to its potent colloid osmotic effects (slightly better than those of hetastarch) but probably also due to its nitric oxide-scavenging properties leading to vasoconstriction.

Drug interactions: Avoid concomitant administration with other plasma-volume expanders. The manufacturer states that no other medications should be added to the infusion line whilst oxyglobin is being administered. No specific interactions are yet reported.

DOSES
Dogs: 20–30 ml/kg i.v. at a rate of 0.5–3 ml/kg/h prn.
Cats: 3–5 ml/kg i.v. at a rate of 0.5–1 ml/kg/h prn (not licensed).

Small mammals: 2 ml/kg as a bolus over approximately 10–15 min followed by a constant rate infusion of 0.2–0.4 ml/kg/h.
Birds: 30 ml/kg i.v., intraosseously divided over 24 hours.
Reptiles: 1–2 ml/kg i.v., intraosseously as a slow bolus injection prn.

Halothane
(Fluothane, Halothane) **POM-V**

Formulations: Inhalational: 250 ml bottle.

Action: Not fully understood.

Use: Induction and maintenance of anaesthesia. Halothane is potent and highly volatile so should only be delivered from a suitable calibrated vaporizer. It is more soluble in blood than isoflurane and sevoflurane therefore induction and recovery from anaesthesia are slower than with the other agents. The concentration of halothane required to maintain anaesthesia depends on the other drugs used in the anaesthesia protocol; the concentration should be adjusted according to clinical assessment of anaesthetic depth. MAC approximately 0.9% in most species.

Safety and handling: Unstable when exposed to light and corrodes certain metals. It dissolves into rubber and may leach out into breathing circuits after the vaporizer is turned off. Thymol 0.01% is included as a preservative; as halothane vaporizes, the concentration of thymol increases and this can cause vaporizer controls to stick and ports to be occluded. Periodic servicing and recalibration of precision vaporizers is essential to ensure delivery of known concentration of halothane vapour. Measures should be adopted to prevent contamination of the environment with halothane during anaesthesia and handling of the agent.

Contraindications: Do not use in patients with liver disease.

Adverse reactions: Dose-dependent hypotension through depression of heart rate and myocardial contractility, although these adverse effects wane with time. Reduces blood flow in the liver. Halothane facilitates the generation of ventricular arrhythmias in the presence of other arrhythmogenic factors, e.g. catecholamines, hypoxia and hypercarbia. Halothane crosses the placental barrier and will effect neonates delivered by caesarean section. Up to 25% of inhaled halothane undergoes oxidative metabolism by hepatic cytochrome.

Drug interactions: Opioid agonists, benzodiazepines and N_2O reduce the concentration of halothane required to achieve surgical anaesthesia.

DOSES
Dogs, Cats, Small mammals: The expired concentration required to maintain surgical anaesthesia in 50% of recipients is 0.8–1.0% in animals (minimum alveolar concentration). Administration of other

anaesthetic agents and opioid analgesics reduces the dose requirement of halothane, therefore the dose should be adjusted according to individual requirement. Halothane at 3–4% concentration is required to induce anaesthesia in unpremedicated patients.

Birds: Do not use due to the risk of catecholamine-induced arrhythmias.

Reptiles: Snakes, Lizards: 3–5% with 100% oxygen for induction, 1–3% in 100% oxygen for maintenance.

Heparin (low molecular weight) (Dalteparin, Enoxaparin)

(Clexane (enoxaparin)*, Fragmin (dalteparin)*) **POM**

Formulations: Injectable: 2,500 IU/ml, 100,000 IU/ml ampoules (dalteparin); 25,000 IU/ml multidose vial plus various pre-filled syringes at concentrations of 12,500 IU/ml and 25,000 IU/ml (dalteparin); pre-filled syringes of 100 mg/ml (enoxaparin). 100 mg enoxaparin is equivalent to 10,000 IU of anti-Factor Xa activity.

Action: Low molecular weight heparin (LMWH) is an anticoagulant that inhibits factor Xa and thrombin. When compared with unfractionated heparin (UFH), LMWH has reduced anti-IIa activity relative to anti-Xa activity (ratio of anti-Xa to anti-IIa is 2–4:1 compared to UFH 1:1) Thus at therapeutic doses LMWH has minimal effect on APTT. Therapeutic monitoring of LMWH is by anti-Xa activity (but this may not be practical).

Use: Treatment of thromboembolic complications and hypercoagulable syndromes (e.g. pulmonary thromboembolism, disseminated intravascular coagulation (DIC)). LMWH is also used in treatment of myocardial infarction, atrial fibrillation, deep vein thrombosis and pulmonary thromboembolism in humans. Its use in DIC is controversial as no beneficial effect has been shown in controlled clinical trials in humans. LMWH is no longer used to try to prevent DIC. Heparins are only effective if sufficient AT III is present. Heparin therapy is only one aspect of the management of DIC: addressing the precipitating cause, administration of fluids, fresh whole blood, aspirin and diligent monitoring of coagulation tests (APTT, PT), fibrin degradation products and fibrinogen are all important factors. The doses of heparin are controversial, with some texts recommending lower or higher doses, the use of constant i.v. infusions, or preincubation with plasma. The aim of therapy is to achieve anti-Factor Xa activity of 0.35–0.7 IU/ml (though in many cases it may not be possible to measure this). This therapeutic target is extrapolated from humans but no data are available to determine if this decreases risk for thromboembolic complications in dogs or cats. Cats appear to require higher dosages of LMWH to achieve proposed therapeutic targets. LMWH has better pharmacokinetic properties than UFH and its actions are more predictable in humans. It is considerably more expensive than UFH.

Safety and handling: Normal precautions should be observed.

Contraindications: Bleeding disorders or severe renal dysfunction.

Adverse reactions: If an overdosage occurs protamine can be used as an antidote. Heparin should not be administered i.m. as it may result in haematoma formation. Its use in DIC may worsen haemorrhage especially if the patient is thrombocytopenic. Heparin-induced thrombocytopenia syndrome is a serious concern in human patients but has not been reported in dogs or cats.

Drug interactions: Use with caution with other drugs that can cause changes in coagulation status (e.g. aspirin, NSAIDs). Heparin may antagonize ACTH, corticosteroids or insulin. Heparin may increase plasma levels of diazepam. The actions of heparin may be partially counteracted by antihistamines, digoxin and tetracyclines. Do not mix other drugs in the same syringe as heparin.

DOSES
Dogs, Cats: 80–150 IU/kg s.c. q4–8h.
Small mammals: No information available.
Birds: PTFE toxicosis: 300 IU/kg i.v. once.
Reptiles: No information available.

Heparin (unfractionated) (UFH)
(Heparin*, Hepsal*) **POM**

Formulations: Injectable: 1,000–25,000 IU/ml solutions; 10 IU/ml in saline, 100 IU/ml in saline.

Action: Heparin is an anticoagulant that exerts its effects primarily by enhancing the binding of antithrombin III (AT III) to factors IIa, IXa, Xa, XIa and XIIa; it is only effective if adequate AT III is present. The AT III/clotting factor complex is subsequently removed by the liver. Heparin inactivates thrombin and blocks the conversion of fibrinogen to fibrin. The inhibition of factor XII activation prevents the formation of stable fibrin clots. Heparin does not significantly change the concentrations of clotting factors, nor does it lyse pre-existing clots.

Use: Treatment of DIC and thromboembolic disease (for more details see low molecular weight heparin (LMWH) above). Therapy must be carefully monitored as the activity of UFH is somewhat less predictable than LMWH. In veterinary medicine it is mainly used to maintain the patency of catheters/cannulae.

Safety and handling: Normal precautions should be observed.

Contraindications: Major bleeding disorders, increased risk of haemorrhage, thrombocytopenia.

Adverse reactions: If an overdosage occurs protamine can be used as an antidote. Heparin should not be administered i.m. as it may result in haematoma formation. Its use in DIC may worsen haemorrhage especially if the patient is thrombocytopenic. Heparin-induced thrombocytopenia syndrome is a serious concern in human patients but has not been reported in dogs or cats.

Drug interactions: Use with caution with other drugs that can cause changes in coagulation status (e.g. aspirin, NSAIDs). Heparin may antagonize ACTH, corticosteroids and insulin. Heparin may increase plasma levels of diazepam. The actions of heparin may be partially counteracted by antihistamines, digoxin and tetracyclines. Do not mix other drugs in the same syringe as heparin.

DOSES
Dogs:
- Catheter maintenance: 1250 IU in 100 ml water for injection.
- Treatment of DIC: 200 IU/kg q6h provided patient is not thrombocytopenic (see LMWH for more information).
- Treatment of pulmonary thromboembolism: 200–500 IU/kg s.c. q6–8h; adjust dosage so that the APTT is 1.5–2.0 times normal or anti-Factor Xa activity between 0.35 and 0.7 IU/ml (see LMWH for more information).

Cats: Feline arterial thromboembolism: 250–300 IU/kg s.c. q8h.
Small mammals: Catheter maintenance: 1250 IU in 100 ml water for injection.
Birds, Reptiles: No information available.

Human chorionic gonadotrophin see Chorionic gonadotrophin

Hyaluronate
(Hyabak*, Hylo-Care*, Hylo-Forte*, Hylo-Tear*, Oxyal*, Vismed Multi*) **P**

Formulations: Ophthalmic: 0.1%, 0.15%, 0.18%, 0.3%, 0.4% solution in 10 ml bottle.

Action: Viscoelastic fluid with mucomimetic properties. Sodium hyaluronate is also available in different formulations as a viscoelastic for intraocular surgery.

Use: Used as a tear replacement and is beneficial for the management of quantitative (keratoconjunctivitis sicca (KCS) or dry eye) and qualitative tear film disorders. It has longer corneal contact time than the aqueous tear substitutes.

Safety and handling: Normal precautions should be observed.

Contraindications: No information available.

Adverse reactions: It is tolerated well and ocular irritation is unusual.

Drug interactions: No information available.

DOSES

Dogs, Cats, Small mammals: 1 drop per eye q4–6h, although it can be used hourly if required.

Birds, Reptiles: No information available.

Hydralazine
(Apresoline*, Hydralazine*) **POM**

Formulations: Oral: 25 mg, 50 mg tablets.

Action: Hydralazine acts chiefly on arteriolar smooth muscle causing vasodilation; it is able to decrease systemic vascular resistance to about 50% of the baseline value. The effects of hydralazine are to reduce afterload and increase heart rate, stroke volume and cardiac output.

Use: Afterload reducer as adjunctive therapy of congestive heart failure in dogs secondary to severe or refractory mitral value insufficiency. It can be used to treat systemic hypertension. Hospitalization with frequent monitoring of blood pressure is advised during its use. It is not typically used as a first-line drug in hypertension. As hydralazine may cause sodium and water retention, concomitant use of diuretic therapy is often necessary. Give with food if possible.

Safety and handling: Normal precautions should be observed.

Contraindications: Hypovolaemia, hypotension, renal impairment or cerebral bleeding.

Adverse reactions: Reflex tachycardia, severe hypotension (monitor and adjust doses as necessary), anorexia and vomiting (the latter two effects commonly seen in cats).

Drug interactions: The hypotensive effects of hydralazine may be enhanced by ACE inhibitors (e.g. enalapril), anaesthetics, beta-blockers (e.g. propranolol), calcium-channel blockers (e.g. diltiazem, verapamil), corticosteroids, diuretics and NSAIDs. Sympathomimetics (e.g. phenylpropanolamine) may cause tachycardia. The pressor response to adrenaline may be reduced.

DOSES

Dogs: 0.5–3 mg/kg p.o. q8–12h. Start at low dose (0.5–1 mg/kg q12h), monitor blood pressure regularly and increase to 2 mg/kg or even 3 mg/kg q12h if necessary.

Cats: 2.5–10 mg/cat p.o. q12h. Start at low dose and titrate upwards cautiously as above if necessary.

Small mammals: Guinea pigs: 1 mg/kg i.v. prn.

Birds, Reptiles: No information available.

Hydrochlorothiazide

(Co-amilozide*, Moduret*, Moduretic*) **POM**

Formulations: Oral: 25 mg hydrochlorothiazide + 2.5 mg amiloride, 50 mg hydrochlorothiazide + 5 mg amiloride tablets.

Action: Thiazide diuretic that inhibits reabsorption of sodium and chloride in the distal convoluted tubule, resulting in sodium, chloride and water loss in the urine. It also causes excretion of potassium, magnesium and bicarbonate. It is formulated with a potassium-sparing diuretic (amiloride).

Use: Additional therapy for congestive heart failure when the clinical signs have become refractory to furosemide. However, furosemide therapy should still be continued when using hydrochlorthiazide. It may also be used in the prevention of calcium oxalate urolithiasis. Thiazides have antihypertensive effects, although the exact mechanism is unclear.

Safety and handling: Normal precautions should be observed.

Contraindications: Renal impairment, as it tends to reduce glomerular filtration rate.

Adverse reactions: Hyperglycaemia, hypokalaemia, hyponatraemia, hypochloraemia and volume contraction. It enhances the effects of the renin-angiotensin-aldosterone system in heart failure.

Drug interactions: Increased possibility of hypokalaemia developing if thiazides are used concomitantly with corticosteroids or loop diuretics (furosemide). Thiazide-induced hypokalaemia may increase the risk of digoxin toxicity. Thus, concomitant use of potassium-sparing diuretics (e.g. spironolactone) or potassium supplementation may be necessary during prolonged administration. The concurrent administration of vitamin D or calcium salts with thiazides may exacerbate hypercalcaemia.

DOSES

Dogs: 12.5–25 mg/dog i.m. or 0.5–4 mg/kg p.o. q12–24h. Start at low dose and titrate upwards every 5–10 days, to effect. Monitor urea, creatinine, electrolytes and blood pressure before increasing dose.

Cats: 12.5 mg/cat i.m. or 1–4 mg/kg p.o. q12–24h with a salt-restricted diet. Start at low dose and titrate upwards cautiously as above.

Small mammals, Birds: No information available.

Reptiles: 1 mg/kg q24–72h.

Hydrocortisone

(Efcortesol*, Solu-cortef*) **POM**

Formulations: Topical: 0.5%, 1% creams, 1% solution (Hydrocortisone). Injectable: 25 mg/ml solution; 100 mg, 500 mg powders for reconstitution (Solu-cortef). Oral: 10 mg, 20 mg tablets (Hydrocortisone).

Action: Alters the transcription of DNA, leading to alterations in cellular metabolism. It has both glucocorticoid and mineralocorticoid activity.

Use: Topical anti-inflammatory drug also used in the management of hypoadrenocorticism. It has only a quarter of the glucocorticoid potency of prednisolone and one thirtieth that of dexamethasone. On a dose basis 4 mg of hydrocortisone is equivalent to 1 mg prednisolone. Animals on chronic therapy should be tapered off steroids when discontinuing the drug (even following topical administration). The use of steroids in most cases of shock or spinal cord injury is of no benefit and may be detrimental. Use corticosteroids with care in rabbits as even single small doses can cause severe adverse effects.

Safety and handling: Wear gloves when applying topically as the cream is absorbed through skin.

Contraindications: Do not use in pregnant animals. Systemic corticosteroids are generally contraindicated in patients with renal disease and diabetes mellitus.

Adverse reactions: Catabolic effects of glucocorticoids lead to weight loss and cutaneous atrophy. Iatrogenic hyperadrenocorticism may develop (PU/PD, elevated liver enzymes). Vomiting and diarrhoea, or GI ulceration may develop. Glucocorticoids may increase urine glucose levels and decrease serum T3 and T4 values. Prolonged use of glucocorticoids suppresses the hypothalamic-pituitary axis and causes adrenal atrophy. Impaired wound healing and delayed recovery from infections may be seen.

Drug interactions: Increased risk of GI ulceration if used concurrently with NSAIDs. Glucocorticoids antagonize the effect of insulin. Antiepileptic drugs (phenobarbital) may accelerate the metabolism of corticosteroids and antifungals (e.g. itraconazole) may decrease it. There is an increased risk of hypokalaemia when corticosteroids are used with acetazolamide, amphotericin and potassium-depleting diuretics (furosemide, thiazides).

DOSES
Dogs:
- Topically: Apply a thin layer of cream to affected area q6–12h.
- Hypoadrenocorticism: 2–4 mg/kg i.v., i.m. q4–6h in acute Addisonian crisis and 0.125 mg/kg p.o. q12h for maintenance.
- Anti-inflammatory: 0.5 mg/kg p.o. q12h.

Cats: Topical use as for dogs. Its use in feline hypoadrenocorticism has not been documented.
Small mammals: Ferrets: 25–40 mg/kg i.v.
Birds, Reptiles: No information available.

Hydrocortisone aceponate
(Cortavance, Easotic) **POM-V**

Formulations: Topical: 76 ml spray (0.584 mg/ml) (Cortavance); suspension for ears: 1.11 mg/ml combined with 15.1 mg/ml miconazole and 1505 IU/ml gentamicin (Easotic).

Action: Hydrocortisone aceponate is a pro-drug that is biotransformed in the epidermis to its active form hydrocortisone 17-propionate.

Use: Treatment of inflammatory and pruritic dermatoses including acute otitis externa and acute exacerbations of recurrent otitis externa associated with bacteria and *Malassezia*. Minimizes systemic side effects (such as increases in liver enzymes, depression of cortisol response to ACTH stimulation). Microbial infections should be treated appropriately prior to use. Patients should be monitored appropriately during long-term use. Use with caution in dogs <7 months old as glucocorticoids are known to slow growth.

Safety and handling: Normal precautions should be observed.

Contraindications: Do not use on ulcerated skin (Cortavance). Do not use if the ear drum is perforated (Easotic).

Adverse reactions: Protracted use of any topical glucocorticoid can result in epidermal atrophy.

Drug interactions: No information available.

DOSES
Dogs: Cortavance: 2 pumps of spray per 10 cm x 10 cm square of skin for 7 days. This delivers 1.52 µg (micrograms) of hydrocortisone aceponate per cm^2 square. Easotic: 1 pump (1 ml) per ear q24h for 5 days.
Cats: Dose not established.
Small mammals, Birds, Reptiles: No information available.

Hydroxycarbamide (Hydroxyurea)   CIL
(Hydrea*) **POM**

Formulations: Oral: 500 mg capsule.

Action: Inhibits ribonucleotide reductase, which converts ribonucleotides to deoxyribonucleotides (important precursors for DNA synthesis and repair). It acts primarily in the S-phase, but may also arrest cells at the G_1-S border.

Use: Treatment of polycythaemia vera, chronic myeloid leukaemia (and sometimes other forms), mast cell tumours and in the adjunctive treatment of canine meningiomas. Once in remission, reduce dosage frequency as required to maintain remission. Haematology should be monitored weekly at the start of drug therapy in cats, as they are at greater risk of myelosuppression compared with dogs. Use with caution in patients with renal dysfunction; dosage reduction may be required.

Safety and handling: Cytotoxic drug; see Appendix and specialist texts for further advice on chemotherapeutic agents.

Contraindications: Patients with bone marrow suppression.

Adverse reactions: Myelosuppression, GI signs (nausea, vomiting, diarrhoea, anorexia), dysuria and skin reactions (stomatitis, sloughing of nails, alopecia). Myelosuppression is dose-limiting; monitor haematological parameters at regular intervals. In cats given very high doses (>500 mg) methaemoglobinaemia is reported. Normal doses are associated with increased diastolic blood pressure and heart rate but decreased systolic blood pressure, QT and PR intervals, maximum left ventricular systolic and end diastolic pressures.

Drug interactions: No information available but advisable not to use with other myelosuppressive agents.

DOSES
See Appendix for chemotherapy protocols and conversion of body weight to body surface area.
Dogs:
- CML: 50 mg/kg p.o. q24h for 1–2 weeks then q48h.
- Polycythaemia vera or CML: 50–80 mg/kg p.o. q3d or 1 g/m^2 p.o. q24h until haematology is normal.

Cats: 10 mg/kg q24h until remission; then taper to lowest effective frequency by monitoring haematocrit; or 25 mg/kg p.o. three times a week.
Small mammals, Birds, Reptiles: No information available.

Hydroxyurea see **Hydroxycarbamide**

Hydroxyzine
(Atarax*, Ucerax*) **POM**

Formulations: Oral: 10 mg, 25 mg tablets; 2 mg/ml syrup.

Action: Binds to H1 histamine receptors preventing histamine from binding. Hydroxyzine is metabolized to cetirizine.

Use: Management of allergic disease in dogs and cats, though specific doses have not been determined by pharmacokinetic studies. Also used in feather plucking in birds. Use with caution in cases with urinary retention, angle-closure glaucoma and pyloroduodenal obstruction.

Safety and handling: Normal precautions should be observed.

Contraindications: No information available.

Adverse reactions: May cause mild sedation. May reduce seizure threshold.

Drug interactions: No information available.

DOSES
Dogs, Cats: 2.0–2.2 mg/kg q8–12h.
Small mammals: Ferrets, Rabbits: 2 mg/kg p.o. q8–12h.
Birds: 2.2 mg/kg q8h.
Reptiles: No information available.

Hyoscine see Butylscopolamine

Hypromellose
(Hypromellose*, Isopto*, Tears Naturale*) **P**

Formulations: Ophthalmic: 0.3%, 0.5%, 1% solutions in 10 ml dropper bottle; 0.32% (single-use vial). Large variety of other formulations also available.

Action: Cellulose based tear substitute (lacrimomimetic).

Use: Lubrication of dry eyes. In cases of keratoconjunctivitis (KCS or dry eye) it will improve ocular surface lubrication, tear retention and patient comfort while lacrostimulation therapy (e.g. topical ciclosporin) is initiated. It may also be used as a vehicle base for compounding ophthalmic drugs. Patient compliance is poor if used >q4h, consider using a longer acting tear replacement.

Safety and handling: Normal precautions should be observed.

Contraindications: No information available.

Adverse reactions: No information available.

Drug interactions: No information available.

DOSES
Dogs, Cats: 1 drop per eye q1h.
Small mammals: 1 drop per eye q1h during anaesthesia.
Birds, Reptiles: No information available.

Ibafloxacin
(Ibaflin) **POM-V**

Formulations: Oral: 3% gel (30 mg/g), 7.5% gel (75 mg/g) in a metered dose applicator; 30 mg, 150 mg, 300 mg, 900 mg tablets.

Action: Inhibits the enzyme DNA gyrase. Its bactericidal action is concentration-dependent as reflected by the once daily dosing regime.

Use: Ideally fluoroquinolone use should be reserved for infections where culture and sensitivity testing predicts a clinical response and where first- and second-line antimicrobials would not be effective. Ibafloxacin has a broad spectrum of activity. It is active against mycoplasmas, many Gram-negative organisms and some Gram-positive organisms, including *Pasteurella*, *Staphylococcus*, *Pseudomonas aeruginosa*, *Klebsiella*, *Escherichia coli*, *Proteus* and *Salmonella*. It is effective against beta-lactamase-producing bacteria but ineffective against obligate anaerobes. It is highly lipophilic, attaining high concentrations within cells in many tissues and is particularly effective in the management of soft tissue, urogenital (including prostatic) and skin infections. Ibafloxacin is specifically authorized for the treatment of pyoderma caused by susceptible strains of *Staphylococcus*, *E. coli* and *Proteus*, for the management of soft tissue infections and of upper respiratory tract infections. Administer at the time of feeding as food enhances the absorption. Avoid using fluoroquinolones as first-line antimicrobials. Caution should be exercised before using dose rates above those recommended by the manufacturer.

Safety and handling: Each syringe should be dedicated to treatment of a single animal and used within 8 weeks of opening.

Contraindications: Do not use in combination with NSAIDs in animals with a history of seizures.

Adverse reactions: Some animals may show GI signs following use of fluoroquinolones (nausea, vomiting, diarrhoea or soft faeces). The drug should be used with caution in epileptics as fluoroquinolones potentiate CNS adverse effects when administered concurrently with NSAIDs in humans. The potential adverse effects of ibafloxacin on the canine retina have not been studied (see Enrofloxacin). Cartilage abnormalities have been reported following the use of other fluoroquinolones in growing animals. Such abnormalities have not been specifically reported following the use of ibafloxacin but the drug is not authorized for use in cats and dogs <8 months of age and in giant breeds this is extended to 18 months.

Drug interactions: Absorbents and antacids containing cations (Mg^{2+}, Al^{3+}) may bind fluoroquinolones, preventing their absorption from the GI tract. The absorption of fluoroquinolones may be inhibited by sucralfate and zinc salts; separate doses of these drugs by at least 2 hours. Cimetidine may reduce the clearance of fluoroquinolones and so should be used with caution with these drugs. Antagonism may be observed with nitrofurantoin.

DOSES
See Appendix for guidelines on responsible antibacterial use.
Dogs, Cats: 15 mg/kg p.o. q24h.
Small mammals, Birds, Reptiles: No information available.

Imepitoin
(Pexion) **POM-V**

Formulations: Oral: 100 mg, 400 mg tablets.

Action: Imepitoin inhibits seizures via potentiation of the $GABA_A$ receptor-mediated inhibitory effects on the neurons. Imepitoin also has a weak calcium-channel blocking effect, which may contribute to its anticonvulsive properties.

Use: Imepitoin and phenobarbital are the initial medications of choice for the management of epileptic seizures due to idiopathic epilepsy in dogs. The choice of initial medication is guided by patient requirements: imepitoin has a more rapid onset of action than phenobarbital (a steady state does not need to be achieved), does not require the determination of serum concentrations and has a less severe adverse effect profile; however, phenobarbital is less expensive and more efficacious.

Safety and handling: Normal precautions should be observed.

Contraindications: The medication should not be used with severely impaired liver, kidney and heart function.

Adverse reactions: The most frequent adverse effect reported is sedation, particularly in dogs on higher doses or already on phenobarbital therapy. Other adverse effects are generally mild and transient and include polyphagia, hyperactivity, polyuria, polydipsia, somnolence, hypersalivation, emesis, ataxia, apathy, diarrhoea, prolapsed nictitating membrane, decreased sight and sensitivity to sound.

Drug interactions: Imepitoin has been used in combination with phenobarbital in a small number of cases and no harmful clinical interactions were reported.

DOSES
Dogs: 10–30 mg/kg p.o. q12h.
Cats: No information available.
Small mammals: Mice: experimental doses have been reported of 25–60 mg/kg.
Birds, Reptiles: No information available.

Imidacloprid

(Advantage, Advantix, Advocate, Bob Martin Double
Action Dewormer) **POM-V, AVM-GSL**

Formulations: Topical: 100 mg/ml imidacloprid in spot-on pipettes
of various sizes (Advantage, Bob Martin). Topical for cat: 100 mg/ml
imidacloprid with moxidectin in spot-on pipette (Advocate). Topical
for dog: 100 mg/ml imidacloprid + 500 mg/ml permethrin in spot-on
pipettes of various sizes (Advantix); 100 mg/ml imidacloprid with
moxidectin in spot-on pipette (Advocate). Numerous GSL and
non-authorized formulations.

Action: Binds to post-synaptic nicotinic receptors resulting in
paralysis and death of fleas and their larvae. Permethrin is a sodium
'open channel blocker' that causes prolongation of the action
potential and therefore paralysis and death of fleas. It also acts as a
tick repellent.

Use: Treatment and prevention of flea and tick infestations in dogs
and cats, and flea infestations in rabbits. Formulations with
permethrin also have repellant activity against sandflies, mosquitoes
and stable flies in dogs. For the treatment of flea infestations the
additional use of an approved insect growth regulator is
recommended and the product should be applied every 4 weeks to
all in-contact cats, dogs and rabbits. May be used in nursing bitches
and queens. The recommended minimum dose of Advantix is 10 mg/
kg imidacloprid + 50 mg/kg permethrin. Treated dogs should not
swim in surface water for 48 hours.

Safety and handling: Permethrin is dangerous to aquatic
organisms. Treated dogs should not swim in surface water for 48
hours.

Contraindications: Do not use the permethrin-containing product
on cats.

Adverse reactions: Transient pruritus and erythema at the site of
application may occur. Permethrin is dangerous to aquatic
organisms.

Drug interactions: No information available.

DOSES

Dogs: 0.4 ml, 1.0 ml, 2.5 ml, 4 ml pipettes. In dogs >40kg the
appropriate combination of pipettes should be applied.
Cats: 0.4 ml, 0.8 ml pipettes (use the smaller size in cats <4 kg). Do
not use the permethrin-containing product.
Small mammals: Ferrets: 0.4 ml pipette q30d; Rabbits 0.4 ml, 0.8 ml
pipettes (use the smaller size in rabbits <4 kg).
Birds, Reptiles: No information available.

Imidapril
(Prilium) **POM-V**

Formulations: Oral: 75 mg, 150 mg, 300 mg powders for reconstitution.

Action: Angiotensin converting enzyme (ACE) inhibitor. It inhibits conversion of angiotensin I to angiotensin II and inhibits the breakdown of bradykinin. Overall effect is a reduction in preload and afterload via venodilation and arteriodilation, decreased salt and water retention via reduced aldosterone production and inhibition of the angiotensin-aldosterone-mediated cardiac and vascular remodelling. Efferent arteriolar dilation in the kidney can reduce intraglomerular pressure and therefore glomerular filtration. This may decrease proteinuria.

Use: Treatment of congestive heart failure caused by mitral regurgitation or dilated cardiomyopathy in dogs and cats. Often used in conjunction with diuretics when heart failure is present as most effective when used in these cases. Can be used in combination with other drugs to treat heart failure (e.g. pimobendan, spironolactone, digoxin). May be beneficial in cases of chronic renal insufficiency, particularly protein-losing nephropathies. May reduce blood pressure in hypertension. ACE inhibitors are more likely to cause or exacerbate prerenal azotaemia in hypotensive animals and those with poor renal perfusion (e.g. acute, oliguric renal failure). Use cautiously if hypotension, hyponatraemia or outflow tract obstruction are present. Regular monitoring of blood pressure, serum creatinine, urea and electrolytes is strongly recommended with ACE inhibitor treatment. The use of ACE inhibitors in cats with cardiac disease stems from extrapolation from theoretical benefits and studies showing a benefit in other species with heart failure and different cardiac diseases (mainly dogs and humans).

Safety and handling: Normal precautions should be observed.

Contraindications: Do not use in animals with acute renal failure, congenital heart disease, haemodynamically relevant stenoses (e.g. aortic stenosis), obstructive hypertrophic cardiomyopathy or hypovolaemia.

Adverse reactions: Potential adverse effects include hypotension, hyperkalaemia and azotaemia. Monitor blood pressure, serum creatinine and electrolytes when used in cases of heart failure. Dosage should be reduced if there are signs of hypotension (weakness, disorientation). Anorexia, vomiting and diarrhoea are rare. Doses of up to 5 mg/kg/day have been well tolerated in healthy dogs. It is not recommended for breeding, pregnant or lactating bitches, as safety has not been established. The safety of imidapril has not been established in dogs <4 kg.

Drug interactions: Concomitant use of potassium-sparing diuretics (e.g. spironolactone) or potassium supplements could result in hyperkalaemia. However, in practice, spironolactone and ACE inhibitors appear safe to use concurrently. There may be an increased risk of nephrotoxicity and decreased clinical efficacy when used with NSAIDs. There is a risk of hypotension with concomitant administration of diuretics, vasodilators (e.g. anaesthetic agents, antihypertensive agents) or negative inotropes (e.g. beta-blockers).

DOSES
Dogs: 0.25 mg/kg p.o. q24h (for dogs weighing >4 kg).
Cats: 0.5 mg/kg p.o. q24h.
Small mammals, Birds, Reptiles: No information available.

Imidocarb dipropionate
(Imizol*) **POM**

Formulations: Injectable: 85 mg/ml solution.

Action: Interferes with parasite nuclear acid metabolism.

Use: Treatment of *Babesia canis* infection in dogs. The safety and effectiveness of imidocarb have not been fully determined in puppies or in breeding, lactating or pregnant animals. Reduce dose with renal, hepatic or pulmonary compromise. Clinical/parasitological cure is often not achieved with other smaller *Babesia* species.

Safety and handling: Normal precautions should be observed.

Contraindications: Do not administer i.v.

Adverse reactions: Cholinergic signs (e.g. salivation, vomiting and occasionally diarrhoea, panting, restlessness) may develop after dosing. These may be alleviated by atropine. Mild injection site inflammation lasting one to several days and which may ulcerate has been reported. Anaphylactoid reactions have been reported in cattle but not in dogs.

Drug interactions: Avoid concurrent use of anticholinesterases.

DOSES
Dogs: 6.6 mg/kg i.m., s.c. once, repeated in 2–3 weeks.
Cats: Do not use.
Small mammals, Birds, Reptiles: No information available.

Imipenem
(Primaxin*) **POM**

Formulations: Injectable: 500 mg powder with cilastatin (as sodium salt) 500 mg for reconstitution (i.v. and i.m. preparations that are not interchangeable).

Action: As other beta-lactams, acts as an antimicrobial through inhibiting cell wall synthesis. It remains very stable in the presence of beta-lactamase produced by a variety of bacteria, and is resistant to beta-lactamases from some Gram-negatives that can destroy most other beta-lactam antibiotics.

Use: Very broad spectrum of activity against aerobic and anaerobic Gram-positive and Gram-negative bacteria. It is particularly important for its activity against *Pseudomonas aeruginosa* and *Enterococcus*. However it is not active against meticillin-resistant *Staphylococcus aureus*. Imipenem should not be considered for routine use in veterinary medicine and increased use will contribute to resistant infections and superinfections. In human medicine use is restricted to highly resistant infections and imipenem should therefore only be used when indicated by bacterial culture and sensitivity testing and when no other options are available. Due to the reported development of resistance during treatment of *Pseudomonas aeruginosa* infections there is some suggestion that imipenem should be combined with an aminoglycoside. Imipenem is partially inactivated in the kidney by enzymatic activity and is therefore administered in combination with cilastatin, a specific enzyme inhibitor, which blocks its renal metabolism.

Safety and handling: Normal precautions should be observed.

Contraindications: Renal disease.

Adverse reactions: Nausea and vomiting are common in humans. Imipenem can also cause seizures. Neurotoxicity has been observed when used at high doses in humans or in renal failure. If administered i.v. then do so slowly, at least over 30 minutes, as rapid administration is associated with seizures.

Drug interactions: May have additive or synergistic effects with aminoglycosides when treating some bacterial infections. Antagonism may occur with other beta-lactam antibacterials.

DOSES
See Appendix for guidelines on responsible antibacterial use.
Dogs: Empirical, but doses of 5–10 mg/kg i.v., i.m., s.c. q8h have been suggested.
Cats, Small mammals, Birds, Reptiles: No information available.

Imipramine
(Imipramine*) **POM**

Formulations: Oral: 10 mg, 25 mg tablets.

Action: Imipramine blocks noradrenaline and serotonin re-uptake in the brain, resulting in antidepressive activity.

Use: Can be used in the management of panic-related, generalized and separation anxieties, especially when these conditions are associated with urine elimination. It may also be used to aid control of supersubmissive urination and excitatory urination, narcolepsy, and may assist learning in anxious subjects. It has been suggested that it may be particularly useful for the control of panic disorders. The atypical tricyclic antidepressant clomipramine is authorized for use in dogs and so may be preferable for use, although it is not authorized for all of these indications. It is suggested that imipramine is less sedating than amitriptyline. Use with caution in young animals.

Safety and handling: Normal precautions should be observed.

Contraindications: Glaucoma, history of seizures or urinary retention, severe liver disease, hypersensitivity to tricyclic antidepressants.

Adverse reactions: Sedation, dry mouth, diarrhoea, vomiting, excitability, arrhythmias, hypotension, syncope and increased appetite are reported in humans.

Drug interactions: Should not be used with monoamine oxidase inhibitors or drugs that are metabolized by cytochrome P450 2D6 (e.g. chlorphenamine, cimetidine).

DOSES
Dogs: 1–2 mg/kg p.o. q12h or 2–4 mg/kg p.o. q24h.
Cats: 0.5–1 mg/kg p.o.q12–24h.
Small mammals, Birds, Reptiles: No information available.

Immunoglobulins
(Gammagard*, Kiovig*) **POM**

Formulations: Injectable: 2.5 g, 5 g 10 g vials for reconstitution.

Action: Has both immediate and long-term effects; however, the exact modes of action are unclear. Binding to Fc receptors and providing anti-idiotype antibodies may explain the immediate effects. The longer term effects on immune system autoregulation may be associated with a reaction with a number of membrane receptors on T cells, B cells and monocytes, which are pertinent to autoreactivity and induction of tolerance to self.

Use: Treatment of severe immune-mediated diseases in dogs where other treatments have failed. Efficacy has been demonstrated in immune-mediated thrombocytopenia; however, the use in immune-mediated haemolytic anaemia is more controversial. Its use has not been investigated for other immune-mediated diseases. Expensive: use should therefore be reserved for exceptional cases.

Safety and handling: Vials may be stored at room temperature but once reconstituted must be used immediately.

Contraindications: Avoid in patients with increased plasma protein levels.

Adverse reactions: Anaphylactic reactions are a risk but have not been recorded in dogs.

Drug interactions: None known but use with care in patients receiving drugs with strong protein binding action and vaccines.

DOSES
See Appendix for immunosuppression protocols.
Dogs: 0.5–1.0 g/kg i.v. over 6–8h.
Cats, Small mammals, Birds, Reptiles: No information available.

Indoxacarb

(Activyl, Activyl Tick Plus) **POM-V**

Formulations: Topical: Spot-on solution for dogs and cats containing 195 mg/ml in pipettes of various sizes (Activyl); spot-on solution for dogs and cats containing 150 mg/ml indoxacarb and 480 mg/ml permethrin (Activyl Tick Plus).

Action: Acts on voltage-dependent sodium channels in susceptible insects.

Use: Treatment of flea infestations (*Ctenocephalides felis*). Developing stages of fleas in the immediate environment are killed on contact. Formulations with permethrin also provide prevention of tick infestations (*Ixodes ricinus* and *Rhipicephalus sanguineus*). If ticks are present on the dog at the time of application they may not be killed within 48 hours. As indoxacarb is a pro-drug bioactivated by insect enzymes and the active component has a much higher affinity for insect sodium channels, it is very specific for insect cells.

Safety and handling: Normal precautions should be observed.

Contraindications: Do not use on dogs and cats <8 weeks old or on dogs <1.5 kg or on cats <0.6 kg.

Adverse reactions: May be harmful to aquatic organisms.

Drug interactions: No information available.

DOSES
Dogs: 15 mg/kg (equivalent to 0.077 ml/kg Activyl or 0.1 ml/kg Activyl Tick Plus). Treatment lasts at least 4 weeks.
Cats: 25 mg/kg (equivalent to 0.128 ml/kg Activyl). Treatment lasts at least 4 weeks. The combined formulation is not authorized for cats.
Small mammals, Birds, Reptiles: No information available.

Insulin

(Caninsulin, Prozinc, Actrapid*, Humulin*, Hypurin*, Insulatard*, Lantus*) **POM-V, POM**

Formulations: Injectable: 40 IU/ml, 100 IU/ml suspensions (for s.c. injection) or 100 IU/ml solutions (for s.c., i.v. or i.m. injection). There are many preparations (including soluble) authorized for use in humans; however, veterinary authorized preparations (lente and PZI), when available, are preferential for both legal and medical reasons.

Action: Binds to specific receptors on the cell surface which then stimulate the formation of glycogen from glucose, lipid from free fatty acids, protein from amino acids and many other metabolic effects.

Use: Treatment of insulin-dependent diabetes mellitus (IDDM) and occasionally as adjunctive therapy in the management of hyperkalaemia associated with urinary tract obstruction. There are various formulations of insulins from various species (see tables).

Neutral (soluble) insulin is the normal crystalline form. Lente insulins rely on different concentrations of zinc and size of zinc-insulin crystals to provide different durations of activity. Glargine insulin (Lantus) is a pH sensitive, long-acting formulation that precipitates at the site of injection. Further advice on the use of insulin should be obtained from an authoritative source such as the *BSAVA Manual of Canine and Feline Endocrinology*. Hyperkalaemia associated with hypoadrenocorticism is often associated with hypoglycaemia and insulin should be avoided in those cases.

Type	Route	Onset	Peak effect in dog (hours)	Peak effect in cat (hours)	Duration of action in dog (hours)	Duration of action in cat (hours)
Soluble (neutral)	i.v.	Immediate	0.5–2	0.5–2	1–4	1–4
	i.m.	10–30 min	1–4	1–4	3–8	3–8
	s.c.	10–30 min	1–5	1–5	4–8	4–8
Semilente (amorphous IZS)	s.c.	30–60 min	1–5	1–5	4–10	4–10
Isophane (NPH)	s.c.	0.5–3 h	2–10	2–8	6–24	4–12
Lente (mixed IZS)	s.c.	30–60 min	2–10	2–8	8–24	6–14
Ultralente (crystalline IZS)	s.c.	2–8 h	4–16	4–16	8–28	8–24
PZI	s.c.	1–4 h	4–14	3–12	6–28	6–24
Glargine	s.c.	1–4 h	Unknown	3–12	Unknown	12–24

IZS = Insulin zinc suspension; NPH = Neutral protamine Hagedorn; PZI = Protamine zinc insulin. Note that all times are approximate averages and insulin doses need to be adjusted for individual patients.

Trade name	Species of insulin	Types available
Actrapid*	Human	Neutral
Caninsulin	Porcine	Lente
Lantus*	Human	Glargine
Humulin*	Human	Neutral, Isophane
Hypurin*	Bovine	Neutral, Isophane, Lente, PZI
	Porcine	Neutral, Isophane
Insulatard*	Human or porcine	Isophane
Prozinc	Human	PZI

* = Not authorized for veterinary use.

Safety and handling: Normal precautions should be observed.

Contraindications: Hypoglycaemia.

Adverse reactions: Overdosage results in hypoglycaemia and hypokalaemia.

Drug interactions: Corticosteroids, ciclosporin, thiazide diuretics and thyroid hormones may antagonize the hypoglycaemic effects of insulin. Anabolic steroids, beta-adrenergic blockers (e.g. propranolol), phenylbutazone, salicylates and tetracycline may increase insulin's effect. Administer with caution and monitor patients closely if digoxin is given concurrently. Beta-adrenergic agonists, such as terbutaline, may prevent or lessen insulin-induced hypoglycaemia in humans. This effect has not been investigated in dogs or cats.

DOSES

Dogs:
- IDDM: Initially 0.25–0.5 IU/kg (dogs >25 kg) or 0.5–1 IU/kg (dogs <25 kg) of lente insulin s.c. q12–24h. Adjust dose and frequency of administration by monitoring clinical effect, urine results, blood glucose and/or fructosamines.
- Diabetic ketoacidosis: 0.2 IU/kg soluble insulin i.m. initially followed by 0.1 IU/kg i.m. q1h. Alternatively i.v. infusions may be given (though are not reported to be better) at 0.025–0.06 IU/kg/h of soluble insulin. Run approximately 50 ml of i.v. solution through tubing as insulin adheres to glass and plastic; change insulin/saline solution q6h.
- Hyperkalaemic myocardial toxicity (not in hypoadrenocorticism): give a bolus of 0.5 IU/kg of soluble insulin i.v. followed by 2–3 g of dextrose/unit of insulin. Half the dextrose should be given as a bolus and the remainder administered i.v. over 4–6h.

Cats:
- IDDM: Initially 0.25 IU/kg of lente insulin s.c. q12h or 0.25 IU/kg of glargine insulin (or PZI if available) s.c. q12–24h. Adjust dose and frequency of administration by monitoring clinical effect, urine results, blood glucose and/or fructosamine levels.
- Diabetic ketoacidosis: Doses as for dogs.
- Hyperkalaemic myocardial toxicity: Doses as for dogs.

Small mammals: Ferrets: Lente insulin 0.5–1.0 IU/ferret q12h.

Birds: No information available.

Reptiles: Chelonians, Snakes: 1–5 IU/kg i.m. q24–72h; Crocodilians, Lizards: 5–10 IU/kg i.m. q24–72h; adjust doses according to serial glucose measurement.

Interferon omega
(Virbagen omega) **POM-V**

Formulations: 10 million units/vial powder with solvent for reconstitution.

Action: Interferons are cytokines that have many effects on immunity and immune cell function.

Use: Has been shown to reduce mortality and clinical signs of the enteric form of parvovirus infection in dogs. Has also been used to treat early-stage FeLV infection, albeit with limited success as shown by a reduction in mortality. The effect of treatment on cats with an FeLV-associated tumour is not known. No reduction in mortality is seen if the drug is used to treat FIV-infected cats. Limited reports of use in feline infectious peritonitis, acute feline calicivirus infection and feline chronic gingivostomatitis. In refractory and severe cases of feline herpesvirus-1 infection, combined therapy including oral or topical antiviral medication, topical interferon and oral lysine, can be used. Has also been used topically in the management of herpetic keratitis in cats. Although used frequently with beneficial results, there are limited clinical data about the appropriate concentration and frequency of treatment and the efficacy in treating ocular disease. For ophthalmic use, reconstitute a 10 million unit vial with 1 ml of the solvent supplied and make up to 4 ml with sterile saline; decant into 0.2 ml aliquots and keep in freezer. To use, take a 0.2 ml aliquot of the diluted solution and add to 0.8 ml hypromellose.

Safety and handling: In case of accidental self-injection, seek medical advice immediately and show the package insert or the label to the physician.

Contraindications: No information available.

Adverse reactions: Transient fatigue, hyperthermia, vomiting and mild diarrhoea may be observed (i.v. administration to cats increases the risk of these). In addition, a slight decrease in white blood cells, platelets and red blood cells, and increases in the concentration of liver enzymes may be observed. Side effects such as the induction of immune-mediated diseases have been reported with long-term administration in humans. Ocular irritation has been seen in cats.

Drug interactions: Vaccines should not be administered concurrently until the animal has clinically recovered. The use of supplementary supportive treatments such as antibiotics and NSAIDs improves prognosis, and no interactions have been observed with these.

DOSES
Dogs: 2.5 million units/kg i.v. q24h for 3 days.
Cats:
- Parenteral: 1–2.5 million units/kg i.v., s.c. q24–48h for up to 5 doses; then reduced, according to clinical effect, to twice weekly and then once weekly. Specific protocols within this dose range have been published for FeLV, FIP, FCV and chronic gingivostomatitis; users should consult the manufacturer for further advice.
- Ophthalmic: 1 drop (50 microlitres) of a diluted (500,000 units/ml) solution per eye up to q6h for 10 days, then 1 drop q8–12h for a further 3 weeks.

Small mammals, Birds, Reptiles: No information available.

Iron salts (Ferrous sulphate, Ferrous fumarate, Ferrous gluconate, Iron dextran)

(CosmoFer, Scordex, Venofer) **POM-VPS, POM, GSL**

Formulations: Injectable: 50 mg/ml iron dextran (CosmoFer), 200 mg/ml iron dextran (Scordex), 20 mg/ml iron sucrose (Venofer). Oral: 200 mg $FeSO_4$ tablet (ferrous sulphate), ferrous gluconate and other formulations in variable tablet and liquid preparations; ferrous fumarate preparations also typically contain folic acid.

Action: Essential for oxygen-binding in haemoglobin, electron transport chain and oxidative phosphorylation, and other oxidative reactions in metabolism.

Use: Treatment of iron deficiency anaemia and conditions where red blood cell synthesis is high and iron stores are depleted. The oral route should be used if possible. Iron absorption is complex and dependent in part on physiological demand, diet composition, current iron stores and dose. Valid reasons for administering iron parenterally are failure of oral therapy due to severe GI adverse effects, continuing severe blood loss, iron malabsorption, or a non-complaint patient. Modified-release preparations should be avoided as they are ineffective. Iron is absorbed in the duodenum and the release of iron from modified-release preparations occurs lower down the GI tract. Absorption is enhanced if administered 1 hour before or several hours after feeding. Reduce dosage if GI side effects occur.

Safety and handling: Normal precautions should be observed.

Contraindications: Severe infection or inflammation, intolerance to the oral preparation, any anaemia other than iron deficiency anaemia, presence of GI ulcers. Also contraindicated in patients with hepatic, renal (particularly pyelonephritis) or cardiac disease, and untreated urinary tract infections.

Adverse reactions: Parenteral iron may cause arrhythmias, anaphylaxis, shunting of iron to reticuloendothelial stores and iron overload. Oral iron may cause nausea, vomiting, constipation and diarrhoea. The faeces of animals treated with oral iron may be dark in appearance. High doses may be teratogenic and embryotoxic (injectable iron dextran).

Drug interactions: Chloramphenicol can delay the response to iron dextran and its concurrent use should be avoided. Oral preparations bind to tetracyclines and penicillamine causing a decrease in efficacy. Antacids, milk and eggs significantly decrease the bioavailability of oral iron.

DOSES

Dogs: 100–600 mg/dog p.o. q24h or 10–20 mg/kg i.m. once only, followed by oral therapy.

Cats: Chronic renal failure: 50 mg/cat i.m. iron dextran every 3–4 weeks in conjunction with erythropoietin in chronic renal failure or

20–25 mg/cat i.m. once followed by 50–100 mg/cat p.o. q24h. Note that the majority of cats do not tolerate oral iron therapy and require parenteral treatment.

Small mammals: 10 mg/kg i.m. of iron dextran once weekly or prn.
Birds: 10 mg/kg i.m. of iron dextran.
Reptiles: No information available.

Isoflurane

(Isoba, Isocare, Isofane, IsoFlo, Isoflurane Vet, Vetflurane)
POM-V

Formulations: Inhalational: 250 ml bottle of liquid isoflurane.

Action: Halogenated ethyl methyl ether and structural isomer of enflurane. The mechanism of action of volatile anaesthetic agents is not fully understood.

Use: Induction and maintenance of anaesthesia. Isoflurane is potent and highly volatile so should only be delivered from a suitable calibrated vaporizer. It is less soluble in blood than halothane but more soluble than sevoflurane, therefore induction and recovery from anaesthesia are quicker than halothane but slower than sevoflurane. The concentration of isoflurane required to maintain anaesthesia depends on the other drugs used in the anaesthesia protocol; the concentration should be adjusted according to clinical assessment of anaesthetic depth. MAC approximately 1.2–1.7% in most species. Isoflurane has a pungent smell and induction to anaesthesia using chambers or masks may be less well tolerated in small dogs and cats compared with halothane and sevoflurane.

Safety and handling: Measures should be adopted to prevent contamination of the environment with isoflurane during anaesthesia and when handling of the agent.

Contraindications: Avoid gaseous induction in rabbits and chelonians as they can breath-hold and develop serious complications.

Adverse reactions: Isoflurane causes dose-dependent hypotension by causing vasodilation, particularly in skeletal muscle. This adverse effect does not wane with time. Isoflurane is a more potent respiratory depressant than halothane, respiratory depression is dose-dependent. Isoflurane does not sensitize the myocardium to catecholamines to the extent that halothane does, but can generate arrhythmias in certain conditions. Assertions that isoflurane is safer than halothane in certain high-risk cases should be discounted. Isoflurane is not metabolized by the liver (0.2%) and has less effect on liver blood flow compared with halothane. In ferrets isoflurane can cause marked depression in haematological parameters (especially haematocrit, RBC count, Hb concentration) rapidly after induction, so care should be taken in interpreting blood results if isoflurane is used for restraint, or in anaemic or debilitated ferrets.

Drug interactions: Opioid agonists, benzodiazepines and N$_2$O reduce the concentration of isoflurane required to achieve surgical anaesthesia. The duration of action of non-depolarizing neuromuscular blocking agents is longer with isoflurane compared with halothane anaesthetized animals.

DOSES
Dogs: The expired concentration required to maintain surgical anaesthesia in 50% of dogs is 1.2% (minimum alveolar concentration). Administration of other anaesthetic agents and opioid analgesics reduces the dose requirement of isoflurane, therefore the dose should be adjusted according to individual requirement. 3–5% isoflurane concentration is required to induce anaesthesia in unpremedicated patients.
Cats: The expired concentration required to maintain surgical anaesthesia in 50% of cats is 1.6% (minimum alveolar concentration).
Small mammals: Ferrets, Rabbits: Doses as for dogs. The expired concentration required to maintain surgical anaesthesia in 50% of rabbits is 2.05%.
Birds: Doses as for dogs.
Reptiles: 3–5% in 100% oxygen for induction in snakes and lizards; 2–4% in 100% oxygen for maintenance.

Ispaghula (Psyllium)
(Isogel*, Ispagel*, Regulan*) **GSL**

Formulations: Oral: granules, powder.

Action: Bulk-forming agent that increases faecal mass and stimulates peristalsis. Moderately fermentable in the colon and the resultant volatile fatty acids exert an osmotic laxative effect.

Use: Management of impacted anal sacs, diarrhoea and constipation, and the control of stool consistency after surgery. Available preparations are for humans and often fruit-flavoured and may be effervescent when mixed with water. They can be added to food for animals.

Safety and handling: Normal precautions should be observed.

Contraindications: Bowel obstruction.

Adverse reactions: Constipation or, if excess is given, diarrhoea and bloating may occur.

Drug interactions: No information available.

DOSES
Dogs: 1–2 teaspoonfuls with meals (anecdotal).
Cats: ½–1 teaspoonful with meals (anecdotal).
Small mammals, Birds, Reptiles: No information available.

Itraconazole

(Fungitraxx, Itrafungol, Sporanox*) **POM, POM-V**

Formulations: Oral: 100 mg capsule, 10 mg/ml oral solution.

Action: Triazole antifungal agent that inhibits the cytochrome systems involved in the synthesis of ergosterol in fungal cell membranes, causing increased cell wall permeability and allowing leakage of cellular contents.

Use: Treatment of aspergillosis, candidiasis, blastomycosis, coccidioidomycosis, cryptococcosis, sporotrichosis, histoplasmosis, dermatophytosis and *Malassezia*. Itraconazole is authorized in the form of an oral solution for the treatment of *Microsporum canis* dermatophytosis in cats and has been used successfully to treat ringworm in Persian cats without the need for clipping. It is widely distributed in the body, although low concentrations are found in tissues with low protein contents, e.g. CSF, ocular fluid and saliva. Itraconazole extends the activity of methylprednisolone. In humans, antifungal imidazoles and triazoles inhibit the metabolism of antihistamines, oral hypoglycaemics and antiepileptics. Concomitant use of itraconazole is likely to increase blood levels of ciclosporin.

Safety and handling: Normal precautions should be observed.

Contraindications: Pregnancy. Avoid use if liver disease is present.

Adverse reactions: Vomiting, diarrhoea, anorexia, salivation, depression and apathy, abdominal pain, hepatic toxicosis, drug eruption, ulcerative dermatitis and limb oedema have been reported. It has a narrow safety margin in birds and should be discontinued if emesis or anorexia occurs. Not well tolerated by Grey Parrots.

Drug interactions: In humans antifungal imidazoles and triazoles inhibit the metabolism of antihistamines (particularly terfenadine), oral hypoglycaemics, antiepileptics, cisapride, ciclosporin and glucocorticoids). Although not as well studied in veterinary species, itraconazole is known to increase the bioavailability of ciclosporin in cats. Antacids, omeprazole, H2 antagonists and adsorbents may reduce the absorption of itraconazole. Plasma concentrations of digoxin, benzodiazepines, glucocorticoids and vincristine may be increased by itraconazole.

DOSES

Dogs, Cats: 5 mg/kg p.o. q24h. 4–20 weeks of treatment may be needed, dependent upon culture results. Pulse dosing (7 days on, 7 days off) has been described for dermatophytosis in cats.

Small mammals: Ferrets: dermatophytosis: 15 mg/kg p.o q24h or 25–33 mg/ferret p.o. q24h; Rabbits: dermatophytosis: 10 mg/kg p.o. q24h for 15 days; pulmonary aspergillosis: 20–40 mg/kg p.o. q24h; Guinea pigs: 5 mg/kg p.o. q24h.

Birds:

- Aspergillosis treatment: 5–10 mg/kg p.o. q12–24. Grey Parrots: use with great care and only at lowest dose and longest interval (voriconazole at 12–18 mg/kg p.o. q12h or terbinafine may be better); Raptors: higher doses of up to 20 mg/kg p.o. q12–24h may be used.

- Aspergillosis prophylaxis: 10–20 mg/kg p.o. q24h in susceptible species (e.g. Gyrs (and their hybrids), Goshawks, Snowy Owls, Golden Eagles) during stressful events (e.g. manning) where drug therapy should be started 5 days before the stressful event starts.

Reptiles: 23.5 mg/kg p.o. q24h for 3d (spiny lizard pharmacokinetic study maintained systemic itraconazole levels for a further 6 days); 1.5 mg/kg p.o. q36h (corn snake fungal granuloma) for minimum 4 weeks; 5 mg/kg p.o. q24h (panther chameleon periodontal fungal osteomyelitis).

Ivermectin

(Alstomec, Animec, Bimectin, Ivomec, Panomec, Qualimec, Qualimintic, Virbamec, Xeno 450, Xeno 50-mini, Xeno 200 spray) **POM-V, POM-VPS, ESPA**

Formulations: Injectable: 1% w/v solution. Topical: 100 µg/g, 800 µg/g spot-on tubes; 1 µg/ml, 10 µg/ml drops; 200 µg/ml spray (Xeno).

Action: Interacts with GABA and glutamate-gated channels leading to flaccid paralysis of parasites.

Use: Treatment of dogs with generalized demodicosis, sarcoptic acariasis or cheyletiellosis, and cats with cheyletiellosis or otoacariasis when approved treatments have failed or cannot be employed. Prevention and treatment of internal and external parasites in small mammals and birds.

Safety and handling: Normal precautions should be observed.

Contraindications: Administration to collies and related breeds is not recommended. Consider multiple drug resistance gene testing in these breeds before use. Highly toxic to aquatic organisms. Do not use in chelonians.

Adverse reactions: Neurotoxicity may be seen if it crosses mammalian blood-brain barrier. Dose adjustments may be required when administered concurrently with other therapeutic agents transported by P-glycoprotein.

Drug interactions: Dose adjustments may be required when administered concurrently with other therapeutic agents transported by P-glycoprotein.

DOSES
Dogs:
- Generalized demodicosis 300–600 µg (micrograms)/kg p.o. daily.
- Effective for sarcoptic mange (200–400 µg (micrograms)/kg p.o., s.c. q2w for 4–6 weeks) and cheyletiellosis (200–300 µg (micrograms)/kg p.o., s.c. q1–2w for 6–8 weeks) but other options (selamectin, moxidectin) are available.

Cats: Otoacariasis (*Otodectes cynotis* infestation): 1% w/v ivermection diluted 1:9 with propylene glycol topically (in affected ears) 1 drop daily for 21 days.

Small mammals: 0.2–0.5 mg/kg s.c., p.o. q7–14d; Ferrets, Rabbits, Guinea pigs: apply 450 μg (micrograms)/kg (1 tube Xeno 450) topically; Ferrets, small rodents <800 g: 50 μg (micrograms)/250 g (15 drops Xeno 50-mini) q7–14d.

Birds: 200 μg (micrograms)/kg i.m., s.c., p.o. q7–14d; Raptors: capillariasis: 0.5–1 mg/kg i.m., p.o. q7–14d; *Serratospiculum*: 1 mg/kg p.o., i.m. q7–14d (moxidectin or doramectin may be given at same dose rates); Passerines and small psittacids: systemic dosing as above or 0.2 mg/kg applied topically to skin using 0.02% solution (in propylene glycol) q7–14d; Pigeons: 0.5 ml applied topically to bare skin using 0.02% solution q7–14d; Ornamental birds: mites and lice: 1 drop/50 g body weight weekly for 3 weeks.

Reptiles: 0.2 mg/kg s.c., p.o. once, repeat in 10–14 days until negative for parasites; may use as environmental control for snake mites (*Ophionyssus natricis*) at dilution of 5 mg/l water sprayed in tank q7–10d (if pre-mix ivermectin with propylene glycol this facilitates mixing with water); Chelonians: do not use.

A
B
C
D
E
F
G
H
I
J
K
L
M
N
O
P
Q
R
S
T
U
V
W
X
Y
Z

Kaolin
(Kaogel VP, Prokolin) **AVM-GSL, general sale**

Formulations: Oral: Kaogel VP: aqueous suspension containing Kaolin Light. Combination products with pectin, magnesium trisilicate, aluminium hydroxide and phosphate, bismuth salts, calcium carbonate or tincture of morphine are also available.

Action: Adsorbent antidiarrhoeal agent with possible antisecretory effect.

Use: Treatment of diarrhoea of non-specific origins in cats and dogs. Although stool consistency may improve, studies do not show that fluid balance is corrected or that the duration of morbidity is shortened.

Safety and handling: Normal precautions should be observed.

Contraindications: Intestinal obstruction or perforation.

Adverse reactions: No information available.

Drug interactions: May decrease the absorption of lincomycin, trimethoprim and sulphonamides.

DOSES
Dogs, Cats: 0.5–1.0 ml/kg p.o. as a total daily dose q6–8h.
Small mammals: No information available. The use of kaolin is not advisable in rabbits, guinea pigs and chinchillas due to the risk of decreasing GI motility.
Birds: Kaolin/pectin mixture: 15 ml/kg p.o. once.
Reptiles: No information available.

Ketamine
(Ketaset injection, Narketan-10, Vetalar-V) **POM-V CD SCHEDULE 4**

Formulations: Injectable: 100 mg/ml solution.

Action: Antagonizes the excitatory neurotransmitter glutamate at *N*-methyl-D-aspartate (NMDA) receptors in the CNS. It interacts with opioid receptors in a complex fashion, antagonizing mu receptors, whilst showing agonist actions at delta and kappa receptors. It does not interact with GABA receptors.

Use: Provision of chemical restraint or dissociative anaesthesia. Ketamine may also provide profound visceral and somatic analgesia and inhibits central sensitization through NMDA receptor blockade and is used to provide perioperative analgesia as an adjunctive agent, although optimal doses to provide analgesia have not been elucidated. Dissociative anaesthesia is associated with mild stimulation of cardiac output and blood pressure, modest respiratory depression and the preservation of cranial nerve reflexes. For example, the eyes remain open during anaesthesia and should be protected using a bland ophthalmic ointment. Used alone at doses adequate to provide general anaesthesia ketamine causes skeletal muscle hypertonicity and movement may occur that is unrelated to surgical stimulation. These effects are normally controlled by the co-administration of alpha-2 adrenergic agonists and/or benzodiazepines. When ketamine is combined with alpha-2 agonists (such as medetomidine or dexmedetomidine) reversal of the alpha-2 agonist should be delayed until 45 min after ketamine administration.

Safety and handling: Normal precautions should be observed.

Contraindications: Not recommended for animals whose eyes are at risk of perforation or who have raised intraocular pressure.

Adverse reactions: Cardiovascular depression, rather than stimulation, and arrhythmias may arise in animals with a high sympathetic nervous system tone (e.g. animals in shock or severe cardiovascular disease). Tachycardias can also arise after administration of high doses i.v. Respiratory depression may be marked in some animals. Ketamine may result in spacey, abnormal behaviour for 1–2 hours during recovery. Prolonged administration of ketamine by infusion may result in drug accumulation and prolong recovery. Higher doses may be dangerous in debilitated reptiles.

Drug interactions: No information available.

DOSES
When used for sedation is generally given as part of a combination. See Appendix for sedation protocols in all species.
Dogs:
- Perioperative analgesia: Intraoperatively: 10 μg (micrograms)/kg/min, postoperatively: 2–5 μg (micrograms)/kg/min, both preceded by a 250–500 μg (micrograms)/kg loading dose. There is some evidence to suggest that a 10 μg/kg/min dose may be too low to provide adequate analgesia continuously, although other evidence-based dose recommendations are lacking.
- Induction of anaesthesia (combined with diazepam or midazolam) as part of a volatile anaesthetic technique: 2 mg/kg i.v.
- Induction of general anaesthesia combined with medetomidine or dexmedetomidine to provide a total injectable combination: ketamine (5–7 mg/kg i.m.) combined with medetomidine (40 μg (micrograms)/kg i.m.) or dexmedetomidine (20 μg (micrograms)/kg i.m.).

Cats:
- General anaesthesia: combinations of ketamine (5–7.5 mg/kg i.m.) combined with medetomidine (80 μg (micrograms)/kg i.m.) or dexmedetomidine (40 μg (micrograms)/kg i.m.) will provide 20–30 min general anaesthesia. Reduce the doses of both drugs when given i.v.
- Perioperative analgesia: Doses are the same as those for dogs.

Small mammals:
- Ferrets: 10–30 mg/kg i.m., s.c. alone gives immobilization and some analgesia but there is poor muscle relaxation and prolonged recovery. For general anaesthesia, sedate first and then induce with isoflurane or sevoflurane. Alternatively, combinations of ketamine (10–15 mg/kg) with medetomidine (0.08–0.1 mg/kg i.m., s.c.) or dexmedetomidine (0.04–0.05 mg/kg i.m., s.c.) will provide a short period of heavy sedation or general anaesthesia in most ferrets. The duration and depth of anaesthesia is increased by the addition of butorphanol at 0.2–0.4 mg/kg i.m., s.c. or buprenorphine at 0.02 mg/kg i.m., s.c. which also provides analgesia.
- Rabbits: 15–30 mg/kg i.m., s.c. alone gives moderate to heavy sedation with some analgesia but there is poor muscle relaxation and prolonged recovery. Alternatively, 5 mg/kg i.v. or 10–15 mg/ kg i.m., s.c. in combination with medetomidine (0.05–0.1 mg/kg i.v., 0.1–0.3 mg/kg s.c., i.m.) or dexmedetomidine (0.025–0.05 mg/kg i.v. or 0.05–0.15 mg/kg s.c., i.m.) and butorphanol (0.1–0.5 mg/kg i.v., s.c., i.m.) or buprenorphine (0.02–0.05 mg/kg i.m., i.v., s.c.) will give a short duration of heavy sedation or anaesthesia in most rabbits. Intravenous combinations are ideally given incrementally to effect.
- Guinea pigs: 10–50 mg/kg i.m., s.c. will provide immobilization, with little muscle relaxation and some analgesia, however it is suggested to use the lower end of the dose range to sedate first and then induce with isoflurane or sevoflurane; alternatively, a combination of ketamine (3–5 mg/kg i.m., s.c.) with medetomidine (0.10 mg/kg i.m., s.c.) or dexmedetomidine (0.05 mg/kg i.m., s.c.) will provide a short period of anaesthesia.
- Other rodents: 10–50 mg/kg i.m., s.c. will provide immobilization, however it is suggested to use the lower end of the dose range and to induce anaesthesia with isoflurane or sevoflurane or use in combination with other agents.

Birds: Largely superseded by gaseous anaesthesia.
Reptiles: Chelonians: 20–60 mg/kg i.m., i.v.; Lizards: 25–60 mg/kg i.m., i.v.; Snakes: 20–80 mg/kg i.m., i.v.; all doses given alone.

Ketoconazole is not available at the time of publication.
Itraconazole is an alternative for most uses.

Ketoprofen
(Ketofen) **POM-V**

Formulations: Injectable: 1% solution. Oral: 5 mg, 20 mg tablets.

Action: COX-1 inhibition reduces the production of prostaglandins, while lipoxygenase enzyme inhibition has a potent effect on the vascular and cellular phases of inflammation. It has antipyretic, analgesic and anti-inflammatory effects.

Use: Relief of acute pain from musculoskeletal disorders and other painful disorders in the dog and cat. Management of chronic pain from osteoarthritis in the dog. Ketoprofen is not COX-2 selective and is not authorized for preoperative administration to cats and dogs. Do not administer perioperatively until the animal is fully recovered from anaesthesia and normotensive. Liver disease will prolong the metabolism of ketoprofen, leading to the potential for drug accumulation and overdose with repeated dosing. Accurate dosing of ketoprofen in cats is essential. Administration of ketoprofen to animals with renal disease must be carefully evaluated.

Safety and handling: Normal precautions should be observed.

Contraindications: Do not give to dehydrated, hypovolaemic or hypotensive patients or those with GI disease or blood clotting problems. Do not give to pregnant animals or animals <6 weeks of age. Do not use in vultures.

Adverse reactions: GI signs may occur in all animals after NSAID administration. Stop therapy if this persists beyond 1–2 days. Some animals develop signs with one NSAID and not another. A 1–2-week wash-out period should be allowed before starting another NSAID after cessation of therapy. Stop therapy immediately if GI bleeding is suspected. There is a small risk that NSAIDs may precipitate cardiac failure in animals with cardiovascular disease.

Drug interactions: Do not administer concurrently or within 24 hours of other NSAIDs and glucocorticoids. Do not administer with other potentially nephrotoxic agents, e.g. aminoglycosides.

DOSES
Dogs: 2 mg/kg s.c., i.m., i.v. q24h, may be repeated for up to 3 consecutive days; 0.25 mg/kg p.o. q24h for up to 30 days in total or 1 mg/kg p.o. q24h for up to 5 days. Oral dosing for 4 days may follow a single injection of ketoprofen on day 1.
Cats: 2 mg/kg s.c. q24h, may be repeated for up to 3 consecutive days; 1 mg/kg p.o. q24h for up to 5 days. Oral dosing for 4 days may follow a single injection of ketoprofen on day 1.
Small mammals: Ferrets: 1 mg/kg p.o., s.c., i.m. q24h; Rabbits: 1–3 mg/kg i.m., s.c. q24h; Hamsters, Gerbils, Rats: Up to 5 mg/kg p.o., i.m., s.c. q24h; Other rodents: 1–3 mg/kg s.c., i.m. q12–24h.
Birds: 1–5 mg/kg i.m. q8–24h. Do not use in vultures.
Reptiles: No information available.

Ketorolac
(Acular*) **POM**

Formulations: Ophthalmic: 0.5% drops in 5 ml bottle.

Action: COX inhibitor that reduces the production of prostaglandins and therefore reduces inflammation.

Use: Treatment of anterior uveitis and ulcerative keratitis when topical corticosteroids are contraindicated. Topical NSAIDs have the potential to increase intraocular pressure and should be used with caution in dogs predisposed to glaucoma.

Safety and handling: Normal precautions should be observed.

Contraindications: No information available.

Adverse reactions: As with other topical NSAIDs, ketorolac trometamol may cause local irritation. Topical NSAIDs can be used in ulcerative keratitis but with caution as they can delay epithelial healing. Topical NSAIDs have been associated with an increased risk of corneal 'melting' (keratomalacia) in humans, although this has not been reported in the veterinary literature. Regular monitoring is advised.

Drug interactions: Ophthalmic NSAIDs may be used safely with other ophthalmic pharmaceuticals although concurrent use of drugs which adversely affect the corneal epithelium (e.g. gentamicin) may lead to increased corneal penetration of the NSAID. The concurrent use of topical NSAIDs with topical corticosteroids has been identified as a risk factor in humans for precipitating corneal problems.

DOSES
Dogs, Cats, Small mammals: 1 drop per eye q6–24h depending on severity of inflammation.
Birds: 1 drop per eye q12h.
Reptiles: No information available.

Lactulose

(Lactugal*, Lactulose*) **P**

Formulations: Oral: 3.1–3.7 g/5 ml lactulose in a syrup base.

Action: Metabolized by colonic bacteria resulting in the formation of low molecular weight organic acids (lactic, formic, acetic acids). These acids increase osmotic pressure, causing a laxative effect, acidifying colonic contents and thereby trapping ammonia as ammonium ions, which are then expelled with the faeces.

Use: Used to reduce blood ammonia levels in patients with hepatic encephalopathy and to treat constipation in dogs, cats and other species. Reduce the dose if diarrhoea develops. Cats and some dogs do not like the taste of lactulose. An alternative is lactitol (β-galactosidosorbitol) as a powder to add to food (500 mg/kg/day in 3 or 4 doses, adjusted to produce two or three soft stools per day), although its efficacy in the management of hepatic encephalopathy has not been extensively evaluated.

Safety and handling: Normal precautions should be observed.

Contraindications: Do not administer orally to severely encephalopathic animals at risk of inhalation.

Adverse reactions: Excessive doses cause flatulence, diarrhoea, cramping and dehydration.

Drug interactions: Synergy may occur when lactulose is used with oral antibiotics (e.g. neomycin). Do not use lactulose with other laxatives. Oral antacids may reduce the colonic acidification efficacy of lactulose. Lactulose syrup contains some free lactose and galactose, and so may alter insulin requirements in diabetic patients.

DOSES

Dogs:
- Constipation: 0.5–1.0 ml/kg p.o. q8–12h. Monitor and adjust therapy to produce two or three soft stools per day.
- Acute hepatic encephalopathy: 18–20 ml/kg of a solution comprising 3 parts lactulose to 7 parts water per rectum as a retention enema for 4–8h.
- Chronic hepatic encephalopathy: 0.5–1.0 ml/kg p.o. q8–12h. Monitor and adjust therapy to produce two or three soft stools per day.

Cats: Constipation and chronic hepatic encephalopathy: 0.5–5 ml p.o. q8–12h. Monitor and adjust therapy to produce two or three soft stools per day.

Small mammals: Ferrets: 0.15–0.75 ml/kg p.o. q12h.

Birds: Appetite stimulant, hepatic encephalopathy: 0.2–1 ml/kg p.o. q8–12h.

Reptiles: 0.5 ml/kg p.o. q24h.

Lanthanum carbonate octahydrate
(Lantharenol)
(Renalzin, Fosrenol*) **POM, general sale**

Formulations: Oral: 200 mg/ml liquid; 500 mg, 750 mg, 1 g chewable tablets (lanthanum carbonate).

Action: Binds ingested phosphate in the gut and the insoluble complexes are not absorbed.

Use: Reduction of serum phosphate in azotaemia. Hyperphosphataemia is implicated in the progression of chronic renal failure. Phosphate-binding agents are usually only used if low phosphate diets are unsuccessful. Monitor serum phosphate levels at 10–14 day intervals and adjust dosage accordingly if trying to normalize serum concentrations. When using lanthanum carbonate octahydrate water should be available at all times.

Safety and handling: Normal precautions should be observed.

Contraindications: It is advisable not to introduce the drug for the first time during an acute crisis: always stabilize the patient before making any dietary alterations to enhance acceptance.

Adverse reactions: None known.

Drug interactions: Should be given at least 1 hour before or 3 hours after other medications.

DOSES
Dogs: 100 mg/kg/day p.o. q12h divided between meals.
Cats: 400–800 mg/cat/day with a recommended starting dose of 400 mg per day. The dose should be divided according to the feeding schedule (it is important to give some with every meal). Dose adjustments should be based on serum phosphate levels.
Small mammals, Birds, Reptiles: No information available.

Latanoprost
(Latanoprost*, Xalatan*) **POM**

Formulations: Ophthalmic: 50 µg/ml (0.005%) solution in 2.5 ml bottle.

Action: Agonist for receptors specific for prostaglandin F. It reduces intraocular pressure by increasing outflow.

Use: Management of primary canine glaucoma and is useful in the emergency management of acute primary glaucoma (superseding mannitol, acetazolamide and dichlorphenamide). May have a profound effect on intraocular pressure in the dog. Its effect in the cat is less predictable and should be avoided in this species. Often used in conjunction with other topical antiglaucoma drugs such as carbonic anhydrase inhibitors. Latanoprost may be useful in the management of lens subluxation despite being contraindicated in anterior lens luxation. Latanoprost has comparable activity to travatoprost.

Safety and handling: Store in refrigerator until opened (then at room temperature).

Contraindications: Uveitis and anterior lens luxation.

Adverse reactions: Miosis in dogs and cats; conjunctival hyperaemia and mild irritation may develop. Increased iridal pigmentation has been noted in humans but not in dogs.

Drug interactions: Do not use in conjunction with thiomersal-containing preparations.

DOSES
Dogs: 1 drop per eye q8–24h.
Cats: Do not use.
Small mammals: Rabbits: 1 drop per eye q8–24h.
Birds, Reptiles: No information available.

Leflunomide
(Arava*) **POM**

Formulations: Oral: 10 mg, 20 mg, 100 mg tablets.

Action: Inhibits T and B lymphocyte proliferation, suppresses immunoglobulin production, and interferes with leucocyte adhesion and diapedesis, usually through inhibition of tyrosine kinases. Also inhibits dihydro-orotate dehydrogenase, an enzyme involved in *de novo* pathway of pyrimidine synthesis.

Use: Treatment of active rheumatoid arthritis in humans. In veterinary medicine has been reported to be effective in treatment of systemic histiocytosis and has also been used in canine immune-mediated diseases. Clinical veterinary experience of this drug is limited.

Safety and handling: Disposable gloves should be worn to handle or administer tablets. Staff and clients should be warned that excreta (including saliva) may contain traces of the parent drug or its metabolites, and should be handled with due care.

Contraindications: Bone marrow suppression, pre-existing infections, liver dysfunction.

Adverse reactions: Anorexia, lethargy, myelosuppression and haematemesis. In humans leflunomide can cause severe hepatotoxicity, myelosuppression and interstitial lung disease.

Drug interactions: In humans live virus vaccines, tolbutamide, rifampin and isoniazid should not be given concomitantly.

DOSES

See Appendix for immunosuppression protocols.

Dogs: 4 mg/kg p.o. q24h.

Dogs, Cats: Rheumatoid arthritis (in combination with methotrexate): 10 mg (total dose) p.o. q24h, after significant improvement reduce to 10 mg p.o. twice weekly.

Small mammals, Birds, Reptiles: No information available.

Lenograstim (rhG-CSF)
(Granocyte*) **POM**

Formulations: Injectable: 33.6 million IU (263 μg) vial for reconstitution.

Action: Recombinant human granulocyte-colony stimulating factor (rhG-CSF). Activates proliferation and differentiation of granulocyte progenitor cells, enhances granulopoiesis.

Use: In humans it is indicated in the management of neutropenia. Neutrophil counts rise within 24 hours. Following discontinuation, neutrophil counts drop to normal after 5 days. There are few reports on the use of G-CSF in dogs and cats; filgrastim is more commonly used. Lenograstim is most likely to be used in the management of febrile patients with neutrophil counts $<1 \times 10^9$/l.

Safety and handling: Normal precautions should be observed.

Contraindications: No information available.

Adverse reactions: Normal dogs produce neutralizing antibodies to rhG-CSF. This limits repeated use and may result in neutropenia. This does not appear to be the case in canine chemotherapy patients. A variety of adverse effects have been reported in humans, including musculoskeletal pain, transient hypotension, dysuria, allergic reactions, proteinuria, haematuria and increased liver enzymes. Reported adverse effects are bone pain at high doses and irritation at the injection site.

Drug interactions: In humans steroids and lithium may potentiate the release of neutrophils during G-CSF therapy. Concurrent administration with chemotherapy may increase incidence of adverse effects. G-CSF should be given at least 24 hours after the last dose of chemotherapy as the stimulatory effects of G-CSF on haemopoietic precursors renders them more susceptible to the effects of chemotherapy.

DOSES

Dogs: 19.2 million IU/m² i.v. (over 30 min), s.c. q24h for 3–5 days. **See Appendix for conversion of body weight to body surface area.**

Cats, Small mammals, Birds, Reptiles: No information available.

Levetiracetam (S-Etiracetam, Levetirasetam)

CIL

(Keppra*) **POM**

Formulations: Oral: 250 mg, 500 mg, 750 mg and 1 g tablets; 100 mg/ml oral 300 ml solution. Injectable: 100 mg/ml intravenous solution (5 ml vial); formulated with sodium chloride for injection at 500 mg/100 ml, 1000 mg/100 ml and 1500 mg/100 ml.

Action: The mechanism of anticonvulsant action is unknown but has been shown to bind to the synaptic vesicle protein SV2A within the brain, which may protect against seizures.

Use: Effective as primary or adjunctive maintenance therapy in dogs and cats for management of epileptic seizures refractory to conventional therapy. Used at a higher dose, in addition to conventional maintenance therapy, as pulse therapy for cluster seizures. Constant intravenous infusion used for emergency control of status epilepticus. Levetiracetam is rapidly absorbed from the GI tract with peak plasma concentrations reached in <2 hours of oral dosing. Steady state is rapidly achieved within 2 days. Plasma protein binding is minimal. The plasma half-life is short, being around 7 hours in human patients. Withdrawal of levetiracetam therapy or transition to or from another type of antiepileptic therapy should be done gradually. Use with caution and in reduced doses in patients with renal and severe hepatic impairment. Levetiracetam has also been used for the management of neuropathic pain (similar to gabapentin) in human patients.

Safety and handling: Normal precautions should be observed.

Contraindications: No information available.

Adverse reactions: The most commonly reported adverse effects in humans are sedation, weakness and dizziness. Blood dyscrasias such as neutropenia, pancytopenia and thrombocytopenia may also develop. In one canine study the only adverse effect reported was sedation in one of the 14 dogs in the study.

Drug interactions: Minimal, although there is some evidence to suggest that enzyme-inducing anticonvulsants (including phenobarbita and phenytoin) may modestly reduce levetiracetam levels, but not by clinically relevant amounts.

DOSES

Dogs, Cats:
- Maintenance therapy (as adjunct or sole anticonvulsant): 10–30 mg/kg p.o. q8–12h.
- Pulse therapy for severe cluster seizures (in addition to maintenance therapy): 30 mg/kg p.o. q6–8h for the duration of the cluster (usually for 2–3 days) and then stopped until the start of the next cluster. Incremental increase in dose if required.

- Status epilepticus: 60 mg/kg i.v. bolus q8h or continuous intravenous infusion of 8 mg/kg/h, incrementally increased to effect if required.

Small mammals, Birds, Reptiles: No information available.

Levothyroxine (T4, L-Thyroxine)
(Leventa, Soloxine, Thyforon) **POM-V**

Formulations: Oral: 0.1 mg, 0.2 mg, 0.3 mg, 0.5 mg, 0.8 mg tablets; 1 mg/ml solution.

Action: Binds to specific intracellular receptors and alters gene expression.

Use: Treatment of hypothyroidism. In birds it is used to induce moult. Cases of pre-existing cardiac disorders require lower doses initially.

Safety and handling: Normal precautions should be observed.

Contraindications: Uncorrected adrenal insufficiency.

Adverse reactions: Clinical signs of overdosage include tachycardia, excitability, nervousness and excessive panting. Can unmask Addison's disease in patients with autoimmune polyglandular syndrome. May cause feather dystrophy if moult induced too quickly in birds.

Drug interactions: The actions of catecholamines and sympathomimetics are enhanced by thyroxine. Diabetic patients receiving thyroid hormones may have altered insulin requirements; monitor carefully during the initiation of therapy. Oestrogens may increase thyroid requirements by increasing thyroxine-binding globulin. The therapeutic effect of ciclosporin, digoxin and digitoxin may be reduced by thyroid hormones. Tachycardia and hypertension may develop when ketamine is given to patients receiving thyroid hormones. In addition many drugs may affect thyroid function tests and therefore monitoring of therapy.

DOSES
Dogs, Cats: 0.02–0.04 mg/kg/day. Alternatively dose at 0.5 mg/m^2 body surface area daily. **See Appendix for conversion of body weight to body surface area.** Dose given with food once or divided twice a day. Monitor serum T4 levels pre-dosing and 4–8 hours after dosing.
Small mammals: No information available.
Birds: 0.02 mg/kg p.o. q12–24h. Dissolve 1 mg in 28.4 ml water and give 0.4–0.5 ml/kg q12–24h.
Reptiles: Tortoises: 0.02 mg/kg p.o. q24–48h.

Lidocaine (Lignocaine)

(EMLA, Intubeaze, Lignadrin, Lignol, Locaine, Locovetic, Lidoderm*) **POM-V**

Formulations: Injectable: 1%, 2% solutions (some contain adrenaline). Topical: 2% solution (Intubeaze), 4% solution (Xylocaine); 2.5% cream with prilocaine (EMLA); 5% transdermal patches (Lidoderm).

Action: Local anaesthetic action is dependent on reversible blockade of the sodium channel, preventing propagation of an action potential along the nerve fibre. Sensory nerve fibres are blocked before motor nerve fibres, allowing a selective sensory blockade at low doses. Lidocaine also has class 1b antiarrhythmic actions, decreasing the rate of ventricular firing, action potential duration and absolute refractory period, and increasing relative refractory period. Lidocaine has a rapid onset of action and intermediate duration of action. Addition of adrenaline to lidocaine increases the duration of action by reducing the rate of systemic absorption.

Use: Provision of local or regional analgesia using perineural, infiltration, local i.v. or epidural techniques. Intratesticular lidocaine has been shown to reduce haemodynamic responses to castration in dogs and cats and is recommended to provide intraoperative analgesia during castration and reduce the requirement for inhalant anaesthetic agents. It is generally recommended that adrenaline-free solutions be used for epidural administration. Also used to provide systemic analgesia when given i.v. by continuous rate infusion. First-line therapy for rapid or haemodynamically significant ventricular arrhythmias. May also be effective for some supraventricular arrhythmias, such as bypass-mediated supraventricular tachycardia, and for cardioversion of acute-onset or vagally-mediated atrial fibrillation. Widely used topically to desensitize mucous membranes (such as the larynx prior to intubation). EMLA cream is used to anaesthetize the skin before vascular cannulation. It must be placed on the skin for approximately 45–60 min to ensure adequate anaesthesia; covering the skin with an occlusive dressing promotes absorption. EMLA is very useful to facilitate venous catheter placement in the ears of conscious rabbits and small puppies and kittens. The pharmacokinetics of transdermal lidocaine patches have been evaluated in dogs and cats; bioavailability of transdermal lidocaine is low in cats and dogs compared to humans. The analgesic efficacy and clinical usefulness of transdermal lidocaine has not yet been evaluated in either species. Infusions of lidocaine reduce the inhaled concentrations of anaesthetic required to produce anaesthesia and prevent central sensitization to surgical noxious stimuli. Systemic lidocaine is best used in combination with other analgesic drugs to achieve balanced analgesia. Lidocaine will accumulate after prolonged administration, leading to a delayed recovery. Cats are very sensitive to the toxic effects of local anaesthetics, therefore it is important that doses are calculated and administered accurately.

Safety and handling: Normal precautions should be observed.

Contraindications: Do not give to cats by continuous rate infusion during the perioperative period due to the negative haemodynamic effects. Do not give lidocaine solutions containing adrenaline i.v. Do not use solutions containing adrenaline for complete ring block of an extremity because of the danger of ischaemic necrosis. Do not use preparations with adrenaline in birds.

Adverse reactions: Depression, seizures, muscle fasciculations, vomiting, bradycardia and hypotension. If reactions are severe, decrease or discontinue administration. Seizures may be controlled with i.v. diazepam or pentobarbital. Monitor the ECG carefully during therapy. Cats tend to be more sensitive to the CNS effects. The CFC propellant used in unlicensed aerosol preparations (e.g. Xylocaine spray) is alleged to have caused laryngeal oedema in cats and should not be used to desensitize the larynx prior to intubation.

Drug interactions: Cimetidine and propranolol may prolong serum lidocaine clearance if administered concurrently. Other antiarrhythmics may cause increased myocardial depression.

DOSES
Note: 1 mg/kg is 0.05 ml/kg of a 2% solution.
Dogs:
- Local anaesthesia: Apply to the affected area with a small gauge needle to an appropriate volume. Total dose that should be injected is 4 mg/kg.
- Oesophagitis: 2 mg/kg p.o. q4–6h.
- Topical: Apply thick layer of cream to the skin and cover with a bandage for 45–60 min prior to venepuncture.
- Intraoperative analgesia given by constant rate infusion: 1 mg/kg loading dose (given slowly over 10–15 min) followed by 20–40 µg (micrograms)/kg/min. Postoperatively, similar dose rates can be used but should be adjusted according to pain assessment and be aware of the likelihood of accumulation allowing an empirical reduction in dose rate over time.
- Ventricular arrhythmias: 2–8 mg/kg i.v. in 2 mg/kg boluses followed by a constant rate i.v. infusion of 0.025–0.1 mg/kg/min.
Cats:
- Local anaesthesia, topical, oesophagitis: Doses as for dogs. Avoid systemic lidocaine for analgesia in cats due to the risk of drug accumulation, toxicity and negative haemodynamic effects.
- Ventricular arrhythmias: 0.25–2.0 mg/kg i.v. slowly in 0.25–0.5 mg/kg boluses followed by a constant rate i.v. infusion of 0.01–0.04 mg/kg/min.
Small mammals: Local anaesthesia: apply to the affected area with a small gauge needle to an appropriate volume. Total dose that should be injected is 1–3 mg/kg; doses >4 mg/kg should not be used.
Rabbits: 0.3 ml/kg for epidural anaesthesia; 1–2 mg/ml i.v. bolus for cardiac arrhythmias, 2–4 mg/ml intratracheal for cardiac arrhythmias. Topical: apply thick layer of cream to the skin and cover with a bandage for 45–60 min prior to venepuncture.

Birds: <4 mg/kg as local infusion/nerve block. Do not use preparations with adrenaline.
Reptiles: Local infiltration s.c. to effect. Dilute 1:1 with sterile water prior to injection in small species and do not exceed 5 mg/kg total dose per animal due to cardiotoxic side effects.

Lignocaine see Lidocaine

Lincomycin
(Lincocin, Lincoject) **POM-V**

Formulations: Injectable: 100 mg/ml solution for i.v. or i.m. use. Oral: powder for solution.

Action: Inhibition of bacterial protein synthesis. It is bacteriostatic or bactericidal, depending on the organism and drug concentration. Being a weak base, it is ion-trapped in fluid that is more acidic than plasma and therefore concentrates in prostatic fluid, milk and intracellular fluid.

Use: Active against Gram-positive cocci (including penicillin-resistant staphylococci) and many obligate anaerobes. The lincosamides (lincomycin and clindamycin) are particularly indicated for staphylococcal bone and joint infections. Clindamycin is more active than lincomycin, particularly against obligate anaerobes, and is better absorbed from the gut. Administer slowly if using i.v. route.

Safety and handling: Normal precautions should be observed.

Contraindications: Rapid i.v. administration should be avoided since this can result in collapse due to cardiac depression and peripheral neuromuscular blockade. Do not use lincosamides in rabbits, guinea pigs, chinchillas and hamsters.

Adverse reactions: Human patients on lincomycin may develop colitis. Although not a major veterinary problem, patients developing diarrhoea (particularly if it is haemorrhagic) whilst taking the medication should be monitored carefully. Toxicity is a possibility in patients with liver disease; weigh the risk *versus* the potential benefits before use of this drug in such patients. In rabbits, guinea pigs, chinchillas and hamsters death can occur due to overgrowth of toxin-producing strains of *Clostridium*. May be nephrotoxic in reptiles.

Drug interactions: The action of neuromuscular blocking agents may be enhanced if given with lincomycin. The absorption of lincomycin may be reduced by kaolin. Lincosamide antimicrobials should not be used in combination with chloramphenicols or macrolides as these combinations are antagonistic.

DOSES

See Appendix for guidelines on responsible antibacterial use.

Dogs, Cats: Parenteral: 22 mg/kg i.m. q24h or 11 mg/kg i.m. q12h or 11–22 mg/kg slow i.v. q12–24h. Oral: 22 mg/kg p.o. q12h or 15 mg/kg p.o. q8h.

Small mammals: Ferrets: 11 mg/kg p.o. q8h. Rabbits, Chinchillas, Guinea pigs, Hamsters: Do not use.

Birds: 50–75 mg/kg p.o., i.m. q12h. Pigeons: Lincomycin/spectinomycin preparation: 500–750 mg combined activity/l water.

Reptiles: 5 mg/kg i.m. q12–24h.

Liothyronine (T3, L-Tri-iodothyronine)
POM

Formulations: Oral: 20 µg tablets.

Action: Increases T3 concentrations.

Use: Treatment of hypothyroidism where levothyroxine has been unsuccessful, and in the diagnosis of feline hyperthyroidism (T3 suppression test).

Safety and handling: Normal precautions should be observed.

Contraindications: No information available.

Adverse reactions: Signs of overdosage include tachycardia, excitability, nervousness and excessive panting.

Drug interactions: The actions of catecholamines and sympathomimetics are enhanced by thyroxine. Diabetic patients receiving thyroid hormones may have altered insulin requirements; monitor carefully during the initiation of therapy. Oestrogens may increase thyroid requirements by increasing thyroxine-binding globulin. The therapeutic effect of digoxin and digitoxin may be reduced by thyroid hormones. Tachycardia and hypertension may develop when ketamine is given to patients receiving thyroid hormones. In addition many drugs may affect thyroid function tests and therefore monitoring of therapy.

DOSES

Dogs: Treatment of hypothyroidism: 2–6 µg (micrograms)/kg p.o. q8–12h.

Cats: T3 suppression test: Administer 20 µg (micrograms)/cat p.o. q8h for 7 doses.

Small mammals, Birds, Reptiles: No information available.

Lipid infusions
(ClinOleic*, Intralipid*, Ivelip*, Lipidem*, Lipofundin*, Omegaven*) **POM**

Formulations: Injectable: 10% solution contains soya oil emulsion, glycerol, purified egg phospholipids and phosphate (15 mmol/l) for i.v. use only. Contains 2 kcal/ml (8.4 kJ/ml), 268 mOsm/l. Other human products available and vary in composition.

Action: Support intermediary metabolism, reverse negative energy balance and provide some essential fatty acids.

Use: Used parenterally in animals receiving nutritional support, to provide fat for energy production and essential fatty acids for cellular metabolism and support of the immune system. Can also be used to bind lipid-soluble toxins such as unintentional intravenous administration of bupivacaine or avermectins. Lipid emulsions are isosmolar with plasma and can be infused into a peripheral vein to provide parenteral nutrition. Due to the complex requirements of providing i.v. nutrition, including careful patient monitoring and the need for strict aseptic practice, in all cases product literature and specialist advice should be consulted. Use with caution in patients with known insulin resistance or at risk for developing pancreatitis. See also Amino acid solutions and Glucose.

Safety and handling: Do not use if separation of the emulsion occurs.

Contraindications: Insulin resistance (e.g. diabetes mellitus) and hyperlipidaemia.

Adverse reactions: Reactions include occasional febrile episodes mainly seen with 20% emulsions. 20% and 30% lipid products have a higher rate of complications including vasculitis, thrombosis, fever and other metabolic complications and are not recommended. Rare anaphylactic responses are reported in humans. Early reports of hepatic failure, pancreatitis, cardiac arrest and thrombocytopenia detailed in human literature appear to have been complications of prolonged treatment.

Drug interactions: Consult specific product data sheet(s). Lines for i.v. parenteral feeding (lipid, glucose, amino acids or nutrient admixtures) should be dedicated for that use alone and should not be used for administration of other medications. Interference with biochemical measurements, such as those for blood gases and calcium, may occur if samples are taken before fat has been cleared. Daily checks are necessary to ensure complete clearance from the plasma in conditions where fat metabolism may be disturbed. Additives may only be mixed with fat emulsions where compatibility is known. See Amino acid solutions for additional information.

DOSES

Dogs: The amount required will be governed by the patient's physiological status and whether partial or total parenteral nutrition is provided. Generally lipid infusions are used to supply 30% (partial peripheral) to 40–60% of energy requirements.

Cats: The amount required will be governed by the patient's physiological status and its tolerance of lipids. Generally peripheral parenteral nutrition is provided by amino acids in cats and lipids are used as an energy source in a nutrient admixture for infusion through central venous access (total parenteral nutrition) to supply 40–60% of energy requirements.

Dogs, Cats: For treatment of lipid-soluble toxicosis such as ivermectin or moxidectin toxicosis, administer 1.5–5 ml/kg i.v. of 20% lipid solution as bolus, followed by 0.25–0.50 ml/kg/min i.v. infusion for 30–60 min. Boluses of 1.5 ml/kg can be repeated. Infusions of 0.5 ml/kg/min can be administered for a maximum of 24h.

Small mammals, Birds, Reptiles: No information available.

Lithium carbonate

(Camcolit*, Liskonum*, Priadel*) **POM**

Formulations: Oral: 250 mg, 400 mg tablets.

Action: Stimulates bone marrow stem cells, causing an increase in the production of haemopoietic cell lines, particularly granulocytes.

Use: Treatment of idiopathic aplastic anaemia, cytotoxic drug-induced neutropenia or thrombocytopenia, oestrogen-induced bone marrow suppression and cyclic haemopoiesis. There is a lag phase of up to 4 weeks before its effects may be seen. Experimental studies show that lithium may prevent neutropenia associated with cytotoxic drugs when administered concomitantly; clinical trials showing this are lacking. The recommended serum lithium concentration is 0.5–1.8 mmol/l; assess every 3 months if possible.

Safety and handling: Normal precautions should be observed.

Contraindications: Avoid in patients with renal impairment (nephrotoxic at high doses), cardiac disease and conditions with sodium imbalance (e.g. hypoadrenocorticism). Do not use in cats.

Adverse reactions: Nausea, diarrhoea, muscle weakness, fatigue, polyuria and polydipsia. Seizures are reported. The release of T3 and T4 may be blocked by lithium; assess thyroid status every 6 months. Lithium is toxic to cats.

Drug interactions: The excretion of lithium may be reduced by ACE inhibitors, loop diuretics, NSAIDs and thiazides, thus increasing the risk of toxicity. Lithium toxicity is made worse by sodium depletion; avoid concurrent use with diuretics. The excretion of lithium may be increased by theophylline. Lithium antagonizes the effects of neostigmine and pyridostigmine. Neurotoxicity may occur if lithium is administered with diltiazem or verapamil.

DOSES
Dogs: 10 mg/kg p.o. q12h.
Cats: Do not use.
Small mammals, Birds, Reptiles: No information available.

Liquid paraffin see Paraffin

Lomustine (CCNU)
(Lomustine*) **POM**

Formulations: Oral: 40 mg capsule.

Action: Interferes with the synthesis and function of DNA, RNA and proteins. Antitumour activity correlates best with formation of interstrand crosslinking of DNA. Lomustine is highly lipid-soluble, allowing rapid transport across the blood-brain barrier.

Use: Treatment of primary and metastatic brain tumours in humans. Its use in animals is less well defined but has been reported to have some efficacy in the treatment of brain tumours, mast cell tumours, refractory lymphoma, histiocytic sarcoma and epitheliotrophic lymphoma. *S*-Adenosylmethionine and silybin may be used to prevent or treat lomustine hepatotoxicity.

Safety and handling: Cytotoxic drug: see Appendix and specialist texts for further advice on chemotherapeutic agents.

Contraindications: Bone marrow suppression. Pre-existing liver disease.

Adverse reactions: Myelosuppression is the dose-limiting toxicity, with neutropenia developing 7 days after administration. Neutropenia may be severe and life-threatening at the higher end of the dose range in some dogs. Thrombocytopenia can also be seen, often with no other concurrent cytopenias. GI and cumulative dose-related and potentially irreversible hepatic toxicity have been reported in the dog.

Drug interactions: Do not use with other myelosuppressive agents. Lomustine requires hepatic microsomal enzyme hydroxylation for the production of antineoplastic metabolites. It should be used with caution in dogs being treated with agents that induce liver enzyme activity, e.g. phenobarbital. In humans cimetidine enhances the toxicity of lomustine.

DOSES
See Appendix for chemotherapy protocols and conversion of body weight to body surface area.
Dogs: 60–90 mg/m^2 p.o. q21d.
Cats: A dose of 50–60 mg/m^2 p.o. q21d has been suggested but is not well established. If using this drug in the cat, specialist advise should be sought, as dosing intervals may need to be increased to 6 weeks.

Small mammals: Ferrets: anecdotally used in lymphoma at doses extrapolated from cats.

Birds, Reptiles: No information available.

Loperamide

(Diareze*, Imodium*, Norimode*) **POM, P, GSL**

Formulations: Oral: 2 mg capsule (Diareze, Imodium, Norimode); 0.2 mg/ml syrup (Imodium).

Action: Opioid agonist that alters GI motility by acting on receptors in the myenteric plexus. It normally has no central action.

Use: Management of non-specific acute and chronic diarrhoea, and irritable bowel syndrome. Use with care in cats. Used in birds for cerebral oedema and anuric renal failure.

Safety and handling: Normal precautions should be observed.

Contraindications: Intestinal obstruction. Do not use in dogs likely to be ivermectin-sensitive, e.g. collies. The mutation of the multiple drug resistance (MDR) gene in these dogs allows loperamide (a P-glycoprotein substrate) to penetrate the CNS and cause profound sedation.

Adverse reactions: Constipation will occur in some cases. In cats excitability may be seen.

Drug interactions: No information available.

DOSES

Dogs, Cats: 0.04–0.2 mg/kg p.o. q8–12h.
Small mammals: Ferrets: 0.2 mg/kg p.o. q12h; Rabbits: 0.04–0.2 mg/kg p.o. q8–12h. Should only be used for symptomatic treatment of severe GI motility problems in rabbits and for as short a period as possible to avoid GI stasis.
Birds, Reptiles: No information available.

Loratadine

(Loratadine*) **GSL**

Formulations: Oral: 10 mg tablet; 1 mg/ml syrup.

Action: Binds to H1 histamine receptors preventing histamine from binding.

Use: Management of allergic disease. Specific doses for dogs and cats have not been determined by pharmokinetic studies. Use with caution in cases with urinary retention, angle-closure glaucoma and pyloroduodenal obstruction.

Safety and handling: Normal precautions should be observed.

Contraindications: No information available.

Adverse reactions: May cause mild sedation. May reduce seizure threshold.

Drug interactions: No information available.

DOSES
Dogs: 5–15 mg q24h.
Cats, Small mammals, Birds, Reptiles: No information available.

Lorazepam
(Ativan*, Intensol*) **POM**

Formulations: Oral: 1 mg tablets; 2 mg/ml suspension. Injectable: 4 mg/ml solution.

Action: Increases the activity of GABA (a major inhibitory transmitter) within the CNS, resulting in anxiolysis.

Use: Short-term management of anxiety disorders in dogs and cats. This may be necessary during a long-term behavioural therapy programme to avoid relapses due to exposure to an intensely fear-inducing stimulus during treatment. However, as benzodiazepines may inhibit memory, their routine use as part of a behaviour plan is not recommended unless under careful management. Withdrawal of treatment should be gradual, as acute withdrawal may result in signs of tremor and inappetence.

Safety and handling: Normal precautions should be observed.

Contraindications: Glaucoma, significant liver or kidney disease, hypersensitivity to benzodiazepines. Not recommended in pregnant or lactating animals.

Adverse reactions: A general concern with benzodiazepines concerns disinhibition and the subsequent emergence of aggression. Drowsiness and mild transient incoordination may develop.

Drug interactions: Caution is advised if used in association with antifungals such as itraconazole which inhibit its metabolism.

DOSES
Dogs, Cats: 0.02–0.1 mg/kg p.o. q12–24h; start at lower dose and gradually increase.
Small mammals, Birds, Reptiles: No information available.

Lufenuron
(Program, Program plus) **POM-V**

Formulations: Oral: 67.8 mg, 204.9 mg, 409.8 mg tablets (Program); 46 mg, 115 mg, 230 mg, 460 mg lufeneron with milbemycin (ratio of 20 mg lufeneron: 1 mg milbemycin) tablets (Program plus); 133 mg,

266 mg suspension (Program for cats). Injectable: 40 mg, 80 mg as 100 mg/ml suspension (Program).

Action: Inhibition of chitin synthetase leads to a failure of chitin production which means that flea eggs fail to hatch.

Use: Prevention of flea infestation (*Ctenocephalides felis*, *C. canis*). For treatment of flea infestations the additional use of an approved adulticide is recommended. All animals in the household should be treated. Lufenuron has an additional antifungal action but specific doses for the effective treatment of dermatophytosis are currently unknown. Lufenuron + milbemycin (Program plus) is also indicated for prevention of heart worms (*Dirofilaria immitis* and adult *Ancylostoma caninum*, *Toxacara canis* and *Trichuris vulpis*) in dogs. Tablets/suspension should be administered with food. Can be administered during pregnancy and lactation (Program). Can be administered to puppies from 2 weeks or >1 kg (Program plus); no information about pregnancy or lactation.

Safety and handling: Normal precautions should be observed.

Contraindications: No information available.

Adverse reactions: No information available.

Drug interactions: No information available.

DOSES
Dogs: 10 mg/kg p.o., s.c. q1month (equivalent to a dose of 0.5 mg/kg milbemycin in combined preparations).
Cats: 10 mg/kg s.c. q6months or 30 mg/kg p.o. q1month.
Small mammals: Ferrets: 30–45 mg/kg p.o. q1month.
Birds, Reptiles: No information available.

Lysine (L-Lysine)
(Enisyl) **GSL**

Formulations: Oral: 250 mg/ml paste in 100 ml bottle; 250 mg, 500 mg capsules.

Action: Antagonizes arginine, which is required for viral replication.

Use: Management of human herpes simplex and has been used in the management of feline herpesvirus-1 infection. Dietary lysine supplementation is used in an attempt to suppress FHV-1 infection and reactivation. However, there is limited clinical evidence regarding its efficacy in treating FHV-1. Cats are very sensitive to arginine deficiency and dietary arginine must not be reduced.

Safety and handling: Normal precautions should be observed.

Contraindications: Do not use preparations containing propylene glycol as they may be toxic to cats.

Adverse reactions: Diarrhoea may be seen.

Drug interactions: No information available.

DOSES
Dogs: Not applicable.
Cats: Adults: 500 mg p.o. q12h (equivalent to 2 ml/2 pumps q12h); Kittens: 250 mg p.o. q12h (equivalent to 1 ml/1 pump q12h).
Small mammals, Birds, Reptiles: No information available.

Magnesium salts
(Magnesium sulphate injection BP (Vet) 25% w/v)
POM-VPS, POM

Formulations: Injectable: 25% w/v, 50% w/v solutions containing 1 mEq and 2 mEq magnesium per ml. Dilute to a 20% or lower solution prior to use.

Action: Critical role in muscular excitement and neurological transmission. It is a cofactor in a variety of enzyme systems and maintenance of ionic gradients.

Use: Emergency treatment of serious arrhythmias, especially in the presence of hypokalaemia (when hypomagnesaemia may be present) and severe hypertension in humans. In animals magnesium salts may be used to treat unresponsive ventricular arrhythmias. They have also been used as infusions and orally to treat hypomagnesaemia. Reduce i.v. potassium supplementation to avoid hyperkalaemia. Monitoring of serum magnesium is essential: 30–35% is bound to protein and the remainder is free as the ionized form. Magnesium is compatible in solution with 5% dextrose and calcium gluconate. Treatment of potential overdose or complications should be anticipated and ventilatory support and i.v. calcium gluconate may be required. Product information should be consulted on an individual case basis.

Safety and handling: Normal precautions should be observed.

Contraindications: Do not use in patients with heart block or myocardial damage. Do not use in renal impairment or failure (magnesium is excreted by the kidneys at a rate proportional to serum levels).

Adverse reactions: Somnolence, CNS depression and possibly coma, muscular weakness, bradycardia, hypotension, respiratory depression and prolonged Q-T intervals have been seen, typically following overdosage. Very high levels can cause neuromuscular blockade and cardiac arrest.

Drug interactions: Additive effects can be seen with other CNS depressants including barbiturates and general anaesthetics. Do not use with non-depolarizing neuromuscular blocking agents because of the risk of severe neuromuscular blockage. Because serious conduction disturbances can occur, use with extreme caution with digitalis glycosides.

DOSES
Dogs, Cats:
- Life-threatening ventricular arrhythmia: 0.15–0.3 mEq/kg i.v. administered over 5–15 min.
- Magnesium replacement: 0.75–1.0 mEq/kg/day by continuous rate infusion in 5% dextrose has been advocated for the first 24–48 hours, followed by a lower dose of 0.3–0.5 mEq/kg/day for 3–5 days to allow complete repletion of magnesium stores.

Small mammals, Birds, Reptiles: No information available.

Mannitol (Cordycepic acid)
(Mannitol*) **POM**

Formulations: Injectable: 10%, 20% solutions.

Action: Mannitol is an inert sugar alcohol that acts as an osmotic diuretic.

Use: Reduction of intracranial pressure (most effective in acute elevations of intracranial pressure), treatment of acute glaucoma and may also be used in the treatment of oliguric renal failure. Reduction in intracranial and intraocular fluid pressure occurs within 15 minutes of the start of a mannitol infusion and lasts for 3–8 hours after the infusion is discontinued; diuresis occurs after 1–3 hours. A 5.07% solution in water is isosmotic with serum. It is recommended that an in-line filter be used when infusing concentrated mannitol. There is some evidence that bolus administration (over 20–30 minutes) may be more effective for reduction of intracranial pressure than continuous administration. When used as treatment for raised intracranial pressure, hypovolaemia should be avoided to maintain cerebral perfusion pressure.

Safety and handling: Any crystals that have formed during storage should be dissolved by warming prior to use. The formation of crystals is a particular problem with the 20% formulations, which are supersaturated.

Contraindications: Prolonged administration may lead to the accumulation of mannitol in the brain and worsening of the cerebral oedema and raised intracranial pressure. Use with care in intracranial haemorrhage (except during intracranial surgery), take care to avoid volume overload in generalized oedema, severe congestive heart failure, pulmonary oedema or anuric renal failure (before rehydration).

Adverse reactions: The most common adverse reactions seen are fluid and electrolyte imbalances. Infusion of high doses may result in circulatory overload and acidosis. Thrombophlebitis may occur and extravasation of the solution may cause oedema and skin necrosis. Mannitol causes diarrhoea if given orally. Rarely mannitol may cause acute renal failure in human patients.

Drug interactions: Diuretic-induced hypokalaemia may occur when ACE inhibitors are used with potassium-depleting diuretics. Concurrent use of potassium-depleting diuretics should be used with care in conjunction with beta-blockers. Nephrotoxicity has been described with concurrent use of mannitol and ciclosporin in human patients. Mannitol may result in temporary impairment of the blood-brain barrier for up to 30 min after administration of high doses. Mannitol should never be added to whole blood for transfusion or given through the same set by which the blood is being infused. Do not add KCl or NaCl to concentrated mannitol solutions (20% or 25%) as a precipitate may form.

DOSES

Dogs, Cats:
- Raised intracranial pressure: 0.25–2 g/kg i.v. infusion of 15–20% solution. There is some evidence that higher doses have greater clinical effect, but lower doses allow for repeated boluses. Doses of 0.25–1.0 g/kg are recommended. The dose is given over 20–30 min. The dose may be repeated once or twice after 4–8 h as long as hydration and electrolyte levels are monitored. Rebound increases in intracranial or intraocular pressure may occur.
- Acute glaucoma: 1–2 g/kg i.v. infusion over 30 min. Withhold water for the first few hours after administering. May repeat 2–4 times over next 48 hours; monitor for dehydration.
- Early oliguric renal failure (as an alternative to using furosemide and dopamine): 0.25–0.5 g/kg i.v. infusion over 5–10 min. Rehydrate the patient prior to the use of mannitol.

Small mammals: Ferrets: 0.5–1.0 g/kg i.v. infusion over 20 min.

Birds: Acute renal failure and cerebral oedema: 0.2–2 mg/kg slow i.v.

Reptiles: No information available.

Marbofloxacin

(Aurizon, Efex, Marbocyl, Marboxidin, Marfloquin, Softiflox, Ubiflox) **POM-V**

Formulations: Injectable: 200 mg powder for reconstitution giving 10 mg/ml when reconstituted. Oral: 5 mg, 20 mg, 80 mg tablets. Topical: Compound preparation containing 3 mg/ml of marbofloxacin along with clotrimazole and dexamethasone (aural use).

Action: Broad-spectrum bactericidal antibiotic inhibiting bacterial DNA gyrase. The bactericidal effect is concentration-dependent particularly against Gram-negative bacteria, meaning that pulse-dosing regimens may be effective. Low urinary pH may reduce the activity.

Use: Ideally fluoroquinolone use should be reserved for infections where culture and sensitivity testing predicts a clinical response and where first- and second-line antimicrobials would not be effective. Active against mycoplasmas and many Gram-positive and particularly Gram-negative organisms, including *Pasteurella*, *Staphylococcus*, *Pseudomonas aeruginosa*, *Klebsiella*, *Escherichia coli*, *Proteus* and *Salmonella*. Fluoroquinolones are effective against beta-lactamase-producing bacteria. Marbofloxacin is relatively ineffective in treating obligate anaerobic infections. Fluoroquinolones are highly lipophilic drugs that attain high concentrations within cells in many tissues and are particularly effective in the management of soft tissue, urogenital (including prostatitis) and skin infections.

Safety and handling: Normal precautions should be observed.

Contraindications: The 20 mg and 80 mg tablets should not be administered to cats.

Adverse reactions: Some animals show GI signs (nausea, vomiting). Use with caution in epileptics until further information is available, as fluoroquinolones potentiate CNS adverse effects when administered concurrently with NSAIDs in humans. High doses of enrofloxacin have resulted in reports of retinal blindness in cats. Although not reported with marbofloxacin, caution should be exercised before using dose rates above those recommended by the manufacturer for cats. Cartilage abnormalities have been reported following the use of other fluoroquinolones in growing animals. Such abnormalities have not been specifically reported following the use of marbofloxacin, but the drug is not authorized for use in dogs <12 months of age and cats <16 weeks. In giant breeds should not be administered to animals <18 months.

Drug interactions: Adsorbents and antacids containing cations (Mg^{2+}, Al^{3+}) may bind to fluoroquinolones, preventing their absorption from the GI tract. The absorption of fluoroquinolones may be inhibited by sucralfate and zinc salts; doses should be at least 2 hours apart. Enrofloxacin increases plasma theophylline concentrations. Preliminary data suggest this may not be clinically significant with marbofloxacin unless used in patients with renal insufficiency. Cimetidine may reduce the clearance of fluoroquinolones and should be used with caution in combination.

DOSES
See Appendix for guidelines on responsible antibacterial use.
Dogs: Oral and parenteral: 2 mg/kg i.v., s.c., p.o. q24h. Topical: 10 drops per ear once daily.
Cats: 2 mg/kg i.v., s.c., p.o. q24h.
Small mammals: 2–5 mg/kg p.o., s.c., i.m. q24h.
Birds: 10 mg/kg p.o., i.m., i.v. q24h.
Reptiles: 10 mg/kg s.c., i.m., p.o. q48h.

Maropitant
(Cerenia) **POM-V**

Formulations: Injectable: 10 mg/ml solution. Oral: 16 mg, 24 mg, 60 mg, 160 mg tablets.

Action: Inhibits vomiting reflex by blocking NK-1 receptors in medullary vomiting centre. A high degree of protein binding gives a long duration of activity (24 hours). Maropitant is not known to have any prokinetic effect.

Use: Treatment and prevention of vomiting in dogs, including that caused by chemotherapy and motion sickness. There have been no studies in feline clinical patients. However, the manufacturer has conducted a number of studies on cats from which it can be concluded that maropitant is well tolerated and has potent antiemetic activity in cats. In cases of frequent vomiting, treatment by injection is recommended. Treatment by injection and/or tablets can be given for up to 5 days. If used chronically, a rest period of 2 days after every 5 doses is suggested. In some individual dogs, repeat treatment at a lower dose may be adequate. Maropitant is more effective if used pre-emptively for chemotherapy-induced emesis, but should be given at least 1 hour in advance, and may even be given the night before. For motion sickness, treatment for up to 2 days can be given. If longer periods of treatment are required the recommended interval between the last dose of one course and the first dose of a subsequent course is 72 hours. It should be used in combination with investigation into the cause of vomiting and with other supportive measures and specific treatments.

Safety and handling: Normal precautions should be observed.

Contraindications: No specific contraindications but it would be sensible not to use maropitant where GI obstruction or perforation is present or for longer than 48 hours without a definitive diagnosis.

Adverse reactions: Transient pain reaction during injection is reported as a rare occurrence, but no significant lasting adverse reactions. Very high doses in cats may cause haemolysis.

Drug interactions: No compatibility studies exist, and therefore the injection should not be mixed with any other agent.

DOSES
Dogs, Cats: 1 mg/kg s.c. q24h or 2 mg/kg p.o. q24h. For prevention of motion sickness, tablets at a dose rate of 8 mg/kg q24h for a maximum of 2 days are indicated.
Small mammals, Birds, Reptiles: No information available.

Masitinib mesylate
(Masivet) **POM-V**

Formulations: Oral: 50 mg, 150 mg film-coated tablets.

Action: Protein tyrosine kinase inhibitor, which showed *in vitro* selectively and effectively highest affinity for mutated forms of the c-KIT tyrosine kinase receptor. Tyrosine kinase inhibitors block the TK receptor pathways essential for cell replication.

Use: Treatment of dogs with non-resectable mast cell tumours (grade 2 or 3), preferably with a confirmed mutated c-KIT tyrosine kinase receptor. Studies indicate that masitinib may be useful for the treatment of some dogs with atopic dermatitis. Preliminary studies have investigated safety in healthy cats, but this drug is not licensed in this species and further clinical trials are likely to be required. Patients should be monitored closely during treatment. As a guideline urinalysis, haematology and biochemistry should be undertaken before starting therapy, and then at least once a month (some clinicians may also check these parameters 1 week after drug initiation). Full coagulation profiles and faecal occult blood tests should be undertaken if adverse clinical signs are witnessed. It is good practice to contact owners once a week for the first 6 weeks of therapy to check for potential side effects, so that prompt action can be taken if these occur. Use with caution if pre-existing renal or hepatic dysfunction is present.

Safety and handling: Cytotoxic drug; see Appendix or specialist texts for further advice on chemotherapeutic agents.

Contraindications: Do not use in pregnant or lactating bitches, in dogs <6 months old, in dogs <4 kg, if there are any pre-existing signs of myelosuppression, or if the patient has shown previous hypersensitivity to masitinib.

Adverse reactions: Mild to moderate GI reactions (diarrhoea, vomiting) and hair coat changes/hair loss are common. Renal toxicity, anaemia, protein loss, myelosuppression, increased liver enzyme activity, lethargy, cough and lymphadenomegaly have also been described.

Drug interactions: Concurrent use of drugs that are highly protein bound or interact with the cytochrome P450 enzyme pathway may increase the risk of adverse side effects.

DOSES
See Appendix for chemotherapy protocols.
Dogs: 11–14 mg/kg p.o. q24h.
Cats, Small mammals, Birds, Reptiles: No information available.

Mavacoxib
(Trocoxil) **POM-V**

Formulations: Oral: 6 mg, 20 mg, 30 mg, 75 mg, 95 mg chewable tablets.

Action: Selectively inhibits COX-2 enzyme, thereby limiting the production of prostaglandins involved in inflammation. The prolonged duration of action of mavacoxib means that animals should be carefully evaluated for their suitability for NSAID therapy before the onset of treatment.

Use: Treatment of pain and inflammation associated with degenerative joint disease in dogs at least 12 months old in cases where continuous treatment exceeding 1 month is indicated. Continuous treatment may have the potential to reduce central sensitization and breakthrough pain. Approximately 5% of dogs are poor metabolizers of mavacoxib. The treatment regimen recommended below is designed to prevent drug accumulation in this sub-population of animals. Preliminary clinical evidence suggests that treatment can be re-started after a 1-month break from dosing. No recommendations have yet been made regarding whether to give a loading dose (first and second doses separated by 14 days) each time treatment is re-started. If necessary, analgesia should be provided in the 1-month break from treatment using a different class of drug.

Safety and handling: Normal precautions should be observed.

Contraindications: Do not give to dehydrated, hypovolaemic or hypotensive patients or those with GI disease or blood clotting problems. Administration of mavacoxib to animals with renal disease must be carefully evaluated. Liver disease prolongs the metabolism of mavacoxib, leading to the potential for drug accumulation and overdose with repeated dosing, therefore use is not recommended. Do not give to pregnant animals or animals <12 months or <5 kg.

Adverse reactions: Should an animal require anaesthesia or develop any illness while receiving mavacoxib, then care must be taken to avoid dehydration, hypotension and hypovolaemia, and prompt intervention to manage these conditions should be implemented if they occur. Although the duration of action of mavacoxib is prolonged, symptomatic management of any side effects associated with drug administration is recommended only until the clinical signs resolve. There is a small risk that NSAIDs may precipitate cardiac failure in animals with cardiovascular disease.

Drug interactions: Do not administer concurrently with other NSAIDs and glucocorticoids. Do not administer another NSAID within 1 month of dosing with mavacoxib. Do not administer with other potentially nephrotoxic agents, e.g. aminoglycosides.

DOSES
Dogs: 2 mg/kg p.o. q14d for 2 doses then q1month for a total maximum of 7 doses. Should be given immediately before or with the dog's main meal.
Cats: Do not use.
Small mammals, Birds, Reptiles: Administration is not recommended.

Medetomidine
(Domitor, Dorbene, Dormilan, Medetor, Sedastart, Sedator, Sededorm) **POM-V**

Formulations: Injectable: 1 mg/ml solution.

Action: Agonist at peripheral and central alpha-2 adrenoreceptors producing dose-dependent sedation, muscle relaxation and analgesia.

Use: Provides sedation and premedication when used alone or in combination with opioid analgesics. Medetomidine combined with ketamine is used to provide a short duration (20–30 min) of surgical anaesthesia. Specificity for the alpha-2 receptor is greater for medetomidine than for xylazine, but is lower than for dexmedetomidine. Medetomidine is a potent drug that causes marked changes in the cardiovascular system including an initial peripheral vasoconstriction that results in an increase in blood pressure and a compensatory bradycardia. After 20–30 min vasoconstriction wanes, while blood pressure returns to normal values. Heart rate remains low due to the central sympatholytic effect of alpha-2 agonists. These cardiovascular changes result in a fall in cardiac output; central organ perfusion is well maintained at the expense of redistribution of blood flow away from the peripheral tissues. Respiratory system function is well maintained; respiration rate may fall but is accompanied by an increased depth of respiration. Oxygen supplementation is advisable in all animals. The duration of analgesia from a 10 μg/kg dose is approximately 1 hour. Combining medetomidine with an opioid provides improved analgesia and sedation. Lower doses of medetomidine should be used in combination with other drugs. Reversal of sedation or premedication with atipamezole shortens the recovery period, which may be advantageous. Analgesia should be provided with other classes of drugs before atipamezole. The authorized dose range of medetomidine for dogs and cats is very broad. High doses (>20 μg/kg) are associated with greater physiological disturbances than doses between 5–20 μg/kg. Using medetomidine in combination with other drugs in the lower dose range can provide good sedation and analgesia with minimal side effects. Similarly to dexmedetomidine, medetomidine may be used in low doses to manage excitation during recovery from anaesthesia and to provide perioperative analgesia when administered by continuous rate infusion.

Safety and handling: Normal precautions should be observed.

Contraindications: Do not use in animals with cardiovascular or other systemic disease. Use in geriatric patients is not advisable. Do not use in pregnant animals. Do not use when vomiting is contraindicated. Not recommended in diabetic animals.

Adverse reactions: Causes diuresis by suppressing ADH secretion, a transient increase in blood glucose by decreasing endogenous insulin secretion, mydriasis and decreased intraocular pressure. Vomiting after i.m. administration is common, so medetomidine should be avoided when vomiting is contraindicated (e.g. foreign body, raised intraocular pressure). Due to effects on blood glucose, use in diabetic animals is not recommended. Spontaneous arousal from deep sedation following stimulation can occur with all alpha-2 agonists; aggressive animals sedated with medetomidine must still be managed with caution.

Drug interactions: When used for premedication, medetomidine will significantly reduce the dose of all other anaesthetic agents required to maintain anaesthesia. Drugs for induction of anaesthesia should be given slowly and to effect to avoid inadvertent overdose, the dose of volatile agent required to maintain anaesthesia can be reduced by up to 70%. Do not use in patients likely to require or receiving sympathomimetic amines.

DOSES
When used for sedation is generally given as part of a combination. See Appendix for sedation protocols in all species.
Dogs, Cats: Premedication: 5–20 μg (micrograms)/kg i.v., i.m, s.c. in combination with an opioid. Use lower end of dose range i.v. Doses

of 1–2 µg/kg i.v. can be used to manage excitation in the recovery period, although following administration animals must be monitored carefully. A continuous rate infusion of 2–4 µg/kg/h can be used to provide perioperative analgesia and rousable sedation, particularly when administered as an adjunct to opioid-mediated analgesia.
Small mammals: Ferrets: 80–100 µg (micrograms)/kg i.m., s.c. in combination with an opioid and ketamine; Rabbits: 100–300 µg/kg i.v., i.m., s.c. (use the lower end of the dose range when giving i.v.) in combination with an opioid and ketamine; Rodents: Doses from 100–200 µg/kg i.p., i.m., s.c. in combination with ketamine and/or opioids or as premedication prior to induction with a volatile anaesthetic.
Birds: See Appendix.
Reptiles: 100–200 µg (micrograms)/kg i.m; may be combined with 5–10 mg/kg ketamine to provide light anaesthesia.

Medroxyprogesterone
(Promone-E) **POM-V**

Formulations: Injectable: 50 mg/ml suspension. Oral: 5 mg tablet.

Action: Alters the transcription of DNA leading to alterations in cellular metabolism which mimic progesterone.

Use: Feline psychogenic alopecia, dermatitis and eosinophilic keratitis, to decrease libido in male dogs, to manage prostatic hypertrophy (although other drugs are better and safer), and to control oestrus in the bitch and queen. Used in birds to manage feather plucking. When used in the management of feline skin disease, ensure effective topical and environmental parasite controls are instituted before considering progestogen therapy. Because of adrenocortical suppression, rapid withdrawal of the drug without adequate glucocorticoid cover is not advisable.

Safety and handling: Normal precautions should be observed.

Contraindications: Not recommended for treatment of behavioural disorders in cats and dogs, specifically feline spraying. Do not use in pregnancy or diabetes mellitus.

Adverse reactions: Temperament changes (listlessness and depression), increased thirst or appetite, cystic endometrial hyperplasia/pyometra, diabetes mellitus, adrenocortical suppression, reduced libido (males), mammary enlargement/neoplasia and lactation. As progestogens may cause elevated levels of growth hormone in the dog, acromegaly may develop. Subcutaneous injections may cause a permanent local alopecia, skin atrophy and depigmentation. There are many side effects in birds including liver damage, obesity and diabetes mellitus.

Drug interactions: No information available.

DOSES

Dogs:
- Prevention of oestrus in bitches: 2–3 mg/kg s.c. (>12 kg). Inject 6–8 weeks before oestrus is due. Repeat every 5 months.
- Interruption of oestrus: Once pro-oestral bleeding has started, 10 mg/dog p.o. q24h for 4 days then 5 mg/dog p.o. q24h for 12 days. Use a doubled dose for bitches >15 kg.
- Prostatic hypertrophy: 50–100 mg/dog s.c. every 3–6 months.

Cats:
- Psychogenic dermatitis: 10 mg/kg s.c. q3months prn.
- Prevention of oestrus: 5 mg/cat/week commencing in dioestrus or anoestrus.

Small mammals: No information available.

Birds: Persistent ovulation, Feather plucking, Sexual behavioural problems: 5–50 mg/kg i.m. Repeat in 4–6 weeks if necessary.

Reptiles: No information available.

Megestrol (Megoestrol acetate)
(Ovarid) **POM-V**

Formulations: Oral: 5 mg, 20 mg tablets.

Action: Alters the transcription of DNA, leading to alterations in cellular metabolism which mimic progesterone.

Use: Prevention and postponement of oestrus in the bitch and queen. Management of pseudopregnancy and oestrogen-dependent mammary tumours in the bitch. Management of miliary dermatitis, eosinophilic granuloma and eosinophilic keratitis in the cat. When used in the management of feline skin disease, ensure effective topical and environmental parasite controls are instituted before considering progestogen therapy. Has major glucocorticoid-type effects and, because of adrenocortical suppression, rapid withdrawal of the drug without adequate glucocorticoid cover is not advisable. Largely superseded by other treatments.

Safety and handling: Normal precautions should be observed.

Contraindications: Do not administer on more than 2 consecutive occasions or to animals with diabetes mellitus. Do not administer to bitches with reproductive tract disease, pregnancy or mammary tumours (unless oestrus-dependent). Not recommended for management of behavioural disorders in cats and dogs.

Adverse reactions: Temperament changes (listlessness), increased thirst or appetite, cystic endometrial hyperplasia/pyometra, diabetes mellitus, adrenocortical suppression, mammary enlargement/neoplasia and lactation. As progestogens may cause elevated levels of growth hormone in the dog, acromegaly may develop.

Drug interactions: No information available.

DOSES
Dogs:
- Prevention of oestrus: begin during first 3 days of pro-oestrus at 2 mg/kg p.o. q24h for 8 days or 2 mg/kg p.o. q24h for 4 days followed by 0.5 mg/kg p.o. q24h for 16 days.
- Postponement of oestrus: 0.5 mg/kg p.o. q24h for a maximum of 40 days. Commence treatment preferably 14 days (minimum 7 days) before the effect is required.
- False pregnancy: 2 mg/kg p.o. q24h for 5–8 days commencing when signs of false pregnancy are first seen.
- Treatment of oestrogen-dependent mammary tumours: 2 mg/kg p.o. q24h for 10 days or 2 mg/kg p.o. q24h for 5 days, then 0.5–1 mg/kg p.o. q24h for 10 days.

Cats:
- Progestogen-responsive skin disorders (eosinophilic alopecia, granuloma, miliary dermatitis): 2.5–5 mg p.o. q48–72h until response and then reduce dose to 2.5–5 mg once a week.
- Prevention of oestrus: 2.5 mg/cat p.o. weekly for up to 30 weeks or 5 mg/cat p.o. for 3 days at signs of calling.

Small mammals, Birds, Reptiles: No information available.

Meglumine antimonate
(Glucantime*) **POM**

Formulations: Injectable: 300 mg/ml solution.

Action: Reported to interfere with glucose metabolism of *Leishmania* parasites.

Use: Treatment of canine leishmaniosis. Intolerance is rare but it is recommended to start with half dosage and gradually increase to an effective dose. Animals may be clinically normal after treatment but remain carriers and concurrent treatment with allopurinol may be beneficial. It is advisable to consult specialist texts or seek expert advice when treating leishmaniosis.

Safety and handling: Normal precautions should be observed.

Contraindications: Do not use where severe liver dysfunction, renal dysfunction or heart disease exists.

Adverse reactions: No information available.

Drug interactions: Care with agents that can also cause QT interval prolongation.

DOSES
Dogs: 100 mg/kg s.c., i.m., slow i.v. q24h (or divided doses q12h) until clinical remission achieved. Treat for at least 28 days.
Cats, Small mammals, Birds, Reptiles: No information available.

Megoestrol see Megestrol

Melatonin

(Circadin) **POM**

Formulations: Oral: 2 mg tablets. Melatonin is also available in many over-the-counter formulations of various sizes and often with other drugs added.

Action: Hormone which is involved in the neuroendocrine control of seasonal hair loss.

Use: Treatment of hair cycling disorders in dogs; in particular the treatment of alopecia X and seasonal flank alopecia. A 4–6 week trial is recommended, if no growth is noted then treatment should be discontinued. For seasonal flank alopecia, treatment may have to be repeated the following year. The effect of melatonin on hair re-growth in dogs with non-pruritic alopecia of unknown aetiology is variable and every effort should be made to identify the underlying disorder before starting this therapy. Oral bioavailability of melatonin in dogs is unknown. Also used for palliative treatment of adrenocortical disease in ferrets.

Safety and handling: Normal precautions should be observed.

Contraindications: No information available.

Adverse reactions: No information available.

Drug interactions: No information available.

DOSES
Dogs: 3–6 mg p.o. q8h.
Cats: No information available.
Small mammals: Ferrets: 0.5 mg p.o. q24h.
Birds, Reptiles: No information available.

Meloxicam

(Inflacam, Loxicom, Meloxidyl, Meloxivet, Metacam, Revitacam, Rheumocam) **POM-V**

Formulations: Oral: 0.5 mg/ml suspension for cats, 1.5 mg/ml oral suspension for dogs; 1.0 mg, 2.5 mg tablets for dogs; 5 mg/ml oromucosal spray for dogs. Injectable: 2 mg/ml solution for cats, 5 mg/ml solution.

Action: Preferentially inhibits COX-2 enzyme thereby limiting the production of prostaglandins involved in inflammation.

Use: Alleviation of inflammation and pain in both acute and chronic musculoskeletal disorders and the reduction of postoperative pain and inflammation following orthopaedic and soft tissue surgery. All NSAIDs should be administered cautiously in the perioperative period as they may adversely affect renal perfusion during periods of hypotension. If hypotension during anaesthesia is anticipated, delay meloxicam administration until the animal is fully recovered from anaesthesia and normotensive. Liver disease will prolong the metabolism of meloxicam leading to the potential for drug accumulation and overdose with repeated dosing. The oral dose (standard liquid preparation) may be administered directly into the mouth or mixed with food. An oromucosal spray preparation is available for dogs. The spray should be delivered into the gums/inner cheek of the dog, ensuring that none of the mist leaves the dog's mouth. In the cat, due to the longer half-life and narrower therapeutic index of NSAIDs, particular care should be taken to ensure the accuracy of dosing and not to exceed the recommended dose. Administration to animals with renal disease must be carefully evaluated.

Safety and handling: After first opening a bottle of liquid oral suspension use contents within 6 months. Shake the bottle of the oral suspension well before dosing. The shelf-life of a broached bottle of injectable solution is 28 days. The shelf-life of the oromucosal spray is 6 months after the bottle is first broached. The pump must be primed with the meloxicam liquid before first use (by depressing the pump approximately 10 times) and the pump must be re-primed (by depressing the pump 2–3 times) when it has not been used for at least 2 days after first opening.

Contraindications: Do not give to dehydrated, hypovolaemic or hypotensive patients or those with GI disease or blood clotting problems. Administration of meloxicam to animals with renal disease must be carefully evaluated and is not advisable in the perioperative period. Do not give to pregnant animals or animals <6 weeks of age.

Adverse reactions: GI signs may occur in all animals after NSAID administration. Stop therapy if this persists beyond 1–2 days. Some animals develop signs with one NSAID and not another. A 1–2-week wash-out period should be allowed before starting another NSAID after cessation of therapy. Stop therapy immediately if GI bleeding is suspected. There is a small risk that NSAIDs may precipitate cardiac failure in humans and this risk in animals is not known.

Drug interactions: Do not administer concurrently or within 24 hours of other NSAIDs and glucocorticoids. Do not administer with other potentially nephrotoxic agents, e.g. aminoglycosides.

DOSES

Dogs: Initial dose is 0.2 mg/kg s.c., p.o.; if given as a single preoperative injection effects last for 24 hours. Can be followed by a maintenance dose of 0.1 mg/kg p.o q24h. Specific pack sizes of the oromucosal spray should be used for dogs of different body weight ranges; the number of pumps daily to be given to dogs of different body weights is specified on the product information leaflet.

Cats:
- Initial injectable dose is 0.2 mg/kg s.c.; if given as a single preoperative injection effects last for 24 hours. To continue treatment for up to 5 days, may be followed 24 h later by the oral suspension for cats at a dosage of 0.05 mg/kg p.o.

- Postoperative pain/inflammation: single injection of 0.3 mg/kg s.c. has been shown to be safe and efficacious. It is not recommended to follow this with oral meloxicam 24 hours later.
- Chronic pain: initial oral dose is 0.1 mg/kg p.o. q24h, which can be followed by a maintenance dose of 0.05 mg/kg p.o q24h. Treatment should be discontinued after 14 days if no clinical improvement is apparent.

Small mammals: Rabbits: 0.3–0.6 mg/kg s.c., p.o. q24h; studies have shown that rabbits may require a dose exceeding 0.3 mg/kg q24h to achieve optimal plasma levels of meloxicam over a 24-hour interval and doses of 1.5 mg/kg s.c., p.o. are well tolerated for 5 days; Rats: 1–2 mg/kg s.c., p.o. q24h; Mice: 2 mg/kg s.c. p.o. q24h.
Birds: 0.5–1.0 mg/kg i.m., p.o. q12–24h.
Reptiles: 0.2 mg/kg i.m., p.o. q24h.

Melphalan
(Alkeran*) **POM** `CIL`

Formulations: Oral: 2 mg tablet. Injection: 50 mg powder in vial plus diluent.

Action: Forms inter- and intrastrand crosslinks with DNA, resulting in inhibition of DNA synthesis and function.

Use: Treatment of multiple myeloma and may also be used as a substitute for cyclophosphamide in the treatment of canine lymphoma and in some rescue protocols for lymphoma. Also used to treat some solid tumours (e.g. ovarian carcinoma, osteosarcoma, pulmonary and mammary neoplasia). Take care in dosing small dogs using their body surface area as there is a risk of overdose due to the tablet sizes (tablets should not be split). Give tablets on an empty stomach.

Safety and handling: Cytotoxic drug; see Appendix and specialist texts for further advice on chemotherapeutic agents. Tablets should be stored in a closed, light-protected container under refrigeration (2–8°C).

Contraindications: Bone marrow suppression, concurrent infection and impaired renal function.

Adverse reactions: Myelosuppression is dose-limiting toxicity with leucopenia, thrombocytopenia; effect may be prolonged and cumulative. GI adverse reactions include anorexia, nausea and vomiting. Pulmonary infiltrates or fibrosis can also occur. Oral ulceration is seen in humans.

Drug interactions: Cimetidine decreases the oral bioavailability of melphalan. Steroids enhance the antitumour effects of melphalan. In humans ciclosporin enhances the risk of renal toxicity.

DOSES
See Appendix for chemotherapy protocols and conversion of body weight to body surface area.
Dogs:
- Myeloma: 2 mg/m² p.o. q24h for 1–2 weeks then reduce to

2–4 mg/m² p.o. q48h. Often used with prednisolone 40 mg/m² p.o. q24h for 7–14 days then 20 mg/m² p.o. q48h or 0.05–0.1 mg/kg p.o. q24h until remission, then every other day.
- Lymphoma: 5 mg/m² p.o. q48h or 20 mg/m² q14d.
- Adjunctive treatment of ovarian carcinoma, lymphoreticular neoplasms, osteosarcoma, mammary/pulmonary neoplasia: 2–4 mg/m² p.o. q48h.

Cats:
- Chronic lymphocytic leukaemia: 2 mg/m² p.o. q48h, with or without prednisolone.
- Multiple myeloma: 0.1 mg/kg p.o. q24h for 14 days then q48h until improvement or leucopenia detected. Cats already with leucopenia and anaemia should be treated q72h.
- Maintenance therapy: 0.1 mg/kg p.o. q7d with prednisolone at 0.5 mg/kg p.o. q24h.

Small mammals, Birds, Reptiles: No information available.

Mepivacaine
(Intra-epicaine) **POM-V**

Formulations: Injectable: 2% solution.

Action: Local anaesthetic action is dependent on reversible blockade of the sodium channel, preventing propagation of an action potential along the nerve fibre. Sensory nerve fibres are blocked before motor nerve fibres, allowing a selective sensory blockade at low doses.

Use: Blockade of sensory nerves to produce analgesia following perineural or local infiltration. Instillation into joints to provide intra-articular analgesia. Mepivacaine has less intrinsic vasodilator activity than lidocaine and is thought to be less irritant to tissues. It is of equivalent potency to lidocaine but has a slightly longer duration of action (100–120 minutes). It does not require addition of adrenaline to prolong its effect.

Safety and handling: Normal precautions should be observed.

Contraindications: Mepivacaine should not be injected i.v.

Adverse reactions: Inadvertent i.v. injection may cause convulsions and/or cardiac arrest.

Drug interactions: No information available.

DOSES
Dogs, Cats: Inject the minimal volume required to achieve an effect. Toxic doses of mepivacaine have not been established in companion animals.
Small mammals, Birds, Reptiles: No information available.

Metaflumizone
(Promeris, Promeris Duo) POM-V

Formulations: Topical: 200 mg/ml spot-on pipettes of various sizes (Promeris); 150 mg/ml metaflumizone + 150 mg/ml amitraz in various sizes (Promeris Duo).

Action: Blocks sodium channels, causing flaccid paralysis of parasites. Amitraz increases neuronal activity through its action of octopamine receptors on mites.

Use: Treatment and prevention of flea infestations (*Ctenocephalides canis* and *C. felis*) in cats and dogs >8 weeks of age. The amitraz-containing product is additionally indicated for the treatment and prevention of tick and lice infestations in dogs. For treatment of flea infestations the additional use of an insect growth regulator is recommended.

Safety and handling: The solvent in Promeris may stain fabrics and other surfaces.

Contraindications: Safety has not been established in pregnant and lactating females. Promeris Duo (containing amitraz) should not be used in cats.

Adverse reactions: Hypersalivation may occur if the product is ingested. Sedation, bradycardia, respiratory and CNS depression with amitraz-containing product can be reversed with an alpha-2 agonist such as atipamezole or yohimbine. A pemphigus foliaceus-like drug eruption has been reported in a small number of dogs after application of Promeris Duo.

Drug interactions: No information available.

DOSES
Dogs: 40 mg/kg applied topically once for lice (amitraz-containing product) or every 4 weeks for fleas (both products) and ticks (amitraz-containing product).
Cats: 40 mg/kg applied topically every 4 weeks for fleas. Do not use Promeris Duo in cats.
Small mammals, Birds, Reptiles: No information available.

Metamizole (Dipyrone)
(Buscopan Compositum) POM-V

Formulations: Injectable: 4 mg/ml butylscopolamine + 500 mg/ml metamizole.

Action: Anti-inflammatory effects, which are brought about by a reduction in prostaglandin production at the site of inflammation. It also has antipyretic and analgesic effects which occur through blocking the synthesis of endogenous pyrogens (prostaglandins D and E).

Use: The combination of metamizole and butylscopolamine is indicated for the management of visceral pain, particularly spasmodic colic or pain from urinary obstruction. Metamizole is indicated in humans for the management of pain (both chronic and acute postoperative pain), but it does not have a marketing authorization for animals in the UK. In countries where metamizole is available without hyoscine (butylscopolamine), studies have shown it has good efficacy when administered both i.v. and p.o. with no serious adverse effects noted on short to medium term treatment. Largely superseded by other treatments.

Safety and handling: Avoid self-injection as metamizole can cause reversible but potentially serious agranulocytosis and skin allergies in humans.

Contraindications: No information available.

Adverse reactions: Hepatitis, nephropathy, blood dyscrasia and GI disturbances in common with other NSAIDs. Because of the seriousness of these side effects it should be used as a second-line agent for the treatment of pyrexia and rarely as an anti-inflammatory.

Drug interactions: No information available.

DOSES
Dogs: 0.1 mg/kg i.v., i.m. q12h.
Cats: Not authorized; use is strongly discouraged.
Small mammals: Rabbits: See butylscopolamine.
Birds, Reptiles: No information available.

Methadone
(Comfortan) **POM-V CD SCHEDULE 2**

Formulations: Injectable: 10 mg/ml solution. Oral: 10 mg tablets.

Action: Analgesia mediated by the mu opioid receptor.

Use: Management of moderate to severe pain in the perioperative period. Incorporation into sedative and pre-anaesthetic medication protocols to provide improved sedation and analgesia. Methadone has similar pharmacological properties to morphine, and is useful in similar situations. It provides profound analgesia with a duration of action of 3–4 hours in dogs and cats. Accumulation is likely to occur after prolonged repeated dosing which may allow the dose to be reduced or the dose interval extended. Methadone can be given i.v. without causing histamine release and does not cause vomiting when given to animals preoperatively. Transient excitation may occur when methadone is given i.v. Methadone may be administered epidurally to provide analgesia; the duration of analgesia following methadone at a dose of 0.1–0.3 mg/kg epidurally is approximately 8 hours in dogs. Oral methadone is rarely used in cats and dogs due to a high first pass metabolism leading to low plasma concentrations after administration. Methadone is absorbed into the systemic circulation after oral transmucosal administration to cats and provides pain relief when administered by this route. Respiratory function should be monitored when given i.v. to anaesthetized patients. The response to all opioids appears to vary between individual patients, therefore assessment of pain after administration is imperative. Methadone is metabolized in the liver, and some prolongation of effect may be seen with impaired liver function.

Safety and handling: Normal precautions should be observed.

Contraindications: No information available.

Adverse reactions: In common with other mu agonists methadone can cause respiratory depression, although this is unlikely when used at clinical doses in conscious cats and dogs. Respiratory depression may occur when given i.v. during general anaesthesia due to increased depth of anaesthesia. Vomiting is rare although methadone will cause constriction of GI sphincters (such as the pyloric sphincter) and may cause a reduction in GI motility when given over a long period. Methadone crosses the placenta and may exert sedative effects in neonates born to bitches treated prior to parturition. Severe adverse effects can be treated with naloxone.

Drug interactions: Other CNS depressants (e.g. anaesthetics, antihistamines, barbiturates, phenothiazines, tranquillizers) may cause increased CNS or respiratory depression when used concurrently with narcotic analgesics.

DOSES
When used for sedation is generally given as part of a combination. See Appendix for sedation protocols in all species.
Dogs: Analgesia: 0.1–0.5 mg/kg i.m. or 0.1–0.3 mg/kg i.v. prn.
Cats:
- Analgesia: 0.1–0.6 mg/kg i.v. slow, i.m., s.c.
- Doses in the range of 0.3–0.4 mg/kg are appropriate for oral transmucosal administration.
Small mammals: Analgesia: Rabbits: 0.3–0.7 mg/kg slow i.v., i.m.
Birds, Reptiles: No information available.

Methenamine (Hexamine hippurate)
(Hiprex*) **POM**

Formulations: Oral: 150 mg methenamine + 116 mg monosodium phosphate tablet; 1 g methenamine hippurate (Hiprex) tablet.

Action: Urinary antiseptic.

Use: Long-term control of recurrent urinary tract infections. It should not be used alone as it is only bacteriostatic. It requires an acidic urine to be effective.

Safety and handling: Normal precautions should be observed.

Contraindications: Severe renal or hepatic impairment, dehydration and metabolic acidosis.

Adverse reactions: Methenamine may cause GI disturbances, bladder irritation or a rash.

Drug interactions: Efficacy is reduced when drugs that alkalinize urine (potassium citrate) are used concurrently.

DOSES
Dogs: 1–3 tablets p.o. q24h (methenamine/sodium acid phosphate) or 500 mg/dog p.o. q12h (methenamine).
Cats: 1 tablet p.o. q24h (methenamine/sodium acid phosphate) or 250 mg/cat p.o. q12h (methenamine).
Small mammals, Birds, Reptiles: No information available.

Methimazole (Thiamazole)
(Felimazole) **POM-V**

Formulations: Oral: 1.25 mg, 2.5 mg, 5 mg tablets.

Action: Interferes with the synthesis of thyroid hormones by inhibiting peroxidase-catalysed reactions (blocks oxidation of iodide), the iodination of tyrosyl residues in thyroglobulin, and the coupling of mono- or di-iodotyrosines to form T3 and T4. There is no effect on iodine uptake and it does not inhibit peripheral de-iodination of T4 to T3.

Use: Control of thyroid hormone levels in cats with hyperthyroidism. Two to three weeks of treatment are generally needed to establish euthyroidism. Monitor therapy on the basis of serum thyroxine concentrations (4–6 hours after dosing) and adjust dose accordingly for long-term medical management. Assess haematology, biochemistry and serum total T4 after 3, 6, 10 and 20 weeks and thereafter every 3 months, adjusting dosage as necessary.

Safety and handling: Normal precautions should be observed.

Contraindications: Do not use in pregnant or lactating queens.

Adverse reactions: Vomiting and inappetence/anorexia may be seen but are often transient. Jaundice, cytopenias, immune-mediated diseases and dermatological changes (pruritus, alopecia and self-induced trauma) are reported but rarely seen. Treatment of hyperthyroidism can decrease glomerular filtration rate, thereby raising serum urea and creatinine values, and can occasionally unmask occult renal failure. Animals that have an adverse reaction to carbimazole are likely also to have an adverse reaction to methimazole.

Drug interactions: Phenobarbital may reduce clinical efficacy. Benzimidazole drugs reduce hepatic oxidation and may lead to increased circulating drug concentrations. Methimazole should be discontinued before iodine-131 treatment. Do not use with low-iodine prescription diets.

DOSES
Dogs: 2.5–5 mg/dog p.o. q12h depending on size.
Cats: 2.5 mg/cat p.o. q12h.
Small mammals: Guinea pigs: 0.5–2.0 mg/kg p.o. q24h.
Birds: No information available.
Reptiles: Snakes: 2 mg/kg p.o. q24h for 30 days.

Methionine
(Methionine*) **P**

Formulations: Oral: 250 mg tablets.

Action: Urinary acidifier. Precursor of hepatic glutathione, protecting against oxidative damage resulting from paracetamol ingestion.

Use: Struvite urolithiasis. Paracetamol poisoning if given within 12 hours of ingestion. There is an increased risk of acidosis if used with other urinary acidifying treatments.

Safety and handling: Normal precautions should be observed.

Contraindications: Renal failure or severe hepatic disease. Young age.

Adverse reactions: Overdosage may lead to metabolic acidosis.

Drug interactions: No information available.

DOSES
Dogs:
- Urine acidification: 200 mg/dog to 1 g/dog p.o. q8h. Adjust the dose until urine pH is 6.5 or lower.
- Paracetamol poisoning: 2.5 g/dog p.o., followed by 3 further doses of 2.5 g/dog q4h.

Cats:
- Urine acidification: 200 mg/cat p.o. q8h. Adjust the dose until urine pH is 6.5 or lower.
- Paracetamol poisoning: 2.5 g/cat p.o., followed by 3 further doses of 2.5 g/cat q4h.

Small mammals, Birds, Reptiles: No information available.

Methocarbamol
(Robaxin*) **POM-V**

Formulations: Oral: 500 mg, 750 mg tablets.

Action: Carbamate derivative of guaifenesin that is a CNS depressant with sedative and musculoskeletal relaxant properties. The mechanism of action has not been fully established, it has no direct action on the contractile mechanism of skeletal muscle, the motor endplate or the nerve fibre.

Use: Treatment of tetanus and some toxicities (e.g. pyrethroid, strychnine) and as a general muscle relaxant for muscular spasms. The clearance of methocarbamol is significantly impaired in human patients with renal and hepatic disease. There is very limited literature on the use of methocarbamol in cats; case reports describing the use of methocarbamol by intravenous bolus injection and continuous rate infusion in dogs and cats have been published.

Safety and handling: Normal precautions should be observed.

Contraindications: No information available.

Adverse reactions: Salivation, emesis, lethargy, weakness and ataxia.

Drug interactions: As methocarbamol is a CNS depressant, additive depression may occur when given with other CNS depressant agents.

DOSES
Dogs, Cats: 20–45 mg/kg p.o. q8h. Very high doses may be required for tetanus. It is recommended that the dose does not exceed 330 mg/kg, although serious toxicity or death has not been reported after overdoses.
Small mammals, Birds, Reptiles: No information available.

Methoprene (*S*-Methoprene)
(Acclaim spray, Frontline Combo, R.I.P. fleas, Staykill)
NFA-VPS, GSL

Formulations: Topical: 10% w/v fipronil with *S*-methoprene in spot-on pipettes of various sizes (Frontline). Environmental: *S*-methoprene + permethrin household spray (Acclaim); *S*-methoprene, tetramethrin + permethrin household spray (R.I.P. Fleas).

Action: Juvenile hormone analogue that inhibits larval development.

Use: Treatment and prevention of flea infestations (*Ctenocephalides canis* and *C. felis*) and tick prevention in dogs and cats >8 weeks of age (dogs >2 kg; cats >1 kg). For treatment of flea infestations the product should be applied every 4 weeks to all in-contact cats and dogs (Frontline Combo). Also used for cheyletiellosis and otoacariasis (*Otodectes cynotis*). Bathing between 48 hours before and 24 hours after application is not recommended. Minimum treatment interval 4 weeks. Can be used in pregnant and lactating females. Treat infested household as directed with spray; keep away from birds (and fish). Environmental sprays also have some efficacy against house dust mites *Dermatophagoides farinae* and *D. pteronyssinus*.

Safety and handling: Normal precautions should be observed.

Contraindications: Do not use in rabbits or birds.

Adverse reactions: Local pruritus or alopecia may occur at the site of application. May be harmful to aquatic organisms.

Drug interactions: No information available.

DOSES

Dogs, Cats: 1 pipette per animal monthly according to body weight. Cheyletiellosis, Otoacariasis (*Otodectes cynotis* infestation): two applications 4 weeks apart.
Small mammals: Rabbits: Do not use.
Birds: Do not use.
Reptiles: No information available.

Methotrexate

CIL

(Matrex*, Methotrexate*) **POM**

Formulations: Oral: 2.5 mg, 10 mg tablets.

Action: An S-phase-specific antimetabolite antineoplastic agent; competitively inhibits folic acid reductase which is required for purine synthesis, DNA synthesis and cellular replication. This results in inhibition of DNA synthesis and function.

Use: Treatment of lymphoma, although its use in animals is often limited by toxicity. In humans it is used to treat refractory rheumatoid arthritis; however, data are lacking with regards to its use in canine and feline immune-mediated polyarthritides. Monitor haematological parameters regularly.

Safety and handling: Cytotoxic drug; see Appendix and specialist texts for further advice on chemotherapeutic agents.

Contraindications: Pre-existing myelosuppression, severe hepatic or renal insufficiency, or hypersensitivity to the drug.

Adverse reactions: Particularly with high doses GI ulceration, mucositis, hepatotoxicity, nephrotoxicity and haemopoietic toxicity may be seen. Low blood pressure and skin reactions are seen in humans.

Drug interactions: Methotrexate is highly bound to serum albumin and thus may be displaced by phenylbutazone, phenytoin, salicylates, sulphonamides and tetracycline, resulting in increased blood levels and toxicity. Folic acid supplements may inhibit the response to methotrexate. Methotrexate increases the cytotoxicity of cytarabine. Cellular uptake is decreased by hydrocortisone, methylprednisolone and penicillins, and is increased by vincristine. Concurrent use of NSAIDs increases the risk of haematological, renal and hepatic toxicity.

DOSES

See Appendix for chemotherapy protocols and conversion of body weight to body surface area.
Dogs, Cats: 2.5–5 mg/m^2 p.o. twice weekly. Adjust the frequency of dosing according to toxic effects.
Small mammals, Birds, Reptiles: No information available.

Methylene blue see **Methylthioninium chloride**

Methylprednisolone
(Depo-Medrone, Medrone, Solu-Medrone) **POM-V**

Formulations: Injectable: 40 mg/ml depot suspension (Depo-Medrone); 125 mg, 500 mg powder for reconstitution (Solu-Medrone). Oral: 2 mg, 4 mg tablets (Medrone).

Action: Alters the transcription of DNA leading to alterations in cellular metabolism which result in anti-inflammatory, immunosuppressive and antifibrotic effects. Also acts in dogs as an ADH antagonist.

Use: Anti-inflammatory agent and is authorized for the management of shock. Has 5 times the anti-inflammatory potency of hydrocortisone and 20% more potency than prednisolone. On a dose basis, 0.8 mg methylprednisolone is equivalent to 1 mg prednisolone. The oral formulation of methylprednisolone is suitable for alternate-day use. The use of steroids in shock and acute spinal cord injury is controversial and many specialists do not use them. Any value in administering steroids declines rapidly after the onset of shock or injury, whilst the side effects remain constant and may be substantial. Doses should be tapered to the lowest effective dose. Animals on chronic therapy should be tapered off steroids when discontinuing the drug.

Safety and handling: Normal precautions should be observed.

Contraindications: Do not use in pregnant animals. Systemic corticosteroids are generally contraindicated in patients with renal disease and diabetes mellitus.

Adverse reactions: Prolonged use suppresses the hypothalamic-pituitary axis and causes adrenal atrophy. Catabolic effects of glucocorticoids lead to weight loss and cutaneous atrophy. Iatrogenic hyperadrenocorticism may develop with long-term use. Vomiting and diarrhoea may be seen and GI ulceration may develop. Glucocorticoids may increase urine glucose levels and decrease serum T3 and T4. Impaired wound healing and delayed recovery from infections may be seen. In rabbits, corticosteroids can cause severe immunosuppression. In birds there is a high risk of immunosuppression and side effects, such as hepatopathy and a diabetes mellitus-like syndrome.

Drug interactions: There is an increased risk of GI ulceration if used concurrently with NSAIDs. Hypokalaemia may develop if amphotericin B or potassium-depleting diuretics (furosemide, thiazides) are administered concomitantly with corticosteroids. Insulin requirements are likely to increase in patients taking glucocorticoids. The metabolism of corticosteroids may be enhanced by phenobarbital or phenytoin and decreased by antifungals (e.g. itraconazole).

DOSES

Dogs:
- Inflammation: Initially 1.1 mg/kg i.m. (methylprednisolone acetate depot injection) q1–3wk or 0.2–0.5 mg/kg p.o. q12h.
- Immunosuppression: 1–3 mg/kg p.o. q12h reducing to 1–2 mg/kg p.o. q48h.
- Brain trauma: 30 mg/kg i.v. within 8 hours of trauma, followed by 15 mg/kg i.v. 2 hours and 6 hours later, followed by 2.5 mg/kg as an i.v. infusion for 48h.

Cats:
- Asthma: 1–2 mg/kg (depot injection) i.m. q1-3wk.
- Inflammation/flea allergy: 5 mg/kg i.m. (depot injection) every 2 months or 1 mg/kg p.o. q24h reducing to 2–5 mg/cat p.o. q48h.

Small mammals, Birds: No information available.

Reptiles: 5–10 mg/kg i.m. once.

Methylthioninium chloride
(Methylene blue)

(Methylthioninium chloride*) **AVM-GSL**

Formulations: Injectable: 10 mg/ml (1% solution).

Action: Acts as an electron donor to methaemoglobin reductase.

Use: Methaemoglobinaemia. Use an in-line filter if possible.

Safety and handling: Normal precautions should be observed.

Contraindications: Do not use unless adequate renal function is demonstrated.

Adverse reactions: May cause a Heinz body haemolytic anaemia, especially in cats (relatively contraindicated in this species), and renal failure.

Drug interactions: No information available.

DOSES

Dogs: 1 mg/kg i.v. slowly once; can be repeated if necessary.

Cats, Small mammals, Birds, Reptiles: No information available.

Metoclopramide

(Emeprid, Vomend, Maxolon*, Metoclopramide*) **POM-V, POM**

Formulations: Injectable: 5 mg/ml solution in 10 ml multi-dose vial or clear glass ampoules. Oral: 10 mg tablet; 15 mg capsule; 1 mg/ml solution.

Action: Antiemetic and upper GI prokinetic stimulant; distal intestinal motility is not significantly affected. The antiemetic effect is a result of central dopamine (D2) receptor antagonism, and at higher doses $5HT_3$ antagonism, at the chemoreceptor trigger zone. The gastric prokinetic effect is a result of local D2 antagonism and stimulation of muscarinic acetylcholine and $5HT_4$ receptors leading to increases in oesophageal sphincter pressure, the tone and amplitude of gastric contractions and peristaltic activity in the duodenum and jejunum, and relaxing the pyloric sphincter by sensitizing tissues to acetylcholine. There is no effect on gastric, pancreatic or biliary secretions and nor does metoclopramide depend on an intact vagal innervation to affect motility.

Use: Vomiting of many causes can be reduced by this drug. The prokinetic effect may be beneficial in reflux oesophagitis and in emptying the stomach prior to induction of general anaesthesia. High doses are needed to abolish all reflux during anaesthesia. The prokinetic effect may also help to prevent postoperative ileus in rabbits; however, it is only effective in adult rabbits.

Safety and handling: Injection is light-sensitive. Obscure fluid bag if used in a constant rate infusion.

Contraindications: Do not use where GI obstruction or perforation is present or for >72 hours without a definitive diagnosis. Relatively contraindicated in epileptic patients.

Adverse reactions: Unusual, although more common in cats than dogs, and probably relate to relative overdosing and individual variations in bioavailability. They include changes in mentation (depression, nervousness, restlessness) and behaviour. It may also cause sedation and extrapyramidal effects (movement disorders characterized as slow to rapid twisting movements involving the face, neck, trunk or limbs). Cats may exhibit signs of frenzied behaviour or signs of disorientation. Metoclopramide reduces renal blood flow, which may exacerbate pre-existing renal disease. Very rarely allergic reactions may occur.

Drug interactions: The activity of metoclopramide may be inhibited by antimuscarinic drugs (e.g. atropine) and narcotic analgesics. The effects of metoclopramide may decrease (e.g. cimetidine, digoxin) or increase (e.g. oxytetracycline) drug absorption. The absorption of nutrients may be accelerated, thereby altering insulin requirements and/or timing of its effects in diabetics. Phenothiazines may potentiate the extrapyramidal effects of metoclopramide. The CNS effects of metoclopramide may be enhanced by narcotic analgesics or sedatives.

DOSES

Dogs, Cats: 0.25–0.5 mg/kg i.v., i.m., s.c., p.o. q12h or 0.17–0.33 mg/kg i.v., i.m., s.c., p.o. q8h or 1–2 mg/kg i.v. over 24 hours as a slow constant rate infusion.

Small mammals: Ferrets, Rabbits, Guinea pigs: 0.5–1 mg/kg s.c., p.o. q6–12h.

Birds: 0.3–2.0 mg/kg p.o., i.m. q8–24h.

Reptiles: 0.05–1 mg/kg p.o., i.m. q24h. Higher doses may be needed in desert tortoises.

Metronidazole

CIL

(Stomorgyl, Flagyl*, Metrolyl*, Metronidazole*) **POM-V, POM**

Formulations: Injectable: 5 mg/ml i.v. infusion. Oral: 200 mg, 400 mg, 500 mg tablets; 25 mg metronidazole + 46.9 mg spiramycin tablets, 125 mg metronidazole + 234.4 mg spiramycin tablets, 250 mg metronidazole + 469 mg spiramycin tablets (Stomorgyl 2, 10 and 20, respectively); 40 mg/ml oral solution.

Action: Synthetic nitroimidazole with antibacterial and antiprotozoal activity. Its mechanism of action on protozoans is unknown but in bacteria it appears to be reduced simultaneously under anaerobic conditions to compounds that bind to DNA and cause cell death. Spiramycin is a macrolide antibacterial that inhibits bacterial protein synthesis.

Use: Treatment of anaerobic infections, giardiasis and other protozoal infections, and in the management of hepatic encephalopathy. Metronidazole may have effects on the immune system by modulating cell-mediated immune responses. It is absorbed well from the GI tract and diffuses into many tissues including bone, CSF and abscesses. Spiramycin (a constituent of Stomorgyl) is active against Gram-positive aerobes including *Staphylococcus*, *Streptococcus*, *Bacillus* and *Actinomyces*. Metronidazole has been used as an appetite stimulant in reptiles. In ferrets it is used in combination with amoxicillin, and bismuth subsalicylate, ranitidine or omeprazole (triple therapy) for treatment of *Helicobacter mustelae*. In rabbits it is the treatment of choice for enterotoxaemia due to *Clostridium spiroforme*. Metronidazole is frequently used in combination with penicillin or aminoglycoside antimicrobials to improve anaerobic spectrum. Some texts recommend doses in excess of 25 mg/kg. There is a greater risk of adverse effects with rapid i.v. infusion or high total doses. It is no longer used in dogs and cats for the treatment of giardiasis but may still have a role in chinchillas with this condition (however, use with care in this species).

Safety and handling: Normal precautions should be observed.

Contraindications: Do not administer to Indigo or King snakes due to toxicity. Do not use in very small birds, such as Zebra finches, due to toxicity.

Adverse reactions: Adverse effects in animals are uncommon and are generally limited to vomiting, CNS toxicity (nystagmus, ataxia, knuckling, head tilt and seizures), hepatotoxicity and haematuria. Excessive salivation/foaming is noted in some cats. Prolonged therapy or the presence of pre-existing hepatic disease may predispose to CNS toxicity. Use with caution in the first trimester of pregnancy as it may be teratogenic. Anecdotally has been associated with liver failure in chinchillas.

Drug interactions: Phenobarbital or phenytoin may enhance metabolism of metronidazole. Cimetidine may decrease the metabolism of metronidazole and increase the likelihood of dose-related adverse effects. Spiramycin should not be used concurrently with other antibiotics of the macrolide group as the combination may be antagonistic.

DOSES
See Appendix for guidelines on responsible antibacterial use.
Dogs:
- Flagyl: 15–25 mg/kg p.o. q12h or 10 mg/kg s.c., slow i.v. infusion q12h. Use higher doses, 25 mg/kg p.o. q12h, for protozoal infections. Injectable solution may be given intrapleurally to treat empyema.
- Stomorgyl: 12.5 mg metronidazole + 23.4 mg spiramycin/kg p.o. (equivalent to 1 tablet/2 kg of Stomorgyl 2, 1 tablet/10 kg of Stomorgyl 10 and 1 tablet/20 kg of Stomorgyl 20) q24h for 5–10 days.

Cats:
- 8–10 mg/kg i.v., p.o. q12h. Injectable solution may be given intrapleurally to treat empyema.
- Stomorgyl: 12.5 mg metronidazole + 23.4 mg spiramycin/kg p.o. (equivalent to 1 tablet/2 kg of Stomorgyl 2, 1 tablet/10 kg of Stomorgyl 10 and 1 tablet/20 kg of Stomorgyl 20) q24h for 5–10 days.

Small mammals: Ferrets: 15–20 mg/kg p.o q12h; 50–75 mg/kg p.o. q24h for 14 days with clarithromycin and omeprazole for *Helicobacter*; Rabbits, Chinchillas, Guinea pigs: 10–20 mg/kg p.o. q12h, 40 mg/kg p.o. q24h; 50 mg/kg p.o. q12h for 5 days may be required for giardiasis in chinchillas but use with caution; Rats, Mice: 20 mg/kg s.c. q24h; Other rodents: 20–40 mg/kg p.o. q24h.

Birds: Raptors: 50 mg/kg p.o. q24h for 5 days; Pigeons: 40–50 mg/kg p.o. q24h for 5–7 days or 100 mg/kg p.o. q48h for 3 doses or 200 mg/kg p.o. once; Parrots: 30 mg/kg p.o. q12h; Passerines: 50 mg/kg p.o. q12h or 200 mg/l water daily for 7 days.

Reptiles:
- Anaerobic bacterial infections: Iguanas, Snakes: 20 mg/kg p.o. q24–48h.
- Protozoal infections: Indigo Snake, Kingsnake, Milksnakes: 40 mg/kg p.o., repeat after 14 days; Other snakes: 100 mg/kg p.o., repeat after 14 days; Chelonians: 100–125 mg/kg p.o., repeat after 14 days (use lower doses of 50 mg/kg p.o. q24h for 3–5 days for severe infections); Chameleons: 40–60 mg/kg p.o., repeat after 14 days.

Mexiletine
(Mexitil*) **POM**

Formulations: Oral: 50 mg, 200 mg capsules; 25 mg/ml solution.

Action: Class 1b antiarrhythmic agent similar to lidocaine. It is an inhibitor of the inward sodium current (fast sodium channel), which reduces the rate of rise of the action potential. In the Purkinje fibres it decreases automaticity, the action potential duration and the effective refractory period.

Use: Management of rapid or haemodynamically significant ventricular arrhythmias such as frequent complex ventricular premature complexes or ventricular tachycardia. Also proven to be effective in some dogs with supraventricular tachycardia due to the presence of an accessory conduction pathway (bypass tract). Often effective if there has been a response to i.v. lidocaine. Often given orally at the same time as beta-blockers, such as atenolol at 0.5–1 mg/kg q12–24h. Has been combined with sotalol in dogs not fully responsive to sotalol alone. Not proven to prevent sudden death in dogs with severe ventricular arrhythmias. Use cautiously in patients with severe CHF, sinus node dysfunction, hepatic dysfunction and seizure disorders. Administer oral dose with food to alleviate adverse GI effects.

Safety and handling: Normal precautions should be observed.

Contraindications: 2nd or 3rd degree AV block not treated by pacemaker therapy.

Adverse reactions: Nausea, anorexia, vomiting, depression, convulsions, tremor, nystagmus, bradycardia, hypotension, jaundice and hepatitis.

Drug interactions: The absorption of mexiletine may be delayed by atropine and opioid analgesics. Mexiletine excretion may be reduced by acetazolamide and alkaline urine, and increased by urinary acidifying drugs (e.g. methionine). The action of mexiletine may be antagonized by hypokalaemia. Cimetidine decreases the rate of mexiletine elimination.

DOSES
Dogs: Oral: 4–8 mg/kg p.o. q8–12h. Dose for i.v. not established for dogs.
Cats, Small mammals, Birds, Reptiles: No information available.

Miconazole
(Daktarin, Easotic, Malaseb, Mycozole, Surolan) **POM-V**

Formulations: Topical: 2% cream/powder (Daktarin); 2% shampoo (Malaseb); 23 mg/ml suspension with prednisolone and polymyxin (Surolan).

Action: Inhibits cytochrome P450-dependent synthesis of ergosterol in fungal cells causing increased cell wall permeability and allowing leakage of cellular contents. Miconazole has activity against *Malassezia*, *Cryptococcus*, *Candida* and *Coccidioides*.

Use: Fungal skin and ear infections, including dermatophytosis. Miconazole shampoo is useful in the treatment of dermatophytosis in cats but concurrent itraconazole administration is required.

Safety and handling: Normal precautions should be observed.

Contraindications: No information available.

Adverse reactions: No information available.

Drug interactions: No information available.

DOSES

Dogs:
- Fungal otitis: 2–12 drops in affected ear q12–24h (Surolan).
- Dermatophytosis: apply a thin layer of cream topically to affected area twice daily. Continue for 2 weeks after a clinical cure and negative fungal cultures.
- *Malassezia* dermatitis: shampoo twice weekly until the clinical signs subside and weekly thereafter or as necessary to keep the condition under control (Malaseb).

Cats:
- Fungal otitis: doses as for dogs.
- Dermatophytosis: Topical: doses as for dogs.
- *Microsporum canis*: shampoo twice weekly whilst administering itraconazole for 6–10 weeks or until coat brushings are negative for the culture of *M. canis*, whichever is the longer (Malaseb). The maximum length of the treatment period should not exceed 16 weeks.

Small mammals: Rabbits: fungal otitis: 2–12 drops in affected ear q12–24h; dermatophytosis: apply a thin layer of cream topically to affected area twice daily, continue for 2 weeks after a clinical cure and negative fungal cultures. Avoid preparations containing steroids.

Birds, Reptiles: No information available.

Midazolam
(Hypnovel*) **POM**

Formulations: Injectable: 2 mg/ml, 5 mg/ml solutions. Oral: 10 mg/ml solution for buccal administration.

Action: Causes neural inhibition by increasing the effect of GABA on the $GABA_A$ receptor, resulting in sedation, anxiolytic effects, hypnotic effects, amnesia, muscle relaxation and anticonvulsive effects. Compared with diazepam it is more potent, has a shorter onset and duration of action (<1 h in dogs) and is less irritant to tissues.

Use: Provides sedation with amnesia; as part of a premedication regime, as part of combined anaesthetic protocols, and in the emergency control of epileptic seizures (including status epilepticus). It provides unreliable sedation on its own, although it will sedate depressed animals. It is often used with ketamine to offset the muscle hypertonicity caused by the ketamine. It is used with opioids and/or acepromazine for pre-anaesthetic medication in the critically ill. Midazolam can be diluted with saline, but avoid fluids containing calcium as this may result in precipitation of midazolam. Use with caution in severe hypotension, cardiac disease and respiratory disease.

Safety and handling: Normal precautions should be observed.

Contraindications: Avoid in myasthenia gravis and neonates.

Adverse reactions: In human patients i.v. administration of midazolam has been associated with respiratory depression and severe hypotension. Excitement may occasionally develop.

Drug interactions: Midazolam potentiates the effect of some anaesthetic agents, reducing the dose required, including propofol and some inhalation agents. Concurrent use of midazolam with NSAIDs (in particular diclofenac), antihistamines, barbiturates, opioid analgesics or CNS depressants may enhance the sedative effect. Opioid analgesics may increase the hypnotic and hypotensive effects of midazolam. Erythromycin inhibits the metabolism of midazolam.

DOSES
When used for sedation is generally given as part of a combination. See Appendix for sedation protocols in all species.

Dogs, Cats: Emergency management of seizures including status epilepticus: bolus dose of 0.2–0.3 mg/kg i.v. or intrarectally if venous access is not available. Time to onset of clinical effect is rapid for i.v. use, therefore repeat q10min if there is no clinical effect up to 3 times. Midazolam may be used in conjunction with diazepam for emergency control of seizures. In dogs additional doses may be administered if appropriate supportive care facilities are available (for support of respiration). Once the seizures have been controlled, the dog can be maintained on a constant i.v. infusion of 0.3 mg/kg/h.

Small mammals: Ferrets: 0.25–0.5 mg/kg i.v. or 0.3–1.0 mg/kg s.c., i.m.; Rabbits: 0.2–2 mg/kg i.v., i.m.; general anaesthesia: 0.25–1.0 mg/kg i.v. when used with Fentanyl/Fluanisone; Chinchillas: 1 mg/kg i.v. or 2 mg/kg i.m.; Rodents 2–5 mg/kg i.v., i.m., i.p.

Birds: 0.1–0.5 mg/kg i.m. or 0.05–0.15 mg/kg i.v. (premedicant).

Reptiles: Premedication (single agent): 2 mg/kg i.m. (but more commonly used in combinations).

Mifepristone
(Mifegyne*) **POM**

Formulations: Oral: 200 mg tablet.

Action: Blocks progesterone receptors in the uterus and significantly reduces progesterone levels so that pregnancy cannot be maintained.

Use: Termination of pregnancy in bitches. Other medications are authorized for this in the UK, and so mifepristone should not be considered first choice.

Safety and handling: Normal precautions should be observed.

Contraindications: No information available.

Adverse reactions: Nausea and vomiting may be seen.

Drug interactions: Avoid concurrent use of NSAIDs until 12 days after mifepristone treatment.

DOSES
Dogs: 2.5–3.5 mg/kg p.o. q12h for 5 days after day 32 of pregnancy.
Cats, Small mammals, Birds, Reptiles: No information available.

Milbemycin
(Milbemax, Program plus) **POM-V**

Formulations: Oral: 2.5 mg/25 mg, 12.5 mg/125 mg milbemycin/praziquantel tablets (Milbemax for dogs); 4 mg/10 mg, 16 mg/40 mg (Milbemax for cats); 2.3 mg, 5.75 mg, 11.5 mg, 23 mg milbemycin with lufenuron (ratio 20 mg lufeneron: 1 mg milbemycin) tablets (Program plus).

Action: Interacts with GABA and glutamate gated channels, leading to flaccid paralysis of parasites.

Use: Treatment of adult nematode infestation; roundworms (*Toxocara canis*, *T. cati*), hookworms (*Ancylostoma caninum*, *A. tubaeforme*) and whipworms (*Trichuris vulpis*). The addition of lufeneron provides flea control. For treatment of flea infestations the additional use of an authorized adulticide is recommended. The addition of praziquantel provides control of cestodes (*Dipylidium caninum*, *Taenia* spp., *Echinococcus*, *Mesocestoides*). It is also used for the prevention of heartworm disease (*Dirofilaria immitis*) in countries where this parasite is endemic. Can be used in pregnant and lactating females.

Safety and handling: Normal precautions should be observed.

Contraindications: Do not use in animals suspected of having heartworm disease. Not for use in dogs <2 weeks old or cats <6 weeks old or in any animal <0.5 kg.

Adverse reactions: No information available.

Drug interactions: No information available.

DOSES
Dogs:
- With lufenuron: 0.5 mg milbemycin/kg + 10 mg lufeneron/kg p.o. q30d.
- With praziquantel: 0.5 mg/kg milbemycin + 5 mg/kg praziquantel p.o. q30d. For *Angiostrongylus vasorum*: administer same dose 4 times at weekly intervals.
- Milbemax: Do not use the tablets for small puppies in dogs <2 weeks old or <0.5 kg body weight; do not use the tablets for dogs in dogs <5 kg body weight.
- Program plus: Do not use in dogs <2 weeks old or <1 kg body weight.

Cats: 2 mg/kg milbemycin + 5 mg/kg praziquantel p.o. q30d.
Milbemax: Do not use the tablets for small cats and kittens in cats <6 weeks old or <0.5 kg body weight.

Small mammals: Ferrets: 1.15–2.33 mg/kg p.o. q30d.
Birds, Reptiles: No information available.

Miltefosine
(Milteforan) **POM-V**

Formulations: Oral: 20 mg/ml solution.

Action: Directly toxic to *Leishmania* and also enhances T cell and macrophage activation.

Use: Control of canine leishmaniosis. It is a new alternative to the standard allopurinol/meglumine antimonate protocol and seems to be as effective with fewer serious side effects. However, its efficacy has only been reported in a few studies and until more information is available it should be regarded as second choice. A Special Treatment Authorization is required to obtain this product (it is authorized for veterinary use in Spain and Germany). The clinical signs of the disease start to decrease markedly immediately after the beginning of treatment and are significantly reduced after 2 weeks. The signs continue to improve for at least 4 weeks after completion of the treatment. It is recommended to pour the product on to the animal's feed to reduce digestive side effects. Concurrent administration of antiemetic products could reduce the risk of undesired effects. Underdosing should be avoided to decrease the risk of resistance development, which may ultimately result in ineffective therapy.

Safety and handling: May cause eye and skin irritation and sensitization: personal protective equipment consisting of gloves and glasses should be worn when handling. Do not shake the vial to avoid foaming.

Contraindications: Do not use during pregnancy, lactation or in breeding animals.

Adverse reactions: Moderate and transient vomiting and diarrhoea are very common. These effects generally start within 5–7 days after the beginning of treatment and last for 1–2 days in most of the cases, but can last up to 7 days. The side effects do not affect the efficacy of the product and do not require discontinuation of treatment or change in the dose regimen. They are reversible at the end of treatment. Overdoses may produce uncontrollable vomiting.

Drug interactions: No information available.

DOSES
Dogs: 2 mg/kg q24h for 28 days (it is particularly important that the course is completed and given with allopurinol).
Cats, Small mammals, Birds, Reptiles: No information available.

Mineral oil see Paraffin

Minocycline
(Aknemin*, Minocin*) **POM**

Formulations: Oral: 50 mg, 100 mg capsules or tablets.

Action: Inhibition of bacterial protein synthesis by binding to the 30S subunit of the bacterial ribosome. The effect is bacteriostatic. Minocycline is the most lipid-soluble tetracycline with a broad spectrum of antibacterial activity in addition to antirickettsial, antimycoplasmal and antichlamydial activity. Due to its superior lipid solubility it tends to have greater clinical efficacy compared with other tetracyclines.

Use: Treatment of bacterial, rickettsial, mycoplasmal and chlamydial diseases. Its rate of excretion is not affected by renal function as it is cleared by hepatic metabolism and is therefore recommended when tetracyclines are indicated in animals with renal impairment. Being extremely lipid-soluble, it penetrates well into prostatic fluid and bronchial secretions. Use with care in animals with hepatic disease.

Safety and handling: Normal precautions should be observed.

Contraindications: No information available.

Adverse reactions: Nausea, vomiting and diarrhoea.

Drug interactions: Absorption of minocycline is reduced by antacids, calcium, magnesium and iron salts and sucralfate. Phenobarbital and phenytoin may increase its metabolism, decreasing plasma levels.

DOSES
See Appendix for guidelines on responsible antibacterial use.
Dogs, Cats: 5–10 mg/kg p.o. q12h.
Small mammals, Birds, Reptiles: No information available.

Mirtazapine `CIL`
(Zispin) **POM**

Formulations: Oral: 15 mg tablets, 15 mg/ml solution.

Action: Tricyclic antidepressant that acts on central alpha-2 receptors which leads to increased noradrenaline levels within the brain. Also inhibits several serotonin receptors and histamine (H1) receptors.

Use: Appetite stimulation in dogs and cats. Has been demonstrated to be effective in cats with stable chronic kidney disease. Can also be used as an antiemetic in conjunction with other drugs, but authorized preparations are preferred. Monitor animal carefully when using mirtazapine, particularly if there is also cardiac, hepatic or renal disease.

Safety and handling: Normal precautions should be observed.

Contraindications: Do not use in patients with pre-existing haematological disease.

Adverse reactions: Sedation is common and can be profound. Can affect behaviour in many different ways. Has been associated with blood dyscrasias in humans.

Drug interactions: Several interactions known in humans, principally involving other behaviour-modifying drugs.

DOSES
Dogs: 1.1–1.3 mg/kg p.o. q24h.
Cats: 1.88 mg p.o. q48h (can double dose if needed or increase frequency to q24h but not both).
Small mammals, Birds, Reptiles: No information available.

Misoprostol
(Cytotec*) **POM**

CIL

Formulations: Oral: 200 µg tablet.

Action: Cytoprotection of the gastric mucosa: it inhibits gastric acid secretion and increases bicarbonate and mucus secretion, epithelial cell turnover and mucosal blood flow. It prevents, and promotes healing of, gastric and duodenal ulcers, particularly those associated with the use of NSAIDs. Some reports suggest it may not prevent gastric ulceration caused by methylprednisolone. It may also be useful in the management of canine atopy.

Use: Protection against NSAID-induced gastric ulceration. In humans doses of up to 20 µg/kg p.o. q6–12h are used to manage pre-existing NSAID-induced gastric ulceration, whilst doses of 2–5 µg/kg p.o. q6–8h are used prophylactically to prevent ulceration. Combinations with diclofenac are available for humans, but are not suitable for small animals because of different NSAID pharmacokinetics.

Safety and handling: Women who are or might be pregnant should avoid handling this drug.

Contraindications: Do not use in pregnant animals.

Adverse reactions: Diarrhoea, abdominal pain, nausea, vomiting and abortion.

Drug interactions: Use of misoprostol with gentamicin may exacerbate renal dysfunction.

DOSES
Dogs: 2–7.5 µg (micrograms)/kg p.o. q8–12h.
Cats: 5 µg (micrograms)/kg p.o. q8h.
Small mammals: Ferrets: 1–5 µg (micrograms)/kg p.o. q8h.
Birds, Reptiles: No information available.

Mitotane (o,p'-DDD)

(Lysodren*) **POM**

CIL

Formulations: Oral: 500 mg tablet or capsule.

Action: Necrosis of the adrenal cortex reducing the production of adrenal cortical hormones.

Use: Management of pituitary-dependent hyperadrenocorticism (HAC) in dogs. However, other medications are authorized for this condition (see Trilostane). Has been used in the management of adrenal-dependent HAC, but with variable success. Mitotane is available from Europe for animals that have failed trilostane therapy. It should be given with food to improve its absorption from the intestinal tract. Following the initial 7–10 days therapy, an ACTH stimulation test should be performed to monitor the efficacy of therapy. In diabetic animals the initial dose should be reduced by 30%. The addition of prednisolone is generally not recommended. If switching from trilostane to mitotane, then post-ACTH cortisol concentrations should be >200 nmol/l before starting mitotane.

Safety and handling: Drug crosses skin and mucous membrane barriers. Wear gloves when handling this drug and avoid inhalation of dust.

Contraindications: No information available.

Adverse reactions: Anorexia, vomiting, diarrhoea and weakness, generally associated with too rapid a drop in plasma cortisol levels. They usually resolve with steroid supplementation. Acute-onset of neurological signs may be seen 2–3 weeks after initiation of therapy, possibly due to rapid growth of a pituitary tumour. Provide supplemental glucocorticoids during periods of stress. Approximately 5% of dogs require permanent glucocorticoid and mineralocorticoid replacement therapy if given mitotane overdose.

Drug interactions: Barbiturates and corticosteroids increase the hepatic metabolism of mitotane. There may be enhanced CNS depression with concurrent use of CNS depressants. Spironolactone blocks the action of mitotane. Diabetic animals may have rapidly changing insulin requirements during the early stages of therapy.

DOSES

Dogs: 30–50 mg/kg p.o. q24h to effect (generally 7–10 days) then weekly to fortnightly as required. Higher doses (50–150 mg/kg p.o. q24h) may become necessary for adrenal carcinomas.
Cats: Similar dose to dogs but efficacy in cats is very variable, with many showing no response at non-toxic levels.
Small mammals: Ferrets: Note that mitotane is no longer recommended to treat adrenal disease in ferrets.
Birds, Reptiles: No information available.

Mitoxantrone

(Novantrone*) **POM**

Formulations: Injectable: 2 mg/ml.

Action: Antitumour antibiotic which inhibits topoisomerase II. It is cell cycle non-specific.

Use: Treatment of canine and feline lymphoma, squamous cell carcinoma (SCC), and transitional cell carcinoma. Its use has also been described in renal adenocarcinoma, fibroid sarcoma, thyroid carcinoma, mammary gland adenocarcinoma, haemangiopericytoma and as a radiosensitizer in cats with oral SCC. Renal excretion is minimal, so it is far safer to administer to cats with renal insufficiency than doxorubicin.

Safety and handling: **Potent cytotoxic drug that should only be prepared and administered by trained personnel. See Appendix and specialist texts for further advice on chemotherapeutic agents.** Mitoxantrone should be stored at room temperature. While the manufacturer recommends against freezing, one study demonstrated that the drug maintained cytotoxic effects when frozen and thawed at various intervals over a 12-month period.

Contraindications: Avoid in patients with myelosuppression, concurrent infection, hepatic disease or impaired cardiac function (although it is likely to be much less cardiotoxic than doxorubicin).

Adverse reactions: GI signs (vomiting, anorexia, diarrhoea) and bone marrow depression are the most common signs of toxicity. White blood cell counts are generally lowest 10 days after administration. Seizure activity in cats has been reported. In very rare cases there may be discoloration of the urine and sclera (blue tinge).

Drug interactions: Use with extreme caution if administering other myelosuppressive or immunosuppressive agents. Chemically incompatible with heparin.

DOSES
See Appendix for chemotherapy protocols and conversion of body weight to body surface area.
Dogs: 5–6 mg/m^2 i.v. once every 3 weeks. It should be diluted with up to 50 ml of 0.9% NaCl.
Cats: 6–6.5 mg/m^2 i.v. once every 3 weeks. It should be diluted with up to 50 ml of 0.9% NaCl.
Small mammals, Birds, Reptiles: No information available.

Mitratapide

(Yarvitan) **POM-V**

Formulations: Oral: 5 mg/ml solution.

Action: Causes a reduced uptake of dietary lipids, dose-dependent decreases in serum cholesterol and triglyceride and an increased presence of triglyceride-containing droplets in enterocytes. Mitratapide has no central effect.

Use: Aid in the management of overweight and obesity in adult dogs. Should be used as part of an overall weight management programme which also includes appropriate dietary changes. Introducing appropriate lifestyle changes (e.g. increased exercise) may provide additional benefits. In clinical trials, treated animals rapidly regained weight following cessation of treatment when diet was not restricted. Treatment should be given with food. Mitratapide therapy should be restricted to one treatment course for an individual dog.

Safety and handling: Normal precautions should be observed.

Contraindications: Do not use in dogs that are pregnant, lactating, <18 months of age or that have impaired liver function. Do not use in dogs in which overweight or obesity is caused by a concomitant systemic disease (e.g. hypothyroidism or hyperadrenocorticism).

Adverse reactions: Vomiting, diarrhoea or softened stools may occur during treatment. Reversible decreases in serum albumin, globulin, total protein, calcium and ALP, and increases in ALT, AST and potassium may occur.

Drug interactions: No information available.

DOSES
Dogs: 0.63 mg/kg p.o. q24h (1 ml of the product per 8 kg) given for 2 periods of 21 days with 14 days without treatment in between.
Cats, Small mammals, Birds, Reptiles: No information available.

Montmorillonite (Monmorillonite)
(Diarsanyl*) **GSL**

Formulations: Oral: 10 ml, 24 ml, 60 ml multi-dose syringes (paste); 4.5 g montmorillonite, 2.5 g lactose, 2.5 g dextrose, 2.5 g glycerine, 0.4 g citric acid, 35.8 mg/kg sodium, 3.9 mg/kg potassium, 9.2 mg/kg magnesium, 3.9 calcium, 66.4 mg/kg phosphorus per 10 ml of paste.

Action: Acts in a similar way to kaolin but has superior adsorbent properties; it can bind mycotoxins and bacteria *in vitro*. It is combined in Diarsanyl with simple sugars and electrolytes to help compensate for GI electrolyte loss and energy deficiency. The efficacy has been questioned, but montmorillonite has been shown to have some benefit in humans with irritable bowel syndrome.

Use: Intestinal protectant and adsorbent in dogs with diarrhoea.

Safety and handling: Normal precautions should be observed.

Contraindications: Intestinal obstruction or perforation.

Adverse reactions: No information available.

Drug interactions: Kaolin may decrease the absorption of lincomycin, trimethoprim and sulphonamides, and a similar effect with montmorillonite is possible.

DOSES

Dogs: 1 ml p.o. q12h (dogs <7 kg) or 2 ml p.o. q12h (7–17 kg) or 4 ml p.o. q12h (18–30 kg) or 10 ml p.o. q12h (31–60 kg).
Cats: No information available.
Small mammals: Rabbits, Guinea pigs, Chinchillas: Not recommended in these species due to the risk of GI hypomotility developing.
Birds, Reptiles: No information available.

Morphine

CIL

(Morphine*, Oramorph*) **POM CD SCHEDULE 2**

Formulations: Injectable: 10 mg/ml, 15 mg/ml, 20 mg/ml, 30 mg/ml solution. Oral: 10 mg, 30 mg, 60 mg, 100 mg tablets. In addition there are suspensions, slow-release capsules, and granules in a wide range of strengths. Rectal: Suppositories are available in a wide range of strengths.

Action: Analgesia mediated by the mu opioid receptor.

Use: Management of moderate to severe pain in the perioperative period. Methadone should be used in preference to morphine as the licensed alternative for single or repeated bolus administration to dogs and cats. Morphine can be given as a constant rate infusion to provide analgesia intraoperatively and in the postoperative period. The greater availability of data describing morphine by continuous rate infusion may justify its use over methadone for this method of administration. Incorporation into sedative and pre-anaesthetic medication protocols to provide improved sedation and analgesia. Morphine is the reference opioid with which all others are compared. It provides profound analgesia and forms the mainstay of postoperative analgesic protocols in humans. In dogs it has a short duration of action and needs to be given frequently to be effective. Constant rate infusions can also be used to overcome this limitation. The duration of action in cats has not been rigorously evaluated, but it appears to have a duration of action of 3–4 hours. Accumulation is likely to occur after prolonged repeated dosing, which may allow the dose to be reduced or the dose interval extended. Morphine causes histamine release when given rapidly i.v., so it should be diluted and given slowly i.v. It commonly causes vomiting when given to animals preoperatively that are not in pain, therefore morphine should be avoided when vomiting is contraindicated (e.g. animals with raised intraocular pressure). Transient excitation may occur when morphine is given i.v. Preservative-free morphine can be administered into the epidural space where it will provide analgesia for up to 24 hours. Oral morphine is rarely used in cats and dogs due to a high first pass metabolism, leading to a low plasma concentration after oral administration. Respiratory function should be monitored when morphine is given to anaesthetized patients. The response to all opioids appears to vary between individual patients, therefore assessment of pain after administration is imperative. Morphine is metabolized in the liver, some prolongation of effect may be seen with impaired liver function.

Safety and handling: Normal precautions should be observed.

Contraindications: No information available.

Adverse reactions: In common with other mu agonists morphine can cause respiratory depression, although this is unlikely when used at clinical doses in awake cats and dogs. Respiratory depression may occur when given i.v. during general anaesthesia due to increased depth of anaesthesia. Vomiting is common after morphine administration and it causes constriction of GI sphincters (such as the pyloric sphincter) and may cause a reduction in GI motility when given over a long period. Morphine crosses the placenta and may exert sedative effects in neonates born to bitches treated prior to parturition. Severe adverse effects can be treated with naloxone.

Drug interactions: Other CNS depressants (e.g. anaesthetics, antihistamines, barbiturates, phenothiazines, tranquillisers) may cause increased CNS or respiratory depression when used concurrently with narcotic analgesics.

DOSES
When used for sedation is generally given as part of a combination. See Appendix for sedation protocols in all species.
Dogs:
- Analgesia: A dose of 0.5 mg/kg i.v., i.m. q2h is required to produce analgesia in experimental models. Pain should be assessed frequently and the dose adjusted based on requirement for analgesia.
- Continuous rate infusion: 0.15–0.2 mg/kg/h i.v.
- Epidural morphine (use Duramorph as it is preservative-free): 0.1 mg/kg diluted with 0.26 ml/kg of sterile saline (up to a total maximum volume of 6 ml in all dogs). There is a latent period of 30–60 min following epidural administration; duration of action is 18–24 hours.

Cats:
- Analgesia: 0.1–0.4 mg/kg i.v., i.m. q3–4h. Pain should be assessed frequently and the dose adjusted based on requirement for analgesia.
- Continuous rate infusions of morphine have not been widely evaluated in cats.
- Epidural morphine: dose as for dogs.

Small mammals: Analgesia: Ferrets: 0.5–5 mg/kg i.m., s.c. q6h, 0.1 mg/kg epidural; Rabbits, Guinea pigs: 2–5 mg/kg i.m., s.c. q2–4h; Hamsters, Gerbils, Rats, Mice: 2.5 mg/kg i.m., s.c. q2–4h.

Birds: No information available.
Reptiles: Analgesia: 1–4 mg/kg i.m. May result in significant respiratory depression at higher doses.

Moxidectin
(Advocate) **POM-V**

Formulations: Topical for cat: 10 mg/ml moxidectin with imidacloprid in spot-on pipette. Topical for dog: 25 mg/ml moxidectin with imidacloprid in spot-on pipette.

Action: Interacts with GABA and glutamate gated channels, leading to flaccid paralysis of parasites.

Use: Treatment and prevention of flea infestation (*Ctenocephalides felis*), ear mite infestation (*Otodectes cyanotis*), *Angiostrongylosis* and heartworm (*Dirofilaria immitis*) in dogs. Also used in dogs for treatment of sarcoptic mange, GI nematodes (L4 larvae and adult *Toxocara canis*, *Ancylostoma caninum*, *Uncinaria stenocephala*, adult *Toxascaris leonina*, and *Trichuris vulpis*). For effective treatment of canine sarcoptic mange the product should be applied on 3 occasions at 2-week intervals. Although approved for the treatment of canine demodicosis this product is not uniformly efficacious. Frequent shampooing may reduce the efficacy of the product. In cats it is used for the treatment of GI nematodes (L4 and adult *Toxocara cati* and *Ancylostoma tubaeforme*). Authorized for use in ferrets for treatment and prevention of flea infestation (*Ctenocephalides felis*) and the prevention of heartworm. Used in rabbits for *Psoroptes cuniculi*.

Safety and handling: Normal precautions should be observed.

Contraindications: Not for use in cats <9 weeks old, dogs <7 weeks old. Do not use larger pipette sizes in ferrets.

Adverse reactions: Transient pruritus and erythema at the site of application may occur. Severe effects may be seen if applied to cats with adult heartworm disease. Highly toxic to aquatic organisms.

Drug interactions: No information available.

DOSES
Dogs: 0.4 ml, 1.0 ml, 2.5 ml, 4 ml pipettes according to size of dog. Apply once every month. Minimum dose recommendation 0.1 ml/kg.
Cats: 0.4 ml, 0.8 ml pipettes according to size of cat. Apply once every month. Minimum dose recommendation 0.1 ml/kg.
Small mammals: Ferrets: 0.4 ml pipette monthly. If under heavy flea pressure can repeat once after 2 weeks; Rabbits: 0.2 mg/kg p.o., repeat in 10 days; Rodents: GI nematodes: 1 mg/kg of 2.5% v/w solution once.
Birds: 0.2 mg/kg topically prn.
Reptiles: No information available.

Moxifloxacin
(Moxivig*) **POM**

Formulations: Topical: 0.5% solution (5 mg/ml; 5 ml bottle).

Action: Bactericidal antimicrobial which works by inhibiting the bacterial DNA gyrase enzyme, causing damage to the bacterial DNA. The fluoroquinolones work in a concentration-dependent manner.

Use: Ideally fluoroquinolone use should be reserved for infections where culture and sensitivity testing predicts a clinical response and where first- and second-line antimicrobials would not be effective. Fourth generation fluoroquinolone with broad-spectrum activity against a wide range of Gram-negative and some Gram-positive aerobes. Active against many ocular pathogens, including *Staphylococcus* spp. and *Pseudomonas aeruginosa*.

Safety and handling: Normal precautions should be observed.

Contraindications: No information available.

Adverse reactions: May cause local irritation after application.

Drug interactions: No information available.

DOSES
See Appendix for guidelines on responsible antibacterial use.
Dogs, Cats: 1 drop in affected eye q6h.
Small mammals: No information available.
Birds: 1 drop in affected eye q12h.
Reptiles: 1 drop in affected eye q8–12h.

Mupirocin (Pseudomonic acid A)
(Bactroban*) **POM**

Formulations: Topical: 2% cream, ointment.

Action: Mupirocin has a novel chemical structure unrelated to any other known class of antibiotic. It blocks protein synthesis in bacteria by inhibiting bacterial isoleucyl-tRNA synthetase.

Use: Management of bacterial skin infections, especially those associated with *Staphylococcus*. As a consequence of this unique mode of action, mupirocin lacks cross-resistance with other antibacterial agents and exhibits activity against multiresistant strains of bacteria. Uses for mupirocin include canine pyotraumatic (acute moist) dermatitis, intertrigo (fold pyoderma), callus pyoderma and canine and feline acne. Mupirocin inhibits growth of several pathogenic fungi, including a range of dermatophytes and *Pityrosporum* and topical application may be useful in controlling such infections, although data are currently lacking as to its efficacy *in vivo*. Routine use of this agent cannot be advocated since in human medicine this agent is reserved for the eradication of MRSA within the nasal cavity and low-level resistance to mupirocin is emerging. It is generally indicated for the management of resistant infections. Use only if there are no alternative treatment options and do not use for longer than 7 days to avoid the development of resistance. Anecdotally both safe and useful in small mammals.

Safety and handling: Use impervious gloves for application.

Contraindications: Avoid if renal impairment present.

Adverse reactions: Application in humans has been associated with a stinging sensation.

Drug interactions: No information available.

DOSES
See Appendix for guidelines on responsible antibacterial use.
Dogs, Cats: Apply a thin layer of cream to infected areas q8h.
Small mammals, Birds, Reptiles: No information available.

Mycophenolate mofetil (MMF, Mycophenolic acid) CIL
(CellCept* (MMF), Myfortic* (MPA)) **POM**

Formulations: Oral: 250 mg capsule, 500 mg tablet, 1 g/5 ml powder for oral suspension (MMF); 180 mg, 360 mg tablets. Injectable: 500 mg powder for reconstitution and slow i.v. infusion (mycophenolic acid).

Action: Inhibits the enzyme that controls the rate of synthesis of guanine monophosphate in the *de novo* pathway of purine synthesis. This pathway is important in the proliferation of B and T lymphocytes. This action is similar to azathioprine.

Use: Prevention of organ transplant rejection in humans but it is beginning to be used in a number of immune-mediated conditions. In veterinary medicine MMF use has been reported in a small number of cases of immune-mediated skin disease, myasthenia gravis, immune-mediated haemolytic anaemia and immune-mediated thrombocytopenia. The use of MPA has not been reported in veterinary medicine. Clinical veterinary experience of this drug is limited; however, in humans mycophenolate is more lymphocyte-specific and less bone marrow suppressive than azathioprine.

Safety and handling: Cytotoxic drug; see Appendix and specialist texts for further advice on chemotherapeutic agents.

Contraindications: Bone marrow suppression, pre-existing infections.

Adverse reactions: Bone marrow suppression, nausea, vomiting, diarrhoea and an increased incidence of infections (pyoderma, *Malassezia*).

Drug interactions: Competes with other drugs that undergo active renal tubular secretion resulting in increased concentration of either drug. Concomitant administration of antacids (such as omeprazole) may decrease absorption.

DOSES
See Appendix for immunosuppression protocols.
Dogs:
- Immune-mediated haemolytic anaemia: 10 mg/kg p.o., i.v. q12h (MMF), can be reduced to q24h once clinical control is achieved or if side effects are observed.
- Pemphigus: 7–13 mg/kg p.o. q8h (MMF).

Cats: Immune-mediated haemolytic anaemia: 10 mg/kg p.o. q12h.
Small mammals, Birds, Reptiles: No information available.

Naloxone

(Naloxone*, Narcan*) **POM**

Formulations: Injectable: 0.02 mg/ml, 0.4 mg/ml solutions.

Action: Competitive antagonist for opioid receptors, reversing the effects of opioid agonists.

Use: Treatment of opioid overdose to reverse the adverse effects of opioid agonists. Also used to identify persistent activity of opioid drugs. Onset of action i.v. is very rapid, but duration is short (30–40 min). Repeated doses or an infusion may be required to manage overdose of longer acting opioids such as morphine and methadone or high dose fentanyl. Naloxone will also antagonize the effects of endogenous opioids, therefore it can cause antanalgesic effects in opioid naïve subjects. Administration to animals that could be in pain must therefore be considered carefully. Low dose naloxone i.v. will cause a transient elevation of unconsciousness when persistent opioid activity contributes to an unexpectedly long recovery from anaesthesia.

Safety and handling: Normal precautions should be observed.

Contraindications: No information available.

Adverse reactions: Indiscriminate use in animals that have undergone major surgery or trauma will expose the recipient to acute severe discomfort. In such cases the effects of opioid overdose (respiratory depression) should be managed by endotracheal intubation and artificial ventilation. Naloxone should be reserved for emergency situations when the effects of opioid overdose are severe.

Drug interactions: No information available.

DOSES

Dogs, Cats: 0.01–0.02 mg/kg i.v.; 0.04 mg/kg i.m., s.c., intratracheal. Naloxone can be administered as a continuous rate infusion at 0.02 mg/kg/h i.v. if a longer duration of opioid antagonism is required.
Small mammals: Ferrets: 0.01–0.04 mg/kg i.v., i.m., s.c.; Rabbits: 0.01–0.1 mg/kg i.v., i.m., i.p.; Rodents: 0.01–0.1 mg/kg s.c., i.v., i.p.
Birds: 2 mg/bird i.v.
Reptiles: No information available.

Nandrolone

(Laurabolin, Decadurabolin*) **POM-V, POM**

Formulations: Injectable: 25 mg/ml, 50 mg/ml (in oil).

Action: Binds to testosterone receptors and stimulates protein synthesis.

Use: For use wherever excessive tissue breakdown or extensive repair processes are taking place. Has also been advocated in the management of aplastic anaemia and anaemia associated with renal failure; however, may also have adverse effects on renal failure by increasing protein turnover. Monitor haematology to determine the efficacy of treatment and liver enzymes to monitor for hepatotoxicity.

Safety and handling: Normal precautions should be observed.

Contraindications: Do not use in breeding bitches or queens, in pregnant animals or in those with diabetes mellitus.

Adverse reactions: Androgenic effects may develop. Use in immature animals may result in early closure of epiphyseal growth plates.

Drug interactions: The concurrent use of anabolic steroids with adrenal steroids may potentiate the development of oedema.

DOSES

Dogs: 1–5 mg/kg i.m., s.c. q21d. Maximum dose 40–50 mg/dog.
Cats: 1–5 mg/kg i.m., s.c. q21d. Maximum dose 20–25 mg/cat.
Small mammals: Rabbits: 2 mg/kg s.c., i.m.
Birds: No information available.
Reptiles: 1 mg/kg i.m. q7–14d.

Neomycin

(Auroto, Neopen, Maxitrol*, Nivemycin*) **POM-V, POM**

Formulations: Oral: 500 mg tablets (Nivemycin). Parenteral: 100 mg/ml neomycin combined with 200 mg/ml penicillin G (Neopen). Topical: Many dermatological, ophthalmic and otic preparations contain 0.25–0.5% neomycin.

Action: A bactericidal antimicrobial agent that inhibits bacterial protein synthesis once it has gained access to the bacterial cell via an oxygen-dependent carrier mechanism. As other aminoglycosides, neomycin operates a concentration-dependent cell killing mechanism, leading to a marked post-antibiotic effect.

Use: Active primarily against Gram-negative bacteria, although some *Staphylococcus* and *Enterococcus* species are sensitive. All obligate anaerobic bacteria and many haemolytic streptococci are resistant. Since parenteral neomycin is extremely nephrotoxic and ototoxic it is used topically for infections of the skin, ear or mucous membranes. It is also used orally to reduce the intestinal bacterial population in the management of hepatic encephalopathy. As with other aminoglycosides it is not absorbed after oral administration unless GI ulceration is present. This drug has been used (often combined with antimuscarinic agents) in the treatment of non-specific bacterial enteritides. However, other antibacterial drugs, if required at all, are better indicated for such use. Neomycin is more active in an alkaline environment.

Safety and handling: Normal precautions should be observed.

Contraindications: For systemic use, do not use in animals with pre-existing renal disease. Do not use ear preparations if the tympanum is ruptured.

Adverse reactions: Systemic toxicity, ototoxicity and nephrotoxicity may very occasionally occur following prolonged high-dose oral therapy or where there is severe GI ulceration/inflammatory bowel disease, as sufficient neomycin may be absorbed. Nephrotoxicity and ototoxicity are potential side effects associated with parenteral use. Some patients may develop a severe diarrhoea/malabsorption syndrome and bacterial or fungal superinfections. Topical ophthalmic preparation may cause local irritation.

Drug interactions: Absorption of digoxin, methotrexate, potassium and vitamin K may be decreased. Other ototoxic and nephrotoxic drugs, e.g. furosemide, should be used with caution in patients on oral neomycin therapy as the combinations are likely to be synergistic.

DOSES
See Appendix for guidelines on responsible antibacterial use.
Dogs: Oral: 20 mg/kg p.o. q6h; or per rectum as a retention enema for hepatic encephalopathy. Ophthalmic: 1 drop/eye q6–8h. Otic: 2–12 drops/ear or apply liberally to skin q4–12h.
Cats: Oral: 5.5–10 mg/kg p.o. q12h. Ophthalmic: 1 drop/eye q6–8h. Otic: 2–12 drops/ear or apply liberally to skin q4–12h.
Small mammals: Ferrets: 10–20 mg/kg p.o. q6h; Rabbits 30 mg/kg p.o. q12h; Chinchillas, Guinea pigs: 15 mg/kg p.o. q12h; Rats, Mice: 25 mg/kg p.o q12h; In-water medication: Hamsters: 0.5 mg/ml drinking water; Gerbils, Rats, Mice: 2.6 mg/ml drinking water. Ophthalmic and otic doses as for dogs and cats.
Birds, Reptiles: No information available.

Neostigmine
(Prostigmin*, Robinul-Neostigmine*) **POM**

Formulations: Injectable: 2.5 mg/ml solution. Oral: 15 mg tablets.

Action: Prolongs the action of acetylcholine at the neuromuscular junction, but with low CNS penetration due to its polar structure. In comparison with edrophonium, it has a slower onset but a longer duration of action of approximately 30 minutes to 2 hours.

Use: Treatment of acute myasthenic crises when oral dosing is not possible. Due to its longer duration of effect it is also used in the diagnosis of myasthenia gravis when the collapse episodes are brief. In these cases, instead of injecting the anticholinesterase drug after the collapse episodes, the dog is pre-treated with neostigmine and then exercised to assess whether the collapse episodes have been abolished. If neostigmine is being used to diagnose myasthenia gravis then atropine should be given at an effective dose and demonstrated to have had an effect (dry buccal mucous membranes) prior to the administration of neostigmine. Neostigmine is also used to antagonize non-depolarizing neuromuscular blocking agents. If an overdose of neostigmine has been administered, maintenance of respiration should take priority. Atropine does not antagonize the nicotinic effects, including muscle weakness and paralysis. If muscle twitching is severe, these can be controlled with small doses of a competitive neuromuscular blocker. The cholinesterase reactivator pralidoxime can be used as an adjunct to atropine. Supportive treatment should be provided as required. Use with extreme caution in patients with bronchial disease (especially feline asthma), bradycardia (and other arrhythmias), hypotension, renal impairment or epilepsy.

Safety and handling: Normal precautions should be observed.

Contraindications: Contraindicated in mechanical GI or urinary tract obstruction and in peritonitis.

Adverse reactions: Primarily due to excessive cholinergic stimulation and most commonly include nausea, vomiting, increased salivation and diarrhoea. Overdosage may lead to muscle fasciculations and paralysis. Severe bradyarrhythmias, even asystole, may occur if neostigmine is used to antagonize neuromuscular block without the co-injection of atropine. Overdosage may lead to a 'cholinergic crisis', with both muscarinic and nicotinic effects. These effects may include lacrimation, defecation and urination, miosis, nystagmus, bradycardia and other arrhythmias, hypotension, muscle cramps, fasciculations, weakness and paralysis, respiratory signs and increased bronchial secretion combined with bronchoconstriction. CNS side effects include ataxia, seizures and coma.

Drug interactions: Effect may be antagonized by drugs with neuromuscular blocking activity, including aminoglycosides, clindamycin and halogenated inhalational anaesthetics. Drugs that may increase the clinical severity of myasthenia gravis may reduce the effectiveness of neostigmine treatment in these cases, including quinine and related compounds and beta-blockers. Concurrent use of neostigmine and beta-blockers may result in bradycardia. Neostigmine, as well as other anticholinesterases, inhibits the metabolism of suxamethonium, thereby prolonging and enhancing its clinical effect; combined use is not recommended. Neostigmine antagonizes the effect of non-depolarizing muscle relaxants. Antimuscarinic drugs such as atropine antagonize the muscarinic effects of neostigmine.

DOSES
Dogs:
- Myasthenic crisis: 0.01–0.1 mg/kg i.v., i.m., s.c., interval dependent upon duration of response. For longer term use 0.1–0.25 mg/kg p.o. q4h (total daily dose not to exceed 2 mg/kg).
- Antagonism of non-depolarizing neuromuscular blocking agents: Neostigmine (0.05 mg/kg) is mixed with glycopyrronium (0.01 mg/kg) and injected i.v. over 2 min once signs of spontaneous recovery from 'block', e.g. diaphragmatic 'twitching', are present. Continued ventilatory support should be provided until full respiratory muscles activity is restored. If glycopyrronium is

unavailable, atropine (0.04 mg/kg) is given i.v., followed by neostigmine (0.05 mg/kg) as soon as heart rate rises.

Cats:
* Myasthenic crisis: Use not reported in cats but extrapolation from dogs seems reasonable.
* Antagonism of non-depolarizing neuromuscular blocking agents: Doses as for dogs.

Small mammals, Birds, Reptiles: No information available.

Niacinamide see Nicotinamide

Nicergoline
(Fitergol) **POM-V**

Formulations: Oral: 5 mg freeze-dried tablets.

Action: Blocks serotonin and dopamine receptors and is an alpha-adrenergic antagonist, primarily acting through alpha-1 adrenoceptors. Its reported effects are to promote cerebral vasodilation, thereby improving cerebral oxygenation, and to have a neuroprotective action.

Use: Used to improve ageing-related disorders in dogs, particularly those of behavioural origin: e.g. diminished vigour and vigilance fatigue, sleep disorders, and psychomotor disturbances (such as episodes of ataxia). However, clinically apparent benefits of its pharmacological effects have not been published. Specific age-related diseases should receive appropriate treatment. Demonstrates a wide safety margin: administration of up to 90 times the normal recommended dose in dogs for 6 months has produced no adverse effects.

Safety and handling: The freeze-dried tablets should not be broken in half. For dogs 5–10 kg the drug may be administered in solution. Owners should be instructed to dissolve one tablet in 10 ml of water, stir or shake gently until dissolved, and then immediately administer 5 ml of the solution. The remainder of the solution must be discarded. A 10 ml syringe and suitable container should be provided for this purpose. Owners should be clearly instructed not to use household utensils for preparing the solution.

Contraindications: No information available.

Adverse reactions: No information available.

Drug interactions: Do not use within 24 hours of alpha-2 agonists such as xylazine, medetomidine and romifidine. Do not use before treatment with vasodilators such as acepromazine and prazosin.

DOSES
Dogs: 0.25–0.50 mg/kg p.o. q24h for 30 days. Treatment may be repeated depending on outcome.
Cats, Small mammals, Birds, Reptiles: No information available.

Nicotinamide (Niacinamide, Vitamin B3)
(Numerous trade names) **GSL**

Formulations: Oral: 50 mg, 250 mg tablets.

Action: Blocks antigen-induced histamine release, inhibits phosphodiesterase activity and protease release.

Use: Has been used in combination with oxytetracycline/tetracycline or doxycycline in the management of certain immune-mediated dermatoses such as lupoid onychodystrophy, discoid lupus erythematosus and pemphigus foliaceus.

Safety and handling: Normal precautions should be observed.

Contraindications: Do not use nicotinic acid (niacin) as it causes vasodilation.

Adverse reactions: May cause mild GI irritation.

Drug interactions: No information available.

DOSES
Dogs: 250 mg/dog q8h (dogs up to 25 kg), 500 mg/dog q8h (dogs >25 kg). Taper to effect.
Cats, Small mammals, Birds, Reptiles: No information available.

Nimesulide
(Zolan) **POM-V**

Formulations: Oral: 50 mg, 100 mg tablets.

Action: Nimesulide is an NSAID that preferentially inhibits COX-2 enzyme, thereby limiting the production of prostaglandins involved in inflammation.

Use: To reduce inflammation and pain associated with musculoskeletal disorders in dogs. It may also produce a range of other anti-inflammatory effects, including inhibition of the neutrophil oxidative response, inhibition of the synthesis of platelet activating factor, and a reduction in the synthesis of cartilage degrading enzymes. Administration to animals with renal disease must be carefully evaluated. Nimesulide is not authorized for preoperative administration to cats and dogs.

Safety and handling: Normal precautions should be observed.

Contraindications: Do not give to dehydrated, hypovolaemic or hypotensive patients or those with GI disease or blood clotting problems. Do not administer perioperatively until animal is fully recovered from anaesthesia and normotensive. Do not give to pregnant animals, animals <4 months or <3.5 kg. Liver disease will prolong metabolism, leading to the potential for drug accumulation and overdose with repeated dosing. Do not give to cats.

Adverse reactions: GI signs may occur in all animals after NSAID administration. Stop therapy if this persists beyond 1–2 days. Some animals develop signs with one NSAID and not another. A 1–2-week wash-out period should be allowed before starting another NSAID after cessation of therapy. Stop therapy immediately if GI bleeding is suspected. There is a small risk that NSAIDs may precipitate cardiac failure in animals with cardiovascular disease. A dark yellow discoloration of the serum or urine may be observed.

Drug interactions: Do not administer concurrently or within 24 hours of other NSAIDs and glucocorticoids. Do not administer with other potentially nephrotoxic agents, e.g. aminoglycosides.

DOSES
Dogs: 5 mg/kg q24h for 3–5 consecutive days, given with food.
Cats: Do not use.
Small mammals, Birds, Reptiles: No information available.

Nitenpyram
(Bob Martin Flea Tablets, Capstar, Johnson's 4 Fleas)
AVM-GSL

Formulations: Oral: 11.4 mg, 57 mg tablets.

Action: Post-synaptic binding to insect nicotinic receptors leads to insect paralysis and death. Kills fleas on animal within 30 minutes.

Use: Fleas on dogs and cats. Should be used as part of a fully integrated flea control programme. All animals in the affected household should be treated. Do not use 11.4 mg tablet in animals <1 kg or 4 weeks old. Do not use the 57 mg tablet in dogs <11 kg. Safe in pregnancy and lactation.

Safety and handling: Normal precautions should be observed.

Contraindications: No information available.

Adverse reactions: Transient increase in pruritus may be seen after administration due to fleas reacting to the product.

Drug interactions: No information available.

DOSES
Dogs, Cats: 1 mg/kg once (minimum dose) or q24h.
Small mammals, Birds, Reptiles: No information available.

Nitrofurantoin
(Furadantin*, Nitrofurantoin*) **POM**

Formulations: Oral: 50 mg, 100 mg tablets; 25 mg/5 ml suspension.

Action: Reacts with bacterial nitroreductase enzymes to form products that interact with bacterial DNA and cause strand breakage. It is bacteriostatic at low concentrations and bactericidal at high concentrations.

Use: Active against many Gram-positive and Gram-negative bacteria. Well absorbed following oral administration but is rapidly excreted in urine, thus therapeutic levels are not attained in serum or most tissues but are attained in the urinary tract. The concentration of nitrofurantoin is highest in alkaline urine. However, urine should not be alkalinized as the activity of nitrofurantoin is significantly decreased. Use is limited due to toxicity and concerns about mutagenicity and carcinogenicity. Reserve for infections with confirmed sensitivity.

Safety and handling: Mutagenic so wear gloves when handling.

Contraindications: Do not use in patients with significant renal impairment, as serum levels will rise and give an increased risk of serious toxicity. Since nitrofurans are mutagenic, they should not be given to pregnant animals.

Adverse reactions: In humans may rarely cause a peripheral neuritis, pulmonary complications, hepatotoxicity, emesis, diarrhoea and GI bleeding. High oral doses may cause thrombocytopenia, anaemia and leucopenia, with prolonged bleeding times.

Drug interactions: The bioavailability of nitrofurantoin may be increased by antimuscarinic drugs and food as they delay gastric emptying time and increase absorption of this weak acid from the stomach. Antagonism may be observed with fluoroquinolones.

DOSES
See Appendix for guidelines on responsible antibacterial use.
Dogs, Cats: 4 mg/kg p.o. q8h.
Small mammals, Birds, Reptiles: No information available.

Nitroglycerin(e) see Glyceryl trinitrate

Nitroscanate
(Bob Martin All in One Dewormer, Troscan) **AVM-GSL**

Formulations: Oral: 100 mg, 500 mg tablets.

Action: Unclear but appears to be an uncoupler of oxidative phosphorylation.

Use: Highly effective in a single dose against common canine nematodes and cestodes including *Toxocara canis, Toxascaris leonina, Ancylostoma caninum, Uncinaria stenocephala, Taenia ovis, T. hydatigena, T. pisiformis* and *Dipylidium caninum*. At the recommended dose gives limited control of *Echinococcus granulosus*. Not effective against *Trichuris vulpis*. An adult worming regime of 2–4 times per year is recommended.

Safety and handling: Nitroscanate is irritant and tablets should not be crushed, broken or divided.

Contraindications: Do not administer to sick or convalescing animals. Do not use in cats.

Adverse reactions: Vomiting in dogs. If given mistakenly to cats CNS disturbances (ataxia and disorientation) are seen.

Drug interactions: No information available.

DOSES
Dogs: 50 mg/kg p.o. with one-fifth of the daily food ration in the morning. Tablets should be given whole. Give remaining food ration after 8 hours.
Cats: Do not use.
Small mammals, Birds, Reptiles: No information available.

Nitrous oxide
(Entonox*, Nitrous oxide*) **POM**

Formulations: Inhalational: 100% nitrous oxide (N_2O) gas. Entonox is N_2O plus oxygen.

Action: Causes CNS depression.

Use: Used with oxygen to carry volatile anaesthetic agents such as isoflurane for the induction and maintenance of anaesthesia. N_2O reduces the concentration of inhalant agent required to maintain anaesthesia. Administration of N_2O at the beginning of volatile agent anaesthesia increases the speed of uptake of volatile agent from the alveoli (via the 2nd gas effect and concentration effect), hastening attainment of a stable plane of volatile agent anaesthesia. Oxygen must be supplemented for 5–10 min after N_2O is discontinued to prevent diffusion hypoxia. N_2O causes minimal respiratory and cardiovascular effects and is a useful addition to a balanced anaesthesia technique. A minimum oxygen concentration of 30% is required during anaesthesia. The inspired concentration of oxygen may fall to critically low levels when N_2O is used in rebreathing circuits during low flow rates. Do not use in such systems unless the inspired oxygen concentration can be measured on a breath-by-breath basis.

Safety and handling: Prolonged exposure can have serious adverse effects on human health. Scavenging is essential. N_2O is not absorbed by charcoal in passive scavenging systems utilizing activated charcoal.

Contraindications: Do not give to patients with air-filled spaces within the body, e.g. pneumothorax or gastric dilatation. N_2O will cause a rapid expansion of any gas-filled space, increasing volume or pressure. Do not give to animals with marked respiratory compromise, due to the risks of hypoxia.

Adverse reactions: The cobalt ion present in vitamin B12 is oxidized by N_2O so that it is no longer able to act as the cofactor for methionine synthase. The result is reduced synthesis of methionine, thymidine, tetrahydrofolate and DNA. Exposure lasting only a few hours may lead to megaloblastic changes in bone marrow but more prolonged exposure (a few days) may result in agranulocytosis.

Drug interactions: No information available.

DOSES
Dogs, Cats, Small mammals, Birds: Inspired concentrations of 50–70%.
Reptiles: No information available.

Nizatidine
(Axid*, Nizatidine*) **POM**

Formulations: Injectable: 25 mg/ml solution. Oral: 150 mg, 300 mg capsules, tablets.

Action: Nizatidine is a potent histamine (H2) receptor antagonist blocking histamine-induced gastric acid secretion. It is many times more potent than cimetidine, and does not undergo hepatic metabolism. It also has some prokinetic effect through stimulation of local muscarinic acetylcholine receptors, which may be of benefit when gastric motility is impaired by gastritis or ulceration, and in feline idiopathic megacolon. There is little information on the use of this drug in veterinary medicine. Safety in healthy dogs has been established, and no adverse effects have been reported. However, if used i.v., slow injection is recommended.

Use: Management of gastric and duodenal ulcers, oesophagitis, and hypersecretory conditions secondary to gastrinoma, mast cell neoplasia or short bowel syndrome. Reduction of vomiting due to gastric ulceration is typically achieved in about 2 weeks. Animals should, however, be treated for at least 2 weeks after the remission of clinical signs, so a minimum treatment duration of 28 days is recommended. Absorption is not clinically significantly affected by food intake, anticholinergic agents, or antacids. Currently cimetidine is the only antiulcer drug with a veterinary market authorization. In situations where a GI prokinetic effect is desired, ranitidine may be preferable to nizatidine.

Safety and handling: Normal precautions should be observed.

Contraindications: No information available.

Adverse reactions: No information available.

Drug interactions: No information available.

DOSES
Dogs, Cats: 1 mg/kg i.v. q12h; 2.5 mg/kg p.o. q12–24h.
Small mammals, Birds, Reptiles: No information available.

Nystatin

(Canaural, Nystan*, Nystatin*) **POM-V, POM**

Formulations: Oral: 100,000 IU/ml suspension. Topical: various products.

Action: Binds to ergosterol, a major component of the fungal cell membrane, and forms pores in the membrane that lead to potassium leakage and death of the fungus.

Use: Antifungal agent with a broad spectrum of activity but noted for its activity against *Candida*, particularly *C. albicans*. Not absorbed from the GI tract.

Safety and handling: Normal precautions should be observed.

Contraindications: No information available.

Adverse reactions: No information available.

Drug interactions: No information available.

DOSES

Dogs, Cats: Apply to affected areas q8–12h.
Small mammals: No information available.
Birds: Pigeons: 100,000 IU/kg p.o. q24h for 10 days; Passerines: 5,000–300,000 IU/kg q12h for macrorhabdiasis, though there are many doubts over its efficacy; Other birds: 300,000 IU/kg p.o. q12h.
Reptiles: 100,000 IU/kg p.o. q24h for 10 days.

Oclacitinib
(Apoquel) **POM-V**

Formulations: Oral: 3.6 mg, 5.4 mg, 16 mg tablets.

Action: Inhibits janus-kinases (particularly JAK1), which act as signal transducers that are activated by IL-31 and other cytokines. Elevated IL-31 levels are associated with pruritus in humans and dogs.

Use: For the treatment of pruritus associated with allergic dermatitis in dogs. May increase susceptibility to infection and demodicosis. Oclacitinib may be useful in cats but the optimum dose, pharmakinetics and safety profile have not been studied in detail.

Safety and handling: Normal precautions should be observed.

Contraindications: For use in dogs >12 months old. May exacerbate neoplastic conditions. Not to be used in pregnancy or lactation.

Adverse reactions: Diarrhoea, vomiting, anorexia, new cutaneous or subcutaneous swellings, lethargy and polydipsia have all been reported, but are rare.

Drug interactions: May reduce antibody response to certain vaccinations.

DOSES
Dogs, Cats: 0.4–0.6 mg/kg p.o. q12h for 14 days, then q24h for maintenance.
Small mammals, Birds, Reptiles: No information available.

Octreotide
(Sandostatin*, Sandostatin LAR*) **POM**

Formulations: Injectable: 50 µg/ml, 100 µg/ml, 200 µg/ml, 500 µg/ml solutions; depot preparation: 10 mg, 20 mg, 30 mg vials.

Action: Somatostatin analogue that inhibits the release of several hormones.

Use: May be useful in the management of gastric, enteric and pancreatic endocrine tumours (e.g. insulinoma, gastrinoma) and acromegaly. Variable responses have been reported in veterinary medicine. Most recent research suggests that it is not useful in most insulinomas. Tumours not expressing somatostatin receptors will not respond. There is limited information on the use of this drug in veterinary species. In humans doses up to 200 µg/person q8h are used. Similar doses of the aqueous preparation may be required in animals, but dosages for the depot preparation are not known.

Safety and handling: Normal precautions should be observed.

Contraindications: No information available.

Adverse reactions: GI disturbances (anorexia, vomiting, abdominal pain, bloating, diarrhoea and steatorrhoea), hepatopathy and pain at injection sites have been recorded in humans.

Drug interactions: No information available.

DOSES:
Dogs, Cats: 10–20 μg (micrograms)/animal s.c. q8–12h.
Small mammals: Ferrets: 1–2 μg (micrograms)/kg s.c. q8–12h.
Birds, Reptiles: No information available.

Oestriol see Estriol

Ofloxacin
(Exocin*) **POM**

Formulations: Topical: 0.3% solution.

Action: Bactericidal antimicrobial which works by inhibiting the bacterial DNA gyrase enzyme, causing damage to the bacterial DNA. The fluoroquinolones work in a concentration-dependent manner.

Use: Ideally fluoroquinolone use should be reserved for infections where culture and sensitivity testing predicts a clinical response and where first- and second-line antimicrobials would not be effective. For ophthalmic use when other antibacterial agents are ineffective. Active against many ocular pathogens, including *Staphylococcus* and *Pseudomonas aeruginosa*, although there is increasing resistance amongst some staphylococcal and streptococcal organisms.

Safety and handling: Normal precautions should be observed.

Contraindications: No information available.

Adverse reactions: May cause local irritation after application.

Drug interactions: No information available.

DOSES
See Appendix for guidelines on responsible antibacterial use.
Dogs, Cats, Small mammals: 1 drop to affected eye q6h; loading dose can be used: 1 drop to affected eye q15min for 4 doses.
Birds: 1 drop in affected eye q12h.
Reptiles: 1 drop in affected eye q8–12h.

Olsalazine
(Dipentum*) **POM**

Formulations: Oral: 250 mg capsule, 500 mg tablet.

Action: Olsalazine is a dimer of 5-aminosalicylic acid (5-ASA) that is cleaved by colonic bacteria into free 5-ASA, which has a local anti-inflammatory effect.

Use: Management of colitis, especially in patients sensitive to sulfasalazine. Although the incidence of keratoconjunctivitis sicca is much lower than with sulfasalazine, it is still a potential risk, and periodic Schirmer tear tests should be performed.

Safety and handling: Normal precautions should be observed.

Contraindications: Do not use in patients sensitive to salicylates.

Adverse reactions: Keratoconjunctivitis sicca.

Drug interactions: Activity will be potentiated by administration of other NSAIDs.

DOSES
Dogs: 10–20 mg/kg p.o. q12h.
Cats, Small mammals, Birds, Reptiles: No information available.

Omeprazole

(Gastrogard, Losec*, Mepradec*, Zanprol*) **POM-V, POM**

Formulations: Oral: 10 mg, 20 mg, 40 mg capsules, gastro-resistant tablets, MUPS (multiple unit pellet system) tablets. Injectable: 40 mg vial for reconstitution for i.v. injection; discard remainder after use.

Action: Proton pump inhibitor. Ten times more potent than cimetidine in inhibiting gastric acid secretion and has a longer duration of activity (>24 h).

Use: Management of gastric and duodenal ulcers, oesophagitis, and hypersecretory conditions secondary to gastrinoma (Zollinger-Ellison syndrome) or mast cell neoplasia. Gastrogard is licensed for use in equids, but the formulation (370 mg/g paste) makes accurate dosing of small animals impossible. Lansoprazole, rabeprazole and pantoprazole are similar drugs but have no known clinical advantage over omeprazole. Esomeprazole is a newer preparation containing only the active isomer of omeprazole. Studies have shown that omeprazole produces mild increases in canine gastric pH but that the effects are significantly greater than that produced by cimetidine or ranitidine.

Safety and handling: Normal precautions should be observed.

Contraindications: No information available.

Adverse reactions: Chronic suppression of acid secretion has caused hypergastrinaemia in laboratory animals, leading to mucosal cell hyperplasia, rugal hypertrophy and the development of carcinoids, and so treatment for a maximum of 8 weeks has been recommended. However, such problems have not been reported in companion animals. Adverse effects do include nausea, diarrhoea, constipation and skin rashes. An i.v. preparation of rabeprazole causes pulmonary oedema in dogs at high doses.

Drug interactions: Omeprazole may enhance the effects of phenytoin. There is a risk of interaction with tacrolimus, mycophenolate mofetil, clopidogrel, digoxin and itraconazole.

DOSES
Dogs: 0.5–1.5 mg/kg i.v., p.o. q24h for a maximum of 8 weeks.
Cats: 0.75–1 mg/kg p.o. q24h for a maximum of 8 weeks.
Small mammals: Ferrets: 0.7–4 mg/kg p.o. q24h for a maximum of 8 weeks.
Birds, Reptiles: No information available.

Ondansetron CIL
(Zofran*) **POM**

Formulations: Injectable: 2 mg/ml solution in 2 ml and 4 ml ampoules. Oral: 4 mg, 8 mg tablets; 4 mg/5 ml syrup. Rectal: 16 mg suppositories.

Action: Potent antiemetic effects through action on the GI tract and the chemoreceptor trigger zone. It was developed for, and is particularly useful in, the control of emesis induced by chemotherapeutic drugs. However, recent work suggests its potency at canine 5-HT3 receptors is one tenth that in humans.

Use: Indicated for the management of nausea and vomiting in patients who are unable to tolerate, or whose signs are not controlled by, other drugs (e.g. maropitant, metoclopramide). Dolasetron, granisetron, palanosetron and tropisetron are similar drugs but have yet to be extensively used in companion animals.

Safety and handling: Normal precautions should be observed.

Contraindications: Intestinal obstruction.

Adverse reactions: In humans, constipation, headaches, occasional alterations in liver enzymes and, rarely, hypersensitivity reactions have been reported.

Drug interactions: Ondansetron may reduce the effectiveness of tramadol and so the dose of tramadol may need to be increased.

DOSES
Dogs, Cats: 0.5 mg/kg i.v. loading dose followed by 0.5 mg/kg/h infusion for 6 hours or 0.5–1 mg/kg p.o. q12–24h.
Small mammals: Ferrets: 1 mg/kg p.o. q12–24h.
Birds, Reptiles: No information available.

Orbifloxacin

(Orbax, Posatex) **POM-V**

Formulations: Oral: 30 mg/ml suspension. Otic: Ear drops containing 8.5 mg/ml orbifloxacin combined with mometasone (steroid) and posaconazole (antifungal).

Action: Bactericidal, inhibiting DNA gyrase. Action is concentration-dependent, meaning that pulse dosing regimens may be effective.

Use: Ideally fluoroquinolone use should be reserved for infections where culture and sensitivity testing predicts a clinical response and where first- and second-line antimicrobials would not be effective. Broad spectrum agent. Particularly active against mycoplasmas, many Gram-negative organisms and some Gram-positives including *Pasteurella*, *Staphylococcus*, *Pseudomonas*, *Escherichia coli*, *Proteus* and *Salmonella*. The fluoroquinolones are effective against beta-lactamase-producing bacteria. Orbifloxacin is ineffective in treating obligate anaerobic infections. It is a highly lipophilic drug, attaining high concentrations within cells in many tissues and is particularly effective in the management of soft tissue, urogenital (including prostatic) and skin infections. Caution should be exercised before using dose rates above those recommended by the manufacturer.

Safety and handling: Normal precautions should be observed.

Contraindications: Due to concerns regarding cartilage damage, orbifloxacin is contraindicated in giant-breed dogs <18 months old, large breeds <12 months old, and small and medium-sized breeds <8 months old. Should not be used in pregnant or lactating bitches or animals for breeding. Do not use the otic preparation in animals <4 months of age or if the tympanum is not intact.

Adverse reactions: Cartilage abnormalities have been reported with other fluoroquinolones in growing animals. Such abnormalities have not been specifically reported following the use of orbifloxacin. These drugs should be used with caution in epileptics until further information is available from dogs, as they potentiate CNS adverse effects when administered concurrently with NSAIDs in humans. The potential adverse effects of orbifloxacin on the canine retina have not been studied (see Enrofloxacin).

Drug interactions: Absorbents and antacids containing cations (Mg^{2+}, Al^{3+}) may bind fluoroquinolones, preventing their absorption from the GI tract. Their absorption may also be inhibited by sucralfate and zinc salts; separate dosing by at least 2 hours. Fluoroquinolones increase plasma theophylline concentrations. Cimetidine may reduce the clearance of fluoroquinolones and so should be used with caution with these drugs. Do not use with oral ciclosporin.

DOSES

See Appendix for guidelines on responsible antibacterial use.

Dogs: 2.5–7.5 mg/kg p.o. q24h. For the otic preparation: 2–8 drops per ear q24h. The number of drops is determined by the weight of the dog.
Cats, Small mammals, Birds, Reptiles: No information available.

Osaterone
(Ypozane) **POM-V**

Formulations: Oral: 1.875 mg, 3.75 mg, 7.5 mg, 15 mg tablets.

Action: Competitively prevents the binding of androgens to their prostatic receptors and blocks the transport of testosterone into the prostate.

Use: Treatment of benign prostatic hypertrophy (BPH) in male dogs. In dogs with BPH associated with prostatitis, osaterone can be administered concurrently with antimicrobials. Use with caution in dogs with a history of liver disease.

Safety and handling: Women of child-bearing age should avoid contact with, or wear disposable gloves when administering, the product.

Contraindications: No information available.

Adverse reactions: A transient reduction of plasma cortisol concentration may occur; this may continue for several weeks after administration. Appropriate monitoring should be implemented in dogs under stress (e.g. following surgery) or those with hypoadrenocorticism. The response to an ACTH stimulation test may also be suppressed for several weeks after administration of osaterone. Transient increases in appetite and changes in behaviour occur commonly. Other adverse reactions include transient vomiting and/or diarrhoea, polyuria/polydipsia, lethargy and feminization syndrome including mammary gland hyperplasia. Treatment of some dogs with liver disease has resulted in reversible increases in ALT and ALP.

Drug interactions: No information available.

DOSES:
Dogs: 0.25–0.5 mg/kg q24h for 7 days.
Cats, Small mammals, Birds, Reptiles: No information available.

Oxantel see **Pyrantel**

Oxymetazoline
(Afrazine*) **P**

Formulations: Paediatric nasal drops: 0.025% solution.

Action: A sympathomimetic drug that reduces blood flow to the turbinates and therefore reduces swelling of the nasal mucosa.

Use: Nasal decongestant in cases of allergic (lymphocytic) rhinitis. May also be of some use in 'cat flu'. As the effects of the drug wear off, a rebound phenomenon develops due to secondary vasodilation. This results in a subsequent temporary increase in nasal congestion. Xylometazoline is similar to oxymetazoline.

Safety and handling: Normal precautions should be observed.

Contraindications: No information available.

Adverse reactions: No information available.

Drug interactions: No information available.

DOSES

Dogs, Cats: 1 drop/nostril q12h for maximum 48 hours.
Small mammals, Birds, Reptiles: No information available.

Oxypentifylline see Pentoxifylline

Oxytetracycline
(Engemycin, Oxycare) **POM-V**

Formulations: Injectable: 100 mg/ml solution. Oral: 50 mg, 100 mg, 250 mg tablets. Feed supplement and soluble powders also available.

Action: Inhibits bacterial protein synthesis. The effect is bacteriostatic.

Use: Active against many Gram-positive and Gram-negative bacteria, rickettsiae, mycoplasmas, spirochaetes and other microbes. One of the less lipid-soluble tetracyclines, it is excreted unchanged in urine and bile and undergoes enterohepatic recirculation. Has been used in combination with nicotinamide in the management of immune-mediated conditions, including discoid lupus erythematosus and lupoid onychodystrophy. Resistance to tetracyclines is widespread. Use with care in rabbits as narrow therapeutic range.

Safety and handling: Normal precautions should be observed.

Contraindications: The concentrated injectable depot formulations used for cattle and sheep should never be given to small animals. Avoid oral dosing in birds, other than for prophylaxis, as tetracyclines are poorly absorbed from the GI tract, rapidly lose potency in drinking water and put birds off drinking water due to their taste. Only use in cats when no other agent is suitable.

Adverse reactions: Include vomiting, diarrhoea, depression, hepatotoxicity (rare), fever, hypotension (following i.v. administration) and anorexia (cats). Prolonged use may lead to development of superinfections. Oral tetracyclines may cause GI disturbances and death in guinea pigs. Although not well documented in veterinary medicine, tetracyclines induce dose-related functional changes in renal tubules in several species, which may be exacerbated by dehydration, haemoglobinuria, myoglobinuria or concomitant administration of other nephrotoxic drugs. Severe tubular damage has occurred following the use of outdated or improperly stored products and occurs due to the formation of a degradation product.

Tetracyclines stain the teeth of children when used in the last 2–3 weeks of pregnancy or the first month of life. Although this phenomenon has not been well documented in animals, it does occur in dogs and it is prudent to restrict the use of tetracyclines in all young animals. Injectable preparations in birds may cause toxicity or muscle necrosis. In rabbits, higher doses (30 mg/kg) can be associated with enteritis.

Drug interactions: The bactericidal action of penicillins may be inhibited by oxytetracycline. Antacids containing divalent or trivalent cations (Mg^{2+}, Ca^{2+}, Al^{3+}), food or milk products bind tetracycline, reducing its absorption. Tetracyclines may increase the nephrotoxic effects of methoxyflurane. The GI effects of tetracyclines may be increased if administered concurrently with theophylline products.

DOSES
See Appendix for guidelines on responsible antibacterial use.
Dogs: 7–11 mg/kg i.m., s.c. q24h; 50 mg/kg loading dose, then 25 mg/kg p.o. q12h for up to 5 days. Give oral dose on an empty stomach.
Cats: 7–11 mg/kg i.m., s.c. q24h.
Small mammals: Ferrets, Hamsters, Gerbils: 20–25 mg/kg i.m. q8–12h; Rabbits: 15 mg/kg i.m. q12h; Chinchillas: 15 mg/kg i.m. q12h, 50 mg/kg p.o. q12h; Guinea pigs: 5 mg/kg i.m. q12h; Rats: 20 mg/kg i.m. q8–12h, 10–20 mg/kg p.o. q8h; Mice: 100 mg/kg s.c. q12h, 10–20 mg/kg p.o. q8h.
Birds: Raptors: 25–50 mg/kg p.o. q8h; Parrots: 50 mg/kg i.m. q24h, 200 mg/kg i.m. q24h – long-acting preparations; Passerines: 100 mg/kg p.o. q24h or 4–12 mg/l water for 7 days; Pigeons: 50 mg/kg p.o. q6h or 80 mg/kg i.m. q48h (long-acting preparation) or 130–400 mg/l water.
Reptiles: 6–10 mg/kg p.o., i.m., i.v. q24h.

Oxytocin
(Oxytocin S) **POM-V**

Formulations: Injectable: 10 IU/ml solution.

Action: Synthetic oxytocin.

Use: Induces parturition when uterine inertia is present (as long as there is no uterine obstruction); evacuates uterine contents; decreases haemorrhage following parturition; and promotes milk 'let-down'. Before oxytocin is used in any species it is important to ensure that there is no evidence of obstructive dystocia and that blood calcium levels are adequate. Calcium supplementation should be administered 1 hour prior to oxytocin if ionized or total blood calcium levels are low. Can also be used i.v. (dose at 25% of i.m. dose, diluted in water for injection).

Safety and handling: Store in refrigerator.

Contraindications: Not recommended for use in egg retention in birds.

Adverse reactions: Overstimulation of the uterus can be hazardous to both mother and fetuses. In birds it can cause painful side effects due to stimulation of smooth muscle.

Drug interactions: Severe hypertension may develop if used with sympathomimetic pressor amines.

DOSES
Dogs:
- Obstetric indications: 0.1–0.5 IU/kg i.m., s.c. q30min for up to 3 doses.
- Milk let-down: 2–20 IU/dog i.m., s.c. once.

Cats:
- Obstetric indications: 0.1–0.5 IU/kg i.m., s.c. q30min for up to 2 doses.
- Milk let-down: 1–10 IU/cat i.m., s.c. once.

Small mammals: Ferrets: 0.2-3.0 IU/kg s.c., i.m.; Rabbits: 0.1–3.0 IU/kg s.c., i.m.; Rodents: 0.2–3 IU/kg s.c., i.m., i.v.; Mice (milk let-down) 6.25 IU/kg s.c.

Birds: Do not use.

Reptiles: Egg retention: 2–10 IU/kg i.m. q90min; maximum of 3 doses. Better effect if calcium therapy used first.

Pamidronate

(Aredia*, Pamidronate*) **POM**

Formulations: Injectable: 15 mg, 30 mg, 90 mg powders in vials for reconstitution and i.v. infusion.

Action: Inhibits osteoclast activity and induces osteoclast apoptosis.

Use: Treatment of hypercalcaemia (especially associated with vitamin D toxicosis and hypercalcaemia of malignancy, or if other therapeutic regimens are unsuccessful). In human medicine it is also used to treat osteolytic lesions and bone pain due to bone metastases associated with breast cancer, multiple myeloma and Paget's disease. There may be clinical usefulness in directly treating 'micrometastases' in osteosarcomas but studies are ongoing.

Safety and handling: Normal precautions should be observed.

Contraindications: Renal dysfunction.

Adverse reactions: Can cause renal toxicity, nausea, diarrhoea, hypocalcaemia, hypophosphataemia, hypomagnesaemia and hypersensitivity reactions.

Drug interactions: Concurrent use of aminoglycosides may result in severe hypocalcaemia.

DOSES
Dogs: 0.65–2 mg/kg i.v. slow infusion with NaCl 0.9% over 2h. For cholecalciferol-induced toxicosis, give on days 1 and 4 post-ingestion.
Cats: 1.5–2.0 mg/kg i.v. slow (over 4h) infusion q24h.
Small mammals, Birds, Reptiles: No information available.

Pancreatic enzyme supplements

(Tryplase, Lypex*, Pancreatic Enzyme Supplement for Dogs and Cats*, Panzym*) **AVM-GSL, POM, P**

Formulations: Oral: See BSAVA website for a full list of pancreatic enzyme supplements available in the UK and their contents. Note that Tryplase is the only formulation that is authorized for veterinary use, although others are marketed as nutraceuticals in the veterinary market. Many other formulations on human market.

Action: Exogenous replacement enzymes.

Use: Pancreatic enzymes (lipase, protease, amylase) are used to control signs of exocrine pancreatic insufficiency (EPI). Fresh raw, or fresh-frozen, pig pancreas (approximately 100 g per meal) is also an effective treatment (and is not a Specified Risk Material) but availability is limited and there is a risk of pathogen ingestion by this method. Non-enteric coated powders and enteric coated granules and tablets are available. Lypex enteric coated granules are more effective in increasing body weight in dogs with EPI compared with a non-enteric coated formulation. Tryplase capsules are opened and their contents sprinkled on the food; do not administer whole capsules. Use the manufacturer's recommendations as the minimum required initially; the dose may be reduced empirically once a satisfactory response is achieved. Efficacy may be augmented by antibiotic control of secondary bacterial overgrowth and vitamin B12 therapy for any associated hypocobalaminaemia. Concomitant administration of acid blockers is not cost-effective and there is no requirement for pre-incubation with food. Follow dosing with food or water.

Safety and handling: Powder spilled on hands should be washed off or skin irritation may develop. Avoid inhaling powder as it causes mucous membrane irritation and may trigger asthma attacks in susceptible individuals. These risks are not associated with enteric coated pancreatic granules.

Contraindications: No information available.

Adverse reactions: Contact dermatitis of the lips is occasionally seen with powdered non-coated enzyme and some dogs develop an offensive odour. Non-coated pancreatic enzymes may cause oral or oesophageal ulcers, and so dosing should be followed with food or water. High doses may cause diarrhoea and signs of gastrointestinal cramping.

Drug interactions: The effectiveness may be diminished by antacids (magnesium hydroxide, calcium carbonate).

DOSES
Dogs:
- Lypex: open capsule and sprinkle granules on to food. Dogs <10 kg body weight = 0.5 capsule per meal; dogs >10 kg body weight = 1 capsule per meal. For best results feed at least twice daily.
- Tryplase: the contents of 2–5 capsules per day sprinkled on food; 5 capsules are sufficient to digest 500 g of dog food.
- Alternatively, at least 1–1.5 teaspoonfuls of powdered non-enteric coated pancreatic enzyme per 100 g of food or per 10 kg body weight per meal. Mix thoroughly with food. Best results are usually obtained by feeding only 2 or 3 meals/day.

Cats:
- Lypex: open capsule and sprinkle on to food. Feed 0.5 capsule per meal. For best results feed at least twice daily.
- Tryplase: the contents of 1–2 capsules per day sprinkled on food; 2 capsules are sufficient to digest 250 g of cat food.
- Alternatively, 1 teaspoonful of powdered non-enteric coated pancreatic extract mixed thoroughly with each meal. Adjust dose as necessary.

Birds: Tryplase: 1 capsule/kg body weight q24h mixed in food.
Small mammals, Reptiles: No information available.

Pancuronium

(Pancuronium*) **POM**

Formulations: Injectable: 2 mg/ml solution.

Action: Inhibits the actions of acetylcholine at the neuromuscular junction by binding competitively to the nicotinic acetylcholine receptor on the post-junctional membrane.

Use: Provision of neuromuscular blockade during anaesthesia. This may be to improve surgical access through muscle relaxation, facilitate positive pressure ventilation, or for intraocular surgery. Medium to long duration of action (>45 min), although there is marked variation between individuals. Can also have a modest stimulatory effect on the cardiovascular system, causing an increase in heart rate via a vagolytic effect. Monitoring (using a nerve stimulator) and reversal of the neuromuscular blockade is recommended to ensure complete recovery before the end of anaesthesia. Hypothermia, acidosis and hypokalaemia will prolong the duration of action of neuromuscular blockade. Neostigmine is preferred to edrophonium as the reversal agent because of the potency and duration of action of pancuronium.

Safety and handling: Store in refrigerator.

Contraindications: Do not administer unless the animal is adequately anaesthetized and facilities to provide positive pressure ventilation are available.

Adverse reactions: No information available

Drug interactions: Neuromuscular blockade is more prolonged when pancuronium is given in combination with volatile anaesthetics, aminoglycosides, clindamycin and lincomycin.

DOSES

Dogs, Cats: 0.025–0.075 mg/kg i.v.; initially use a higher dose and repeat doses at increments of 0.01 mg/kg. Repeated doses may be cumulative and lead to difficulty in antagonism.
Small mammals, Birds, Reptiles: No information available.

Papaveretum

(Omnopon*, Papaveretum*) **POM CD SCHEDULE 2**

Formulations: Injectable: 7.7 mg/ml, 15.4 mg/ml papaveretum solutions; 15.4 mg/ml papaveretum and 0.4 mg/ml hyoscine (scopolamine) solution. 7.7 and 15.4 mg/ml solutions provide the equivalent of 5 mg and 10 mg anhydrous morphine per ml, respectively.

Action: Analgesia mediated by the mu opioid receptor.

Use: Management of moderate to severe pain in the perioperative period. Incorporation into sedative and pre-anaesthetic medication protocols to provide improved sedation and analgesia. Papaveretum is a mixture of the alkaloids of opium containing the equivalent of anhydrous morphine 85.5%, anhydrous codeine 6.8% and papaverine 7.8%. It has a similar effect to morphine and is thought to have a duration of action of 4 hours. Papaveretum is not widely used to provide postoperative analgesia in dogs and cats and tends to be used in combination with acepromazine to provide good sedation in aggressive dogs. The comparative sedation produced by papaveretum and other mu agonists combined with acepromazine has not been evaluated in rigorous clinical studies. It has not been widely evaluated in experimental or clinical analgesia studies.

Safety and handling: Normal precautions should be observed.

Contraindications: No information available.

Adverse reactions: In common with other mu agonists papaveretum can cause respiratory depression, although this is unlikely when used at clinical doses in conscious cats and dogs. Respiratory depression may occur when papaveretum is given i.v. during general anaesthesia, due to the increased depth of anaesthesia that accompanies administration. Respiratory function should be monitored when it is given to anaesthetized patients. Vomiting is common after papaveretum administration. It causes constriction of GI sphincters (such as the pyloric sphincter) and may cause a reduction in GI motility when given over a long period. The response to all opioids appears to be very variable between individual patients, therefore assessment of pain after administration is imperative. Papaveretum is metabolized in the liver, some prolongation of effect may be seen with impaired liver function. Papaveretum crosses the placenta and may exert sedative effects in neonates born to bitches treated prior to parturition. Severe adverse effects can be treated with naloxone.

Drug interactions: Other CNS depressants (e.g. anaesthetics, antihistamines, barbiturates, phenothiazines, tranquillizers) may cause increased CNS or respiratory depression when used concurrently with narcotic analgesics.

DOSES
When used for sedation is generally given as part of a combination. See Appendix for sedation protocols in all species.
Dogs: Analgesia: 0.2–0.8 mg/kg i.v., i.m., s.c.; use lower doses i.v.; only use higher doses when deep sedation required.
Cats: Analgesia: 0.2–0.3 mg/kg i.v., i.m., s.c.
Small mammals, Birds, Reptiles: No information available.

Paracetamol (Acetaminophen)
(Paracetamol, Pardale V (paracetamol and codeine phosphate), Perfalgan) **P, POM, POM-V**

Formulations: Oral: 500 mg tablet; 120 mg/5 ml, 250 mg/5 ml suspensions; 400 mg paracetamol and 9 mg codeine phosphate tablet (Pardale V); 10 mg/ml injectable solution.

Action: It has been proposed that its antipyretic actions are due to prostaglandin synthesis within the CNS; however its exact mechanism of action is unclear.

Use: Control of mild to moderate pain and as an antipyretic; however, there are limited data describing the analgesic efficacy of paracetamol in dogs. Paracetamol has poor anti-inflammatory effects. It is believed to produce few GI side effects and therefore is commonly administered to patients with gastric ulceration, particularly if traditional NSAIDs are contraindicated; however, there are limited clinical data to support this practice. Although common practice in human anaesthesia, the combination of an NSAID and paracetamol to provide perioperative analgesia has not undergone rigorous investigation in dogs in terms of either safety or analgesic efficacy. Injectable paracetamol may be useful to provide adjunctive analgesia in dogs during the perioperative period. The licensed oral preparation of paracetamol contains codeine; however, due to a high first pass metabolism of opioids, this codeine is not bioavailable and therefore does not contribute to the analgesia.

Safety and handling: Normal precautions should be observed.

Contraindications: Do not use in cats as they lack the glucuronyl transferase enzymes required to metabolize the drug.

Adverse reactions: Overdose of paracetamol causes liver damage through the production of N-acetyl-p-aminobenzoquinonimine during metabolism, which causes hepatocyte cell death and centrilobular hepatic necrosis. Treatment of overdose with oral methionine or i.v. acetylcysteine is directed at replenishing hepatic glutathione.

Drug interactions: Metoclopramide enhances absorption of paracetamol, thereby enhancing its effects.

DOSES
Dogs: 10 mg/kg p.o., i.v. q12h.
Cats: Do not use.
Small mammals: Rabbits: 200–500 mg/kg p.o.; Rodents: 1–2 mg/ml of drinking water (use flavoured products).
Birds, Reptiles: No information available.

Paraffin (Liquid paraffin, Mineral oil)
(Katalax*, Lacri-Lube*, Liquid paraffin oral emulsion*, Simple Eye Ointment*) **P**

Formulations: Oral: White soft paraffin paste (Katalax); liquid paraffin (50/50 oil/water mix). Topical: 3.5 g, 4 g or 5 g ophthalmic ointment.

Action: Paraffin is a laxative; it softens stool by interfering with intestinal water resorption. It is also a lipid-based tear substitute that mimics the lipid portion of the tear film and helps prevent evaporation of tears.

Use: Paraffin is used to manage constipation. It is beneficial in the management of keratoconjunctivitis sicca, during general anaesthesia and for eyelid paresis. It is a long-acting ocular lubricant and is used when frequency of treatment is not easy.

Safety and handling: Normal precautions should be observed.

Contraindications: Do not give orally in patients with a reduced gag reflex.

Adverse reactions: As paraffin is tasteless, normal swallowing may not be elicited if syringing orally; thus inhalation and subsequent lipoid pneumonia are a significant risk. Paraffin ointment may blur vision, although not often a problem in dogs/cats.

Drug interactions: Reduced absorption of fat-soluble vitamins may follow prolonged use.

DOSES
Dogs:
- Constipation: 1–2 tablespoons per meal as required.
- Ocular: Apply to eye at night or q6–12h prn.

Cats:
- Constipation: Adults 25 mm Katalax paste p.o. q12–24h; kittens 10 mm Katalax paste p.o. q12–24h.
- Ocular: Apply to eye at night or q6–12h prn.

Small mammals, Birds, Reptiles: No information available.

Paroxetine
(Paxil*, Seroxat*) **POM**

Formulations: Oral: 20 mg, 30 mg tablets, 2 mg/ml liquid suspension.

Action: Blocks serotonin re-uptake in the brain, resulting in antidepressive activity and a raising in motor activity thresholds.

Use: Treatment of generalized anxiety in dogs and urine marking with overt aggression in cats. The atypical tricyclic antidepressant clomipramine is authorized for use in dogs.

Safety and handling: Normal precautions should be observed.

Contraindications: Known sensitivity to paroxetine or other SSRIs, history of seizures.

Adverse reactions: Possible reactions include lethargy, decreased appetite and vomiting. Trembling, restlessness, GI disturbance and an apparent paradoxical increase in anxiety may occur in some cases. Owners should be warned of a potential increase in aggression in response to medication and frequency of urination should be monitored when used in cats.

Drug interactions: Paroxetine should not be used within 2 weeks of treatment with an MAOI (e.g. selegiline) and an MAOI should not be used within 6 weeks of treatment with paroxetine. Paroxetine, like other SSRIs, antagonizes the effects of anticonvulsants and so is not recommended for use with epileptic patients or in association with other agents which lower seizure threshold, e.g. phenothiazines. Caution is warranted if paroxetine is used concomitantly with aspirin or other anticoagulants, since the risk of increased bleeding in the case of tissue trauma may be increased.

DOSES
Dogs: 1–2 mg/kg p.o. q24h.
Cats: 0.5–1 mg/kg p.o. q24h; can be increased to 2 mg/kg p.o. q24h but close monitoring is required.
Small mammals: No information available.
Birds: 1–2 mg/kg p.o. q12–24h.
Reptiles: No information available.

Penicillamine
(Distamine*, Penicillamine*) **POM**

Formulations: Oral: 125 mg, 250 mg tablets.

Action: Penicillamine is an orally administered chelating agent that binds copper, mercury and lead. It also binds to cystine.

Use: In dogs, penicillamine is mainly used in the management of copper-associated hepatopathy in Bedlington Terriers and other susceptible breeds, and for the oral treatment of lead poisoning. It is also used in cystinuria as it decreases cystine excretion by combining with cystine to form the soluble complex, cystine-D-penicillamine disulphide. May be used in the management of lead toxicity, especially in birds, when injecting EDTA is too difficult or long-term chelation is required. It has a low therapeutic index in birds. Dogs that fail to tolerate even the lower dose regimes may be pre-treated with antiemetic drugs (phenothiazines or antihistamines) 30–60 min before penicillamine. Penicillamine is used for treating rheumatoid arthritis in humans, but has not yet been used in immune-mediated erosive arthropathies in companion animals.

Safety and handling: Normal precautions should be observed.

Contraindications: Moderate to marked renal impairment and a history of penicillamine-related blood dyscrasias. Penicillamine can reduce gastrointestinal absorption of dietary minerals, including zinc, iron, copper and calcium and, therefore, cause deficiencies with long-term use.

Adverse reactions: Anorexia, vomiting, pyrexia and nephrotic syndrome are seen in dogs. Serious adverse effects that have been described in humans given penicillamine include leucopenia, thrombocytopenia, fever, lymphadenopathy, skin hypersensitivity reactions and lupus-like reactions. May cause vomiting, hypoglycaemia and death in birds.

Drug interactions: The absorption of penicillamine is decreased if administered with antacids, food, or iron or zinc salts. An increase in the renal and haematological effects of penicillamine have been recorded in humans receiving it with cytotoxic drugs.

DOSES

Dogs:
- Copper-associated hepatitis: 10–15 mg/kg p.o. q24h given on an empty stomach 30 min before feeding. Must be given for months to be effective.
- Cystinuria: 10–15 mg/kg p.o. q12h.
- Lead poisoning: Patients commonly receive CaEDTA before receiving penicillamine at 10–15 mg/kg p.o. q24h on an empty stomach for 1–2 weeks. Stop treatment for 1 week and resume until blood lead levels are normal (at end of 'rest' week). If adverse effects occur, the daily dose may be divided and given q6–8h or reduced to 33–55 mg/kg p.o. q24h.

Cats: No information available.

Small mammals: Rabbits: 30 mg/kg p.o. q12h.

Birds: Lead poisoning: 55 mg/kg p.o. q12h.

Reptiles: No information available.

Penicillin G (Benzyl penicillin)

(Crystapen, Depocillin, Duphapen, Neopen) **POM-V**

Formulations: Injectable: comes in a variety of salts (sodium, procaine and benzathine) which affect solubility. Penicillin G sodium (highly soluble): 3 g powder for reconstitution for i.v. use; procaine penicillin (less soluble): 300 mg/ml suspension for s.c. use, slower release.

Action: Binds to penicillin-binding proteins involved in cell wall synthesis, decreasing bacterial cell wall strength and rigidity, and affecting cell division, growth and septum formation. As animal cells lack a cell wall the beta-lactam antibiotics are safe. Kills bacteria in a time-dependent fashion.

Use: A beta-lactamase-susceptible antimicrobial. Narrow spectrum of activity and susceptible to acid degradation in the stomach. Used parenterally to treat infections caused by sensitive organisms (e.g. *Streptococcus*, *Clostridium*, *Borrelia borgderferi*, fusospirochaetes). The sodium salt is absorbed well from s.c. or i.m. sites. Procaine penicillin is sparingly soluble, providing a 'depot' from which it is slowly released. When used for 'blind' therapy of undiagnosed infections, penicillins may be given in conjunction with an aminoglycoside such as gentamicin with or without metronidazole. As penicillin kills in a time-dependent fashion, it is important to maintain tissue concentrations above the MIC for the organism throughout the interdosing interval. Patients with significant renal or hepatic dysfunction may need dosage adjustment.

Safety and handling: After reconstitution penicillin G sodium is stable for 7 days if refrigerated, 24 hours if not.

Contraindications: Do not administer penicillins to hamsters, gerbils, guinea pigs or chinchillas. Use with caution in rabbits, and never orally, though it has been used in injectable forms long term for abscesses and osteomyelitis. Do not use in animals sensitive to beta-lactam antimicrobials. Do not give procaine penicillin to rats and mice.

Adverse reactions: 600 mg of penicillin G sodium contains 1.7 mEq of Na^+. This may be clinically important for patients on restricted sodium intakes. The i.m. administration of >600 mg/ml may cause discomfort.

Drug interactions: Avoid the concomitant use of bacteriostatic antibiotics. The aminoglycosides may inactivate penicillins when mixed in parenteral solutions *in vitro*, but they act synergistically when administered at the same time *in vivo*. Procaine can antagonize the action of sulphonamides and so procaine penicillin G should not be used with them.

DOSES

See Appendix for guidelines on responsible antibacterial use.
Dogs, Cats: Penicillin G sodium: 15–25 mg/kg i.v., i.m. q4–6h; Penicillin G procaine: 30 mg/kg s.c. q24h.
Small mammals: Ferrets: 20 mg/kg s.c., i.m. q12–24h; Rabbits: 40 mg/kg s.c. once every 7 days (x 3 doses) for *Treponema cuniculi*; other infections 40 mg/kg s.c. q24h; Rats (not procaine): 22 mg/kg s.c., i.m. q24h; Chinchillas, Guinea pigs, Hamsters, Gerbils: Do not use.
Birds, Reptiles: No information available.

Pentamidine isethionate
(Pentacarinat*) **POM**

Formulations: Injectable: 300 mg vials of powder for reconstitution.

Action: Kills protozoans by interacting with DNA. It is rapidly taken up by the parasites by a high-affinity energy-dependent carrier.

Use: Treatment of leishmaniosis when resistance to the pentavalent antimony drugs (meglumine antimonate and sodium stibogluconate) has occurred. Pentamidine is a toxic drug and the potential to cause toxic damage to kidney and liver in particular should be carefully considered prior to use. Seek expert advice before treating leishmaniosis.

Safety and handling: Care should be taken by staff handling this drug as it is a highly toxic agent. Similar precautions to those recommended when handling cytotoxic agents used in cancer chemotherapy (see Appendix) should be taken.

Contraindications: Impaired liver or kidney function. Never give by rapid i.v. injection due to cardiovascular effects.

Adverse reactions: Pain and necrosis at the injection site, hypotension, nausea, salivation, vomiting and diarrhoea. Hypoglycaemia and blood dyscrasias are also reported in humans.

Drug interactions: No information available.

DOSES
Dogs: 3–4 mg/kg i.m. on alternate days for a maximum of 10 treatments.
Cats, Small mammals, Birds, Reptiles: No information available.

Pentazocine
(Pentazocine*, Talwin*) **POM CD SCHEDULE 3**

Formulations: Oral: 25 mg tablet, 50 mg capsule. Injectable: 30 mg/ml solution.

Action: Weak agonist effect at kappa receptors and antagonistic effects at the mu receptor.

Use: Short-term management of mild to moderate pain in dogs. Incorporation into sedative and pre-anaesthetic medication protocols to provide improved sedation and analgesia. After i.v. injection it has a rapid onset (2–5 min) and short duration (45–60 min) of action. It will antagonize the effects of morphine and other opioids through an antagonistic effect at the mu receptor, but will also provide analgesia through an action at kappa receptors. Has little effect on the GI tract and causes less respiratory depression than morphine. Unlike most other opioids it can increase heart rate. Oral pentazocine is rarely used in cats and dogs due to a high first pass metabolism leading to a low plasma concentration after oral administration. Avoid in cases with severe pain or where severe pain is anticipated. Full mu agonist opioids are preferred in such cases.

Safety and handling: Normal precautions should be observed.

Contraindications: No information available.

Adverse reactions: Rapid i.v. injection may cause marked excitement.

Drug interactions: In common with other opioids, pentazocine will reduce the doses of other drugs required for induction and maintenance of anaesthesia. Other CNS depressants (e.g. anaesthetics, antihistamines, barbiturates, phenothiazines, tranquillizers) may cause increased CNS or respiratory depression when used concurrently with narcotic analgesics. Administration of pentazocine will reduce analgesia produced from full mu agonists (therefore avoid including pentazocine in premedication when administration of full mu agonist opioids during surgery is anticipated).

DOSES
When used for sedation is generally given as part of a combination. See Appendix for sedation protocols in all species.

Dogs: Analgesia: 1–3 mg/kg i.m., 2–6 mg/kg p.o. repeated q3–4h depending on pain assessment.
Cats: Do not use.
Small mammals: Analgesia: Rodents: 5–10 mg/kg s.c. q2–4h prn.
Birds, Reptiles: No information available.

Pentobarbital (Pentobarbitone)

(Dolethal, Euthasal, Euthatal, Lethobarb, Pentobarbital for euthanasia, Pentoject) **POM-V CD SCHEDULE 3**

Formulations: Injectable: 200 mg/ml, 400 mg/ml, as either a blue or yellow non-sterile aqueous solution.

Action: CNS depressant.

Use: For euthanasia of cats, dogs and other small animals. When it is predicted that euthanasia may be problematical (e.g. aggressive patients) it is recommended that premedication with an appropriate sedative is given. The animal should be restrained in order to forestall narcotic excitement until anaesthesia supervenes. This is particularly important with cats. The route of choice is i.v. if possible, but alternatives such as intraperitoneal (preferred) or intrathoracic are possible when venepuncture is difficult to achieve. The intrathoracic route is usually the last resort. There is a risk of injection into the lungs, which causes coughing and distress. Direct injection into a chamber of the heart is rapid, but it may be difficult to locate the heart chambers accurately and repeated attempts could cause unnecessary pain and distress. There is no authorized pentobarbital product in the UK that is suitable for the emergency control of seizures.

Safety and handling: Normal precautions should be observed.

Contraindications: Should not be given i.m. as it is painful and slow to act. Do not use solutions intended for euthanasia to try to control seizures.

Adverse reactions: Narcotic excitement may be seen with agitated animals. Agonal gasping is sometimes seen.

Drug interactions: Antihistamines and opioids increase the effect of pentobarbital.

DOSES
Dogs, Cats:
- Euthanasia: 80 mg/kg in debilitated animals, up to 120–160 mg/kg in younger and fitter animals, rapid i.v. injection.
- Status epilepticus (no suitable product is available in the UK): Aliquots of 3 mg/kg i.v. q90sec to a maximum of 6 doses until the epileptic seizures have been abolished. Anaesthesia is not necessary and should be avoided as this increases morbidity. Repeat q4–8h if required. Should only be used as part of a balanced seizure protocol.

Small mammals: Euthanasia: 150 mg/kg i.v., i.p. as rapidly as possible or to effect.

Birds: Euthanasia: 150 mg/kg i.v., i.p.

Reptiles: Euthanasia: 60–100 mg/kg i.v. or intracoelomically.

Pentobarbitone see Pentobarbital

Pentosan polysulphate
(Cartrophen) **POM-V**

Formulations: Injectable: 100 mg/ml solution.

Action: Semi-synthetic polymer of pentose carbohydrates with heparin-like properties that binds to damaged cartilage matrix comprising aggregated proteoglycans and stimulates the synthesis of new aggregated glycosaminoglycan molecules. Ability to inhibit a range of proteolytic enzymes may be of particular importance. Modulates cytokine action, stimulates hyaluronic acid secretion, preserves proteoglycan content and stimulates articular cartilage blood flow, resulting in analgesic and regenerative effects.

Use: In dogs, licensed as a disease modifying agent that reduces the pain and inflammation associated with osteoarthritis. Administered by aseptic s.c. injection, using an insulin syringe for accurate dosing. The manufacturer recommends monitoring haematocrit and total solids. It has been suggested that pentosan polysulphate may be of benefit in the management of cats suffering from chronic idiopathic, non-obstructive, lower urinary tract disease because cats suffering from this condition have been shown to have reduced concentrations of gags within the protective mucosal layer of the bladder. However, there is currently no evidence to support this contention. There is good evidence to suggest that this drug is of minimal value in acute cases.

Safety and handling: Normal precautions should be observed.

Contraindications: Do not use if septic arthritis is present or if renal or hepatic impairment exists. As it may induce spontaneous bleeding, do not use in animals with bleeding disorders.

Adverse reactions: Pain at the injection site has been reported. Because of its fibrinolytic action the possibility of bleeding from undiagnosed tumours or vascular abnormalities exists.

Drug interactions: The manufacturers state that pentosan polysulphate should not be used concurrently with steroids or non-steroidal drugs, including aspirin, or used concomitantly with coumarin-based anticoagulants or heparin. However, many dogs suffering from osteoarthritis that might benefit from pentosan polysulphate treatment are concurrently receiving NSAID therapy. The risk of bleeding associated with concurrent administration of pentosan polysulphate and COX-2 preferential and COX-2 selective NSAIDs is probably low in animals with no history of blood clotting disorders.

DOSES
Dogs: 3 mg/kg (0.3 ml/10 kg) s.c. q5–7d on four occasions. 10–20 mg per joint intra-articularly in non-septic joints.
Cats: Oral formulations available in other countries have been used in cats for osteoarthritis and for chronic refractory cases of feline lower urinary tract disease. The use of the injectable form has not been well reported in this species.
Small mammals: Guinea pigs: 3 mg/kg (0.03 ml/1 kg) s.c. q5–7d for 4 doses for osteoarthritis and idiopathic cystitis.
Birds, Reptiles: No information available.

Pentoxifylline (Oxypentifylline) `CIL`
(Trental*) **POM**

Formulations: Oral: 400 mg tablet.

Action: Reduces blood viscosity. Anti-inflammatory through reduction of TNF-alpha production.

Use: Treatment of vasculitis and vasculopathies, and contact dermatitis.

Safety and handling: Normal precautions should be observed.

Contraindications: No information available.

Adverse reactions: GI irritation.

Drug interactions: There is a possible increased risk of bleeding when pentoxifylline is given with NSAIDs. Co-administration of pentoxifylline and sodium thiopental causes death from acute pulmonary oedema in rats.

DOSES
Dogs: 15 mg/kg q8–12h.
Cats, Small mammals, Birds, Reptiles: No information available.

Permethrin see **Imidacloprid**

Pethidine (Meperidine)
(Demerol*, Meperidine*, Pethidine*) **POM CD**
SCHEDULE 2

Formulations: Injectable: 10–50 mg/ml solutions. 50 mg/ml solution is usually used in veterinary practice.

Action: Analgesia mediated by the mu opioid receptor.

Use: Management of mild to moderate pain. Incorporation into sedative and pre-anaesthetic medication protocols to provide improved sedation and analgesia. Pethidine has a fast onset (10–15 min) and short duration (45–60 min) of action. Frequent redosing is used for analgesia. The short duration of action may be desirable in some circumstances (e.g. when a rapid recovery is required or in animals with compromised liver function). It shares common opioid effects with morphine but also has anticholinergic effects, producing a dry mouth and sometimes an increase in heart rate. It causes less biliary tract spasm than morphine, suggesting that it may be useful for the management of pain in dogs and cats with pancreatitis. Due to the concentration of commercially available solutions the injection volume can be 2–3 ml in large dogs, which can cause pain on i.m. injection.

Safety and handling: Normal precautions should be observed.

Contraindications: Do not give i.v. Not advisable to use in animals at risk from histamine release (e.g. some skin allergies, asthma, mast cell tumours).

Adverse reactions: Histamine released during i.v. injection causes hypotension, tachycardia and bronchoconstriction. Histamine-mediated reactions may also occur after i.m. injection, resulting in local urticaria. Pethidine crosses the placenta and may exert sedative effects in neonates born to bitches treated prior to parturition. Severe adverse effects can be treated with naloxone.

Drug interactions: Other CNS depressants (e.g. anaesthetics, antihistamines, barbiturates, phenothiazines, tranquillizers) may cause increased CNS or respiratory depression when used concurrently with narcotic analgesics. Pethidine may produce a serious interaction if administered with monoamine oxidase inhibitors (MAOIs). The mechanism of this interaction is not clear but effects include coma, convulsions and hyperpyrexia.

DOSES
When used for sedation is generally given as part of a combination. See Appendix for sedation protocols in all species.
Dogs: Analgesia: 2–10 mg/kg i.m., s.c. q1–2h depending on pain assessment.
Cats: Analgesia: 5–10 mg/kg i.m., s.c. q1–2h depending on pain assessment.
Small mammals: Analgesia: Ferrets, Rabbits: 5–10 mg/kg i.m., s.c.; Rodents: 10–20 mg/kg i.m. q2–3h.
Birds: No information available.
Reptiles: Analgesia: 20 mg/kg i.m. q12–24h.

Phenobarbital (Phenobarbitone)
(Epiphen, Epityl, Phenobarbital (non-propriety),
Phenoleptil, Gardenal*) **POM-V, POM CD SCHEDULE 3**

Formulations: Oral: 12.5 mg, 15 mg, 25 mg, 30 mg, 50 mg, 60 mg,
100 mg tablets; 4% (40 mg/ml) solution. Injectable: 15 mg/ml, 30 mg/
ml, 60 mg/ml, 200 mg/ml solutions (phenobarbital sodium BP).

Action: Thought to mediate its antiepileptic effect through affinity for
the GABA$_A$ receptor, resulting in a GABA-ergic effect; GABA being
the major inhibitory mammalian neurotransmitter with prolonged
opening of the chloride channel. Phenobarbital also blocks the AMPA
receptor, inhibiting release of the excitatory neurotransmitter
glutamate. This combined potentiation of GABA and inhibition of
glutamate leads to reduced neuronal excitability.

Use: Phenobarbital and imepitoin are the initial medications of choice
for the management of epileptic seizures due to idiopathic epilepsy in
dogs. Phenobarbital is also licensed for the management of epileptic
seizures due to structural brain disease in dogs and is used for the
management of epileptic seizures in cats. The choice of initial
medication is guided by patient requirements: phenobarbital is less
expensive and more efficacious, whilst imepitoin has a more rapid
onset of action than phenobarbital (does not need to achieve a steady
state), does not require the determination of serum concentrations
and has a less severe adverse effect profile. Phenobarbital is rapidly
absorbed after oral administration in dogs; maximal plasma
concentrations reached within 4–8 hours. Wide range of elimination
half-life (40–90 hours) in different dogs. Steady state serum
concentrations are not reached until 7–10 days after treatment is
initiated and the full clinical effect of a dose cannot be ascertained
until this point. Serum concentrations should be determined after
starting treatment or dose alterations, once a steady state has been
reached. If <15 μg/ml the dose should be increased accordingly. If
seizures are not adequately controlled dose may be increased up to a
maximum serum concentration of 45 μg/ml. Plasma concentrations
above this level are associated with increased hepatotoxicity. Blood
samples for serum concentration determination should be collected at
the same time of day relative to the time of dose administration in
dogs on higher daily doses, but timing is not normally important in
dogs on a total daily dose of <8 mg/kg. For accuracy of dosing, dogs
<12 kg should commence therapy with the oral solution formulation.
With chronic therapy, induction of the hepatic microsomal enzyme
system results in a decreased half-life, particularly in dogs during the
first 6 months of therapy. As a result, the dose may need to be
increased. Phenobarbital levels should be assessed every 6–12
months. Any termination of phenobarbital therapy should be
performed gradually with a recommended protocol of: reduce the
dose by 25% of the original dose each month (month 1: 75% of the
original phenobarbital dose; month 2: 50% of the original
phenobarbital dose; month 3: 25% of the original phenobarbital dose).

Safety and handling: Normal precautions should be observed.

Contraindications: Do not administer to animals with impaired hepatic function. Not for use in pregnant animals and nursing bitches, although the risk associated with uncontrolled seizures may be greater than the risk associated with phenobarbital. Do not use to control seizures resulting from hepatic disease (e.g. portosystemic shunt), hypoglycaemia or toxic causes where the clinical signs are mediated through the GABA channels (ivermectin and moxidectin toxicity) as this may exacerbate the seizures. Do not administer high doses by i.v. or i.m. injection in animals with marked respiratory depression.

Adverse reactions: Sedation, ataxia, polyphagia and PU/PD. Polyphagia and PU/PD are likely to persist throughout therapy. Ataxia and sedation occur commonly following initiation of therapy but usually resolve within 1 week, although they may continue if high doses are used. Hepatic toxicity is rare, but may occur at high serum concentrations (or as a rare idiosyncratic reaction within 2 weeks of starting treatment). Hyperexcitability has been reported in dogs on subtherapeutic dose levels. Haematological abnormalities, including neutropenia, anaemia and thrombocytopenia, may occur. Long-term administration in the absence of hepatotoxicity is associated with: moderate increase in liver size on abdominal radiographs; no change in liver echogenicity or architecture on ultrasonography; no evidence of morphological liver damage on histology; significant increase in ALP and, to a lesser extent, ALT activity; transiently decreased albumin (up to 6 months after starting therapy) and increased GGT; and no changes in AST, bilirubin or fasting bile acids. Therefore, liver function should be assessed by other parameters, in particular a bile acid assay, persistent decrease in albumin levels, serum AST, bilirubin and ultrasonographic examination of the liver. Phenobarbital treatment does not affect adrenal function tests (ACTH stimulation test and low dose dexamethasone test) despite acceleration of dexamethasone metabolism. Phenobarbital significantly decreases total T4 and free T4 and cholesterol levels tend to increase towards the upper limits of the normal range.

Drug interactions: The effect of phenobarbital may be increased by other CNS depressants (antihistamines, narcotics, phenothiazines). Phenobarbital may enhance the metabolism of, and therefore decrease the effect of, corticosteroids, beta-blockers, metronidazole and theophylline. Barbiturates may enhance the effects of other antiepileptics. Cimetidine, itraconazole and chloramphenicol increase serum phenobarbital concentration through inhibition of the hepatic microsomal enzyme system.

DOSES

Dogs:
- Initial therapy: 1–2.5 mg/kg p.o. q12h. Only 40% of dogs started on this dose will achieve therapeutic serum concentrations and modification of the dose based on serum concentrations is essential.

- Emergency management of status epilepticus or severe cluster seizures in dogs that have not been on maintenance phenobarbital: aim for a total loading dose of 18–24 mg/kg, followed by a maintenance dose of 2–3 mg/kg q12h. The loading dose is given as an initial 12 mg/kg slow i.v. and then after 20 minutes, two further doses of 4–6 mg/kg slow i.v. 20 minutes apart. Always wait 20 minutes before giving additional doses as CNS levels take 20 minutes to respond, and do not administer if the dog is excessively sedated or has evidence of respiratory depression. Higher doses may be required in very small dogs.
- Emergency management in dogs that have been on maintenance phenobarbital: 4–6 mg/kg i.v. or i.m. to increase the blood levels slightly in case these were subtherapeutic. Always take a blood sample for a phenobarbital level determination first, before giving the top-up dose.

Cats: Initial therapy: 1.5–3 mg/kg p.o. q12h. Emergency management: doses as for dogs.
Small mammals: Ferrets: 1–2 mg/kg p.o. q12–24h, 2–10 mg/kg/h i.v. constant rate infusion; Guinea pigs, Gerbils: 10–25 mg/kg i.v., i.p.
Birds: 3.5–7 mg/kg p.o. q12h.
Reptiles: No information available.

Phenobarbitone see **Phenobarbital**

Phenoxybenzamine

CIL

(Dibenyline*) **POM**

Formulations: Oral: 10 mg capsule. Injectable: 50 mg/ml solution.

Action: An alpha-adrenergic blocker that irreversibly blocks presynaptic and postsynaptic receptors, producing a so-called chemical sympathectomy.

Use: Reflex dyssynergia/urethral spasm and the treatment of severe hypertension in animals with phaeochromocytoma prior to surgery to reduce mortality. If concurrent beta-blockers are also used (for severe tachycardia/arrhythmias), only start these once alpha blockade is in place (to avoid a hypertensive crisis). Use with extreme caution in animals with pre-existing cardiovascular disease.

Safety and handling: Normal precautions should be observed.

Contraindications: No information available.

Adverse reactions: Adverse effects associated with alpha-adrenergic blockade include hypotension, miosis, tachycardia and nasal congestion.

Drug interactions: There is an increased risk of a first dose hypotensive effect if administered with beta-blockers or diuretics. Phenoxybenzamine will antagonize effects of alpha-adrenergic sympathomimetic agents (e.g. phenylephrine).

DOSES

Dogs:
- Reflex dyssynergia: 0.25–1 mg/kg p.o. q8–24h for a minimum of 5 days.
- Hypertension associated with phaeochromocytoma: 0.25 mg/kg p.o. q12h for 10–14 days prior to surgery, titrating up to an effective dose (maximum of 2.5 mg/kg q12h) as required or administer long term for medical management if adrenalectomy not possible.

Cats: 0.5–1 mg/kg p.o. q12h for 5 days before evaluating efficacy.
Small mammals: Ferrets: 0.5–1 mg/kg p.o. q12h (anecdotal).
Birds, Reptiles: No information available.

Phenylbutazone

(Companazone) **POM-V**

Formulations: Oral: 100 mg, 200 mg tablets.

Action: Non-selective COX enzyme inhibitor, limiting prostaglandin production.

Use: Management of mild to moderate pain and inflammation in osteoarthritic conditions. Not selective for COX-2 and likely to cause more adverse effects than more selective COX-2 inhibitors that have superseded the use of phenylbutazone. Not authorized for preoperative administration to dogs. Liver disease will prolong the metabolism of phenylbutazone, leading to the potential for drug accumulation and overdose with repeated dosing. Administration of phenylbutazone to animals with renal disease must be carefully evaluated. Do not use in cats.

Safety and handling: Normal precautions should be observed.

Contraindications: Do not give to dehydrated, hypovolaemic or hypotensive patients or those with GI disease or blood clotting problems. Do not administer perioperatively until the animal is fully recovered from anaesthesia and normotensive. Do not give to pregnant animals or animals <6 weeks of age.

Adverse reactions: GI signs may occur in all animals after NSAID administration. Stop therapy if this persists beyond 1–2 days. Some animals develop signs with one NSAID and not another. A 1–2-week wash-out period should be allowed before starting another NSAID after cessation of therapy. Stop therapy immediately if GI bleeding is suspected. There is a small risk that NSAIDs precipitate cardiac failure in animals with cardiovascular disease. Phenylbutazone may infrequently cause bone marrow suppression, including aplastic anaemias. It may also cause false low T3 and T4 values.

Drug interactions: Do not administer concurrently or within 24 hours of other NSAIDs and glucocorticoids. Do not administer with other potentially nephrotoxic agents, e.g. aminoglycosides.

DOSES
Dogs: 2–20 mg/kg p.o. q8–12h. Maximum dose 800 mg. The manufacturers recommend a starting dose of 10 mg/kg twice daily for 7 days, reducing to 5 mg/kg twice daily thereafter. The 200 mg tablet strength should not be used in dogs weighing <20 kg. The 100 mg tablet strength should not be used in dogs weighing <5 kg.
Cats: Do not use.
Small mammals, Birds, Reptiles: No information available.

Phenylephrine
(Phenylephrine hydrochloride*) **POM**

Formulations: Injectable: 1% (10 mg/ml) solution. Ophthalmic: 2.5%, 10% solution (single-dose vials).

Action: Alpha-1 selective adrenergic agonist that causes peripheral vasoconstriction when given i.v., resulting in increased diastolic and systolic blood pressure, a small decrease in cardiac output and an increased circulation time. Directly stimulates the alpha-adrenergic receptors in the iris dilator musculature.

Use: Used in conjunction with fluid therapy to treat hypotension secondary to drugs or vascular failure. Has minimal effects on cardiac beta-adrenergic receptors. When applied topically to the eye causes vasoconstriction and mydriasis (pupil dilation). Ophthalmic uses include mydriasis prior to intraocular surgery (often in conjunction with atropine), differentiation of involvement of superficial conjunctival vasculature from deep episcleral vasculature (by vasoconstriction). It is also used in the diagnosis of Horner's syndrome (HS) (denervation hypersensitivity) by determining the time to pupillary dilation, following administration of 1% phenylephrine topically to both eyes. Essentially, the shorter the time to pupillary dilation, the closer the lesion to the iris: <20 minutes suggests third-order HS; 20–45 min suggests second-order HS; 60–90 min suggests first-order HS or no sympathetic denervation of the eye. If 10% phenylephrine is used, mydriasis occurs in 5–8 minutes in post-ganglionic (third-order neuron) lesions. Phenylephrine is not a cycloplegic in the dog, so its use in uveitis is limited to mydriasis to reduce posterior synechiae formation. It is inappropriate for diagnostic mydriasis because its onset of action is too slow (2 hours in the dog). Vasoconstrictors should be used with care. Although they raise blood pressure, they do so at the expense of perfusion of vital organs (e.g. kidney). In many patients with shock, peripheral resistance is already high and to raise it further is unhelpful.

Safety and handling: Normal precautions should be observed.

Contraindications: No information available.

Adverse reactions: These include hypertension, tachycardia, and reflex bradycardia. Extravasation injuries can be serious (necrosis and sloughing).

Drug interactions: There is a risk of arrhythmias if phenylephrine is used in patients receiving digoxin or with volatile anaesthetic agents. When used concurrently with oxytocic agents the pressor effects may be enhanced, leading to severe hypertension.

DOSES
Dogs:
- Hypotension: Correct blood volume then infuse 0.01 mg/kg very slowly i.v. q15min. Continuously monitor blood pressure if possible.
- Ophthalmic use: 1 drop approximately 2 hours before intraocular surgery. 1 drop as a single dose for vasoconstriction. 1 drop to both eyes for diagnosis of Horner's syndrome.

Cats: Ophthalmic use: as for dogs.
Small mammals: Ferrets, Guinea pigs: Nasal drops supplied by pharmacies.
Birds, Reptiles: No information available.

Phenylpropanolamine (Diphenylpyraline)
(Propalin, Urilin) **POM-V**

Formulations: Oral: 40 mg/ml syrup.

Action: Increases urethral outflow resistance and has some peripheral vasoconstrictive effects.

Use: Treatment of incontinence secondary to urinary sphincter incompetence. May also be useful in the management of nasal congestion. Incontinence may recur if doses are delayed or missed. The onset of action may take several days.

Safety and handling: Normal precautions should be observed.

Contraindications: No information available.

Adverse reactions: May include restlessness, aggressiveness, irritability and hypertension. Cardiotoxicity has been reported.

Drug interactions: No information available.

DOSES
Dogs, Cats: 0.8 mg/kg p.o. q8h or 1.2 mg/kg p.o. q12h.
Small mammals: Rabbits: 5–10 mg/rabbit q12h.
Birds, Reptiles: No information available.

Phenytoin (Diphenylhydantoin)
(Epanutin*) **POM**

Formulations: Oral: 25 mg, 50 mg, 100 mg, 300 mg capsules; 50 mg chewable tablets; 30 mg/5 ml suspension.

Action: Diminishes the spread of focal neural discharges. Its action appears to be a stabilizing effect on synaptic junctions and it depresses motor areas of the cortex without depressing sensory areas.

Use: Used to control most forms of epilepsy in humans. In dogs it is metabolized very rapidly so that high doses need to be given often, and is associated with hepatic toxicity; cats metabolize the drug very slowly and toxicity easily develops. These undesirable pharmacokinetic properties mean that the drug is not recommended for use in dogs and cats as there are alternative drugs with a better efficacy and fewer adverse effects. If it is used in the dog, then it cannot be recommended for use as the sole anticonvulsant agent and is typically used in combination with other anticonvulsant agents. Hepatic function should be monitored every 6–12 months in patients on chronic therapy.

Safety and handling: Normal precautions should be observed.

Contraindications: Do not use in cats. No longer recommended for use in dogs unless as a last resort medication.

Adverse reactions: Adverse effects include ataxia, vomiting, hepatic toxicity, peripheral neuropathy, toxic epidermal necrolysis and pyrexia.

Drug interactions: A large number of potential drug interactions are reported in human patients, in particular complex interactions with other antiepileptics. The plasma concentration of phenytoin may be increased by cimetidine, diazepam, metronidazole, phenylbutazone, sulphonamides and trimethoprim. The absorption, effects or plasma concentration of phenytoin may be decreased by antacids, barbiturates and calcium. The metabolism of corticosteroids, doxycycline, theophylline and thyroxine may be increased by phenytoin. The analgesic properties of pethidine may be reduced by phenytoin, whereas the toxic effects may be enhanced. Concomitant administration of two or more antiepileptics may enhance toxicity without a corresponding increase in antiepileptic effect.

DOSES
Dogs: 10–35 mg/kg p.o. q6–8h.
Cats: Do not use.
Small mammals, Birds, Reptiles: No information available.

Pheromones see Dog appeasing pheromone, Feline facial fraction F3, Feline facial fraction F4

Pholcodine

(Benylin Children's Dry Cough Mixture, Galenphol)
general sale

Formulations: Oral: 2 mg/5 ml, 5 mg/5 ml, 10 mg/5 ml solutions. Note that many adult cough mixtures contain dextromethorphan (another opiate derivative about which little is known in dogs) and/or guaifenesin (an expectorant).

Action: A derivative of codeine that acts as an antitussive and has mild sedating but no analgesic properties. It depresses the cough reflex by acting on the cough centre in the CNS. It has a lower potential than codeine for inducing dependence.

Use: Cough suppression where the cause of the cough cannot be removed and the coughing is becoming detrimental to the animal's health (e.g. in chronic bronchitis, tracheal or mainstem bronchial collapse). It is not effective in respiratory tract infections in humans and would be unlikely to be effective in kennel cough in dogs. In humans it is effective in reducing the cough associated with lung tumours.

Safety and handling: Normal precautions should be observed.

Contraindications: Respiratory depression, raised intracranial pressure.

Adverse reactions: Sedation, constipation (though less than codeine). Has been associated with anaphylaxis in humans.

Drug interactions: Likely to interact with other opiates (including tramadol).

DOSES
Dogs: 0.1–0.2 mg/kg up to 4 times daily (anecdotal).
Cats, Small mammals, Birds, Reptiles: No information available.

Phosphate (Toldimphos)

(Foston, Phosphate-Sandoz*) **POM-V, GSL**

Formulations: Injectable: 140 mg/ml phosphate (as a 20% w/v solution of toldimphos, an organically combined phosphorus preparation) (Foston), potassium sodium phosphate (contains 40 mmol phosphate, 30 mmol potassium and 30 mmol sodium in 20 ml vials). Oral: Effervescent tablets containing 1.936 g sodium acid phosphate, 350 mg sodium bicarbonate, 315 mg potassium bicarbonate equivalent to 500 mg (16.1 mmol) phosphate, 468.8 mg (20.4 mmol) sodium and 123 mg (3.1 mmol) potassium.

Action: Phosphate is essential for intermediary metabolism, DNA and RNA synthesis, nerve, muscle and red blood cell function.

Use: Hypophosphataemic states, patients on large volume i.v. fluid therapy that have inadequate intake or patients that become hypophosphataemic following administration of parenteral nutrition. Phosphate is filtered by the kidneys but 80% is resorbed. In diabetic ketoacidotic patients a combination of potassium chloride and potassium phosphate in equal parts may be indicated to meet the patient's potassium needs and to treat or prevent significant hypophosphataemia.

Safety and handling: Normal precautions should be observed.

Contraindications: Hyperphosphataemia, hypocalcaemia, oliguric renal failure or if significant tissue necrosis is present.

Adverse reactions: May result in hypotension, renal failure or metastatic calcification of soft tissue. Hyperkalaemia or hypernatraemia may result in patients predisposed to these abnormalities and monitoring of electrolyte profiles is needed. Overdose or administration to patients with renal compromise may lead to hyperphosphataemia.

Drug interactions: Phosphates are incompatible with metals, including calcium and magnesium.

DOSES
Dogs:
- Acute significant hypophosphataemia: 0.06–0.18 mmol/kg of potassium phosphate i.v. over 6h, adjust according to response.
- Chronic hypophosphataemia: 140–280 mg (1–2 ml) i.m., s.c. q48h for 5–10 doses, 0.5–2 mmol phosphate/kg/day p.o.

Cats:
- Acute significant hypophosphataemia: dose as for dogs.
- Chronic hypophosphataemia: 0.5–2 mmol phosphate/kg/day p.o.

Small mammals, Birds, Reptiles: No information available.

Phosphate enema (Sodium acid phosphate)
(Fleet Enema*, Fletchers' Phosphate Enema*) **P**

Formulations: Rectal: 133 ml tube containing 21.4 g sodium acid phosphate and 9.4 g sodium phosphate (Fleet); 128 ml tube containing 12.8 g sodium acid phosphate and 10.24 g sodium phosphate (Fletchers').

Action: Osmotic laxative.

Use: Cathartic used to initiate rapid emptying of the colon in dogs.

Safety and handling: Normal precautions should be observed.

Contraindications: Phosphate enemas are contraindicated for use in cats or small dogs (<5 kg) as they may develop electrolyte abnormalities (hypocalcaemia and hyperphosphataemia) which can be fatal.

Adverse reactions: Electrolyte abnormalities (hypocalcaemia and hyperphosphataemia) which can be fatal.

Drug interactions: No information available.

DOSES
Dogs: 60–118 ml per rectum (dogs 5–10 kg); 128 ml per rectum (dogs >10 kg).
Cats: Do not use.
Small mammals, Birds, Reptiles: No information available.

Phytomenadione see Vitamin K1

Pilocarpine
(Pilocarpine hydrochloride*) **POM**

Formulations: Ophthalmic: 1%, 2%, 4% solutions in 10 ml bottles, single-use vials (2%). Most common concentration used in dogs is 1%.

Action: Direct-acting parasympathomimetic that stimulates cholinergic receptors. It lowers intraocular pressure by causing ciliary body muscle contraction, miosis and improved aqueous humour outflow.

Use: Has been used in the management of glaucoma, although this role has been superseded by other topical drugs such as carbonic anhydrase inhibitors and prostaglandin analogues. Pilocarpine produces miosis in 10–15 min for 6–8 hours in the dog. Oral pilocarpine increases lacrimation and can be used in the management of neurogenic keratoconjunctivitis (KCS or dry eye) in the dog; topical ophthalmic pilocarpine can also be used but can be irritant. Pilocarpine is rarely used for ophthalmic purposes in the cat due to potential toxicity.

Safety and handling: Normal precautions should be observed.

Contraindications: Avoid in uveitis or anterior lens luxation.

Adverse reactions: Conjunctival hyperaemia (vasodilation) and local irritation (due to low pH). Signs of systemic toxicity include hypersalivation, vomiting, diarrhoea and cardiac arrhythmias.

Drug interactions: No information available.

DOSES
Dogs:
- Open-angle glaucoma: 1 drop per eye of 1% solution q8–12h.
- Neurogenic KCS: 1 drop of 1–2% solution per 10 kg p.o. q12h (with food) as initial dose. Dose is increased slowly by 1 drop until signs of systemic toxicity are observed and then lowered to previously tolerated dose.

Cats, Small mammals, Birds, Reptiles: No information available.

Pimobendan
(Cardisure, Vetmedin) **POM-V**

Formulations: Injectable: 0.75 mg/ml solution (5 ml vial, Vetmedin). Oral: 5 mg hard capsules or 1.25 mg, 5 mg or 10 mg chewable tablets (Vetmedin); 1.25 mg, 2.5 mg, 5 mg, 10 mg flavoured tablets (Cardisure).

Action: Inodilator producing both positive inotropic and vasodilatory effects. Inotropic effects are mediated via sensitization of the myocardial contractile apparatus to intracellular calcium and by phosphodiesterase (PDE) III inhibition. Calcium sensitization allows for a positive inotropic effect without an increase in myocardial oxygen demand. Vasodilation is mediated by PDE III and V inhibition, resulting in arterio- and venodilation. It is also a positive lusitrope and has a mild inhibitory action on platelet aggregation in dogs at standard doses.

Use: Management of congestive heart failure due to valvular insufficiency (mitral and/or tricuspid regurgitation) or dilated cardiomyopathy (DCM) in the dog. Indicated for use with concurrent congestive heart failure therapy (e.g. furosemide, ACE inhibitors). Has been shown to be beneficial to delay the onset of heart failure or sudden death in Dobermanns with preclinical DCM. There is evidence of efficacy in the treatment of pulmonary hypertension secondary to mitral valve disease in dogs. Has also been used in cats with heart failure associated with systolic dysfunction, although it is not authorized and available data suggest that the pharmacokinetics in cats differ from that in dogs. The presence of food may reduce bioavailability.

Safety and handling: Normal precautions should be observed.

Contraindications: Do not use in hypertrophic cardiomyopathy and in cases where augmentation of cardiac output via increased contractility is not possible (e.g. aortic stenosis).

Adverse reactions: A moderate positive chronotropic effect and vomiting may occur in some cases, which may be avoided by dose reduction.

Drug interactions: The positive inotropic effects are attenuated by drugs such as beta-blockers and calcium-channel blockers (especially verapamil). No interaction with digitalis glycosides has been noted.

DOSES
Dogs: 0.15 mg/kg i.v. Oral pimobendan can be continued 12 hours after administration of the injection.
Dogs, Cats: 0.1–0.3 mg/kg p.o. q12h one hour before food. The preferable daily dose is 0.25 mg/kg p.o. q12h.
Small mammals, Birds, Reptiles: No information available.

Piperacillin

(Tazocin*) **POM**

Formulations: Injectable: 2.25 g, 4.5 g powder (2 g or 4 g piperacillin sodium + 0.25 g or 0.5 g tazobactam (Tazocin)).

Action: Beta-lactam antibiotics bind penicillin-binding proteins involved in cell wall synthesis, decreasing bacterial cell wall strength and rigidity, and affecting cell division, growth and septum formation. As animal cells lack a cell wall the beta-lactam antibiotics are extremely safe. The effect is bactericidal and killing occurs in a time-dependent fashion.

Use: Piperacillin is a ureidopenicillin, classified with ticarcillin as an antipseudomonal penicillin. It is reserved for life-threatening infections (e.g. endocarditis or septicaemia) where culture and sensitivity testing predict a clinical response. These include infections caused by *Pseudomonas aeruginosa* and *Bacteroides fragilis* in neutropenic patients, although it has activity against other Gram-negative bacilli including *Proteus*. For pseudomonal septicaemias, antipseudomonal penicillins should be given with an aminoglycoside (e.g. gentamicin) as there is a synergistic effect. Piperacillin should usually be combined with a beta-lactamase inhibitor and therefore is co-formulated with tazobactam. Experience in veterinary species is limited, especially cats, and doses are largely empirical. Piperacillin inhibits the excretion of the tazobactam component in the dog.

Safety and handling: Normal precautions should be observed.

Contraindications: Do not administer penicillins to hamsters, gerbils, guinea pigs, chinchillas or rabbits.

Adverse reactions: Nausea, diarrhoea and skin rashes are the commonest adverse effects in humans. Painful if given by i.m. injection. The sodium content of each formulation may be clinically important for patients on restricted sodium intakes.

Drug interactions: Piperacillin enhances the effects of non-depolarizing muscle relaxants. Gentamicin inactivates piperacillin if mixed in the same syringe. Clinical experience with this drug is limited. There is synergism between the beta-lactams and the aminoglycosides.

DOSES

See Appendix for guidelines on responsible antibacterial use.
Dogs: 25–50 mg/kg by slow i.v. injection/infusion q8h.
Cats: No information available.
Small mammals: Rabbits, Chinchillas, Guinea pigs, Hamsters, Gerbils: Do not use.
Birds: 100 mg/kg i.m., i.v. q12h.
Reptiles: 50–100 mg/kg i.m. q24h for 7–14 days; may be nebulized diluted 100 mg piperacillin/10 ml saline for 15–20 min q8–12h for chelonians and lizards with lower respiratory tract infections.

Piperazine
(Biozine, Easy Round Wormer, Piperazine Citrate Worm Tablets, Puppy Easy Worm Syrup, Roundworm, Soluverm)
AVM-GSL

Formulations: Oral: 100 mg, 105 mg, 416 mg, 500 mg tablets; 500 mg/g (50% w/w), 510 mg/g (51% w/w) powder; 58 mg/ml syrup.

Action: An anti-ascaridial anthelmintic that blocks acetylcholine, thus affecting neurotransmission and paralysing the adult worm; it has no larvicidal activity.

Use: Active against *Toxocara cati*, *T. canis*, *Toxascaris leonina* and *Uncinaria stenocephala*. Ineffective against tapeworms and lung worms. High doses are required to treat hookworm infection. Puppies and kittens may be wormed from 6–8 weeks of age and should be weighed accurately to prevent overdosing. Fasting is not necessary. Piperazine may be used in pregnant animals.

Safety and handling: Normal precautions should be observed.

Contraindications: No information available.

Adverse reactions: Uncommon but occasionally vomiting or muscle tremors and ataxia have been reported.

Drug interactions: Piperazine and pyrantel have antagonistic mechanisms of action; do not use together.

DOSES
Dogs, Cats:
- Ascarids: 100 mg/kg p.o. Repeat dose in 2–3 weeks.
- Hookworm: 200 mg/kg p.o. Repeat dose in 2–3 weeks.

Small mammals: Ferrets: 50–100 mg/kg p.o., repeat in 2–3 weeks; Rabbits: 200 mg/kg p.o., repeat in 2–3 weeks; Chinchillas: 100 mg/kg p.o. q24h for two doses. In-water medication (7 days on, 7 days off, 7 days on) at the following doses, is also possible: Guinea pigs, Hamsters: 10 mg/ml; Rats, Mice: 4–5 mg/ml.

Birds: Pigeons: 1.9 g/l water; Passerines: 3.7 g/l water for 12h. Repeat in 2–3 weeks.

Reptiles: No information available.

Piroxicam · CIL
(Brexidol*, Feldene*, Piroxicam*) **POM**

Formulations: Oral: 10 mg, 20 mg capsules, 20 mg dissolving tablet. Injectable: 20 mg/ml solution.

Action: Inhibition of COX enzymes limits the production of prostaglandins involved in inflammation. Also limits tumour growth but the mechanism is still to be determined.

Use: In veterinary medicine, piroxicam has been used to treat certain tumours expressing COX receptors, e.g. transitional cell carcinoma of the bladder, prostatic carcinoma and colonic-rectal carcinoma and polyps. Piroxicam suppositories are available in the human field and may be useful in the management of colorectal polyps/neoplasia. Other NSAIDs are authorized for veterinary use in various inflammatory conditions but there is no information on the effect of these drugs in neoplastic conditions.

Safety and handling: Normal precautions should be observed.

Contraindications: Gastric ulceration, renal disease, concurrent use of corticosteroids.

Adverse reactions: As a non-specific COX inhibitor it may cause general adverse effects associated with NSAIDs, including GI toxicity, gastric ulceration and renal papillary necrosis (particularly if patient is dehydrated).

Drug interactions: Do not use with corticosteroids or other NSAIDs (increased risk of gastric ulceration). Concurrent use with diuretics or aminoglycosides may increase risk of nephrotoxicity. Piroxicam is highly protein bound and may displace other protein bound drugs. The clinical significance of this is not well established.

DOSES
See Appendix for chemotherapy protocols.
Dogs: 0.3 mg/kg p.o. q24–72h; start at least frequent administration and slowly increase if no side effects observed.
Cats: Not recommended.
Small mammals: Mice: 3.4–20 mg/kg p.o. q24h.
Birds: 0.5 mg/kg p.o. q12h.
Reptiles: No information available.

PMSG see **Serum gonadotrophin**

Polymyxin B
(Surolan, Polyfax*) **POM-V, POM**

Formulations: Topical: Surolan 5,500 IU polymyxin/ml suspension combined with miconazole and prednisolone for dermatological and otic use. Polyfax: 10,000 IU polymyxin/g ointment combined with bacitracin for dermatological and ophthalmic use.

Action: Rapidly bactericidal (concentration-dependent mechanism) by disrupting the outer membrane of Gram-negative bacteria through its action as a cationic surface acting agent.

Use: Effective against Gram-negative organisms; Gram-positives usually resistant. Particularly effective in the treatment of external pseudomonal infections, e.g. keratoconjunctivitis, otitis externa. Polymyxins are too toxic for systemic use and because of their strongly basic nature are not absorbed from the GI tract.

Formulations containing corticosteroids should be used with great care in rabbits and birds.

Safety and handling: Normal precautions should be observed.

Contraindications: Do not use if the tympanum is ruptured.

Adverse reactions: Should not be used systemically as is nephrotoxic. Potentially ototoxic.

Drug interactions: Acts synergistically with a number of other antibacterial agents as it disrupts the outer and cytoplasmic membranes, thus improving penetration of other agents into bacterial cells. Cationic detergents (e.g. chlorhexidine) and chelating agents (e.g. EDTA) potentiate the antibacterial effects of polymyxin B against *Pseudomonas aeruginosa*.

DOSES
See Appendix for guidelines on responsible antibacterial use.
Dogs, Cats: Skin: Apply a few drops and rub in well q12h. Otic: Clean ear and apply a few drops into affected ear q12h. Ophthalmic: Apply ointment q6–8h.
Small mammals, Birds, Reptiles: No information available.

Polysulphated glycosaminoglycan
(Adequan) **POM-V**

Formulations: Injectable: 100 mg/ml solution for i.m. injection.

Action: Precursor to mucopolysaccharides, enzyme inhibitor, stimulates chondrocytes and synovial cells. Binds to damaged cartilage matrix consisting of aggregated proteoglycans and stimulates the synthesis of new glycosaminoglycan molecules and inhibits proteolytic enzymes.

Use: Acts as a chondroprotective agent in the adjunctive management of non-infectious and non-immune-mediated arthritides. For intra-articular use surgical preparation of the joint is necessary and for both preparations aseptic technique is mandatory. Not a replacement, but rather an adjunct for other therapies.

Safety and handling: Normal precautions should be observed.

Contraindications: Not for use in patients where arthrotomy is anticipated because of a possible increase in bleeding. Not for use when infection is present or suspected.

Adverse reactions: Intra-articular injection may cause pain and inflammation. Although rare, joint sepsis is possible.

Drug interactions: None described to date.

DOSES
Dogs: 0.5 to 1.0 ml per joint q7d for 5 weeks. For i.m. therapy the manufacturer recommends 500 mg by deep i.m. injection q4d for 7 treatments. Other protocols are: 3–5 mg/kg i.m. q3–5d for 3 weeks or 5 mg/kg i.m. twice weekly.

Cats: 1–5 mg/kg i.m. q4d for six treatments, then as needed.
Small mammals: Rabbits: 2.2 mg/kg s.c., i.m. q3d for 21–28 days, then q14d as needed.
Birds, Reptiles: No information available.

Polyvinyl alcohol
(Liquifilm Tears*, Sno Tears*) **P**

Formulations: Ophthalmic: 1.4%, 10 ml, 15 ml.

Action: Polyvinyl alcohol is a synthetic resin tear substitute (lacromimetic).

Use: It is used for lubrication of dry eyes. In cases of keratoconjunctivitis sicca (KCS or dry eye) it will improve ocular surface lubrication, tear retention and patient comfort while lacrostimulation therapy (e.g. topical ciclosporin) is initiated. It is more adherent and less viscous than hypromellose. Patient compliance is poor if administered >q4h; consider using a longer acting tear replacement.

Safety and handling: Normal precautions should be observed.

Contraindications: No information available.

Adverse reactions: No information available.

Drug interactions: No information available.

DOSES
Dogs, Cats, Small mammals: 1 drop per eye q1h.
Birds, Reptiles: No information available.

Potassium bromide
(Bromilep, Epilease, Libromide, Potassium bromide solution) **POM-V, AVM-GSL**

Formulations: Oral: 325 mg tablets; 100 mg, 250 mg, 1000 mg capsules; 250 mg/ml solution.

Action: Within the CNS it competes with transmembrane chloride transport and inhibits sodium, resulting in membrane hyperpolarization and elevation of the seizure threshold. Bromide competes with chloride in post-synaptic anion channels following activation by inhibitory neurotransmitters and therefore potentiates the effect of GABA. Acts synergistically with other therapeutic agents that have GABA-ergic effects (such as phenobarbital).

Use: Control of seizures in dogs in which the seizures are refractory to treatment with phenobarbital or where the use of phenobarbital or imepitoin is contraindicated. KBr is usually used in conjunction with phenobarbital. Although not authorized for this use, KBr has been used in conjunction with imepitoin. Bromide has a long half-life (>20 days) and steady state plasma concentrations may not be achieved for 3–4 months. Monitoring of serum drug concentrations should be performed and dose levels adjusted accordingly. The serum KBr concentration should reach 0.8–1.5 mg/ml to be therapeutic. In some cases, the dog may need to be started on a loading dose to raise levels in the blood rapidly to therapeutic levels. Loading doses of KBr are associated with an increased incidence of adverse effects (primarily sedation and ataxia) and should only be used in dogs with poorly controlled severe seizures. The loading dose can be administered via enema, but this may result in haemorrhagic diarrhoea. Serum samples should be taken after the end of loading to check the serum concentration. The slow rise of plasma bromide levels after enteral administration limits its usefulness in status epilepticus. Bromide is well absorbed from the GI tract and eliminated slowly by the kidney in competition with chloride. High levels of dietary salt increase renal elimination of bromide. Consequently, it is important that the diet be kept constant once bromide therapy has started. Bromide will be measured in assays for chloride and will therefore produce falsely high 'chloride' results. Use with caution in dogs with renal disease.

Safety and handling: Normal precautions should be observed.

Contraindications: Do not use in the cat due to the development of severe coughing due to eosinophilic bronchitis, which may be fatal. Avoid use in dogs with a history of, or a predisposition for the development of, pancreatitis.

Adverse reactions: Ataxia, sedation and somnolence are seen with overdosage and loading doses. Skin reactions have been reported in animals with pre-existing skin diseases, e.g. flea bite dermatitis. Vomiting may occur after oral administration, particularly if high concentrations (>250 mg/ml) are used. Polyphagia, polydipsia and pancreatitis have also been reported. In the case of acute bromide toxicity, 0.9% NaCl i.v. is the treatment of choice. Less commonly behavioural changes, including irritability or restlessness, may be evident.

Drug interactions: Bromide competes with chloride for renal reabsorption. Increased dietary salt, administration of fluids or drugs containing chloride, and use of loop diuretics (e.g. furosemide) may result in increased bromide excretion and decreased serum bromide concentrations.

DOSES
Dogs: The initial daily maintenance dose is 20–40 mg/kg p.o q24h. It is not necessary to dose more frequently, but more frequent dosing is not detrimental. The loading dose is 200 mg/kg/day p.o. divided into 4–6h doses for 5 days, after which the dose is decreased to the maintenance dose (20–40 mg/kg p.o. q24h). If seizures resolve sooner, it is advisable to decrease the loading dose to maintenance levels earlier to reduce adverse effects. A single loading dose of 600–1000 mg/kg p.o. can be given but this is likely to result in excessive sedation, ataxia and potentially vomiting.

Cats: Do not use.
Small mammals: Ferrets: 22–30 mg/kg p.o. q24h in combination with phenobarbital; 70–80 mg/kg p.o. q24h if used alone.
Birds, Reptiles: No information available.

Potassium chloride see Potassium salts

Potassium citrate
(Cystopurin*, Potassium citrate BP*) **AVM-GSL**

Formulations: Oral: 30% solution. Various preparations are available.

Action: Enhances renal tubular resorption of calcium, and alkalinizes urine.

Use: Management of calcium oxalate and urate urolithiasis, and fungal urinary tract infections. May be used to treat hypokalaemia, although potassium chloride or gluconate is preferred. Used to treat some forms of metabolic acidosis.

Safety and handling: Normal precautions should be observed.

Contraindications: Renal impairment or cardiac disease.

Adverse reactions: Rare, but may include GI signs and hyperkalaemia.

Drug interactions: No information available.

DOSES
Dogs, Cats: 75 mg/kg or 2 mmol/kg p.o. q12h.
Small mammals: Rabbits: 33 mg/kg p.o q8h; Guinea pigs: 10–30 mg/kg p.o. q12h.
Birds, Reptiles: No information available.

Potassium gluconate see Potassium salts
Potassium phosphate see Phosphate

Potassium salts (Potassium chloride, Potassium gluconate)
(Kaminox, Tumil-K) **general sale**

Formulations: Injectable: 20% KCl solution (2 g KCl/10 ml; 26 mmol K+). Before use dilute the solution with at least 70 times its volume of sodium chloride intravenous fluid. Oral: Tablets containing 2 mEq potassium gluconate; Powder (2 mEq per ¼ teaspoon) (Tumil-K); Liquid 1 mEq/ml potassium gluconate formulated with a range of amino acids, B vitamins and iron (Kaminox). Note: 1 mmol/l =1 mEq/l.

Action: Replacement of potassium.

Use: Treatment or prevention of known hypokalaemic states; prolonged anorexia and chronic renal failure are the most common, but can also use with diuretics that are not potassium sparing. If rapid correction is not necessary, may be added to s.c. fluids but do not exceed 30 mEq/l as higher levels are irritating. Because potassium is primarily an intracellular electrolyte, serum concentrations may not immediately reflect clinical effect. Do not give rapid i.v. injections. Concentrated solutions must be diluted before i.v. use. Use with caution in any renal failure patient as 80–90% of excretion is renal. Use with caution in digitalized patients.

Safety and handling: Normal precautions should be observed.

Contraindications: Hyperkalaemia, acute or obstructive renal failure, untreated Addison's disease, acute dehydration and diseases with impaired or obstructed GI motility.

Adverse reactions: Primarily development of hyperkalaemia when administered too rapidly or to patients with impaired renal function. Clinical signs range from muscle weakness to GI disturbances to cardiac arrhythmias and cardiac arrest. Concentrations >60 mmol/l can cause pain, peripheral vein sclerosis and increase the risk of overdose.

Drug interactions: Potassium retention leading to severe hyperkalaemia may develop when used with angiotensin converting enzyme inhibitors (e.g. captopril, enalapril) or potassium-sparing diuretics (e.g. spironolactone). Potassium chloride is not compatible with many drugs especially those in sodium salt form.

Serum potassium	Amount to be added to 250 ml 0.9% NaCl
<2 mmol/l	20 mmol
2–2.5 mmol/l	15 mmol
2.5–3 mmol/l	10 mmol
3–3.5 mmol/l	7 mmol
3.5–5.5 mmol/l	5 mmol (minimum daily need in anorectic patients

DOSES

Dogs: Intravenous: Doses must be titrated for each patient; dilute concentrated solutions prior to use (normally to 20–60 mmol/l). Rate of i.v. infusion should not exceed 0.5 mmol/kg/h, especially when concentration in replacement fluid is >60 mmol/l. Use of fluid pumps is recommended. Oral: Replacement dose needs to be titrated to effect to maintain mid-range normal values in each individual patient. Starting doses are 2 mEq per 4.5 kg in food q12h or 2.2 mEq per 100 kcal required energy intake.

Cats: Intravenous: Doses as for dogs. Oral: Replacement dose needs to be titrated to effect to maintain mid-range normal values in each individual patient. Starting doses are 2.2 mEq per 4.5 kg in food q12h or 2–6 mEq/cat/day p.o. in divided doses q8–12h.
Small mammals, Birds, Reptiles: No information available.

Potentiated sulphonamides see Trimethoprim/ Sulphonamide

Pradofloxacin
(Veraflox) **POM-V**

Formulations: Oral: 15 mg, 60 mg, 120 mg tablets; 25 mg/ml solution.

Action: Broad-spectrum bactericidal antibiotic. Rapidly bactericidal and works in a concentration-dependent manner.

Use: Ideally fluoroquinolone use should be reserved for infections where culture and sensitivity testing predicts a clinical response and where first- and second-line antimicrobials would not be effective. Active against many Gram-negative and Gram-positive organisms. Much improved activity *versus* anaerobes compared with earlier generation fluoroquinolones. Like other members of the class, pradofloxacin has exceptional lipid solubility, attaining high concentrations especially in the urogenital tract including the prostate gland. Specific indications include superficial and deep pyoderms and wound infections associated with susceptible organisms such as *Staphylococcus pseudintermedius*, urinary tract infections associated with susceptible organisms such as *Escherichia coli* and *S. pseudintermedius*, severe periodontal disease associated with anaerobes such as *Porphyromonas* spp. and *Prevotella* spp. and acute severe upper respiratory tract infections associated with organisms such as *E.coli*, *Staphylococcus* spp. and *Pasteurella multocida*.

Safety and handling: Normal precautions should be observed.

Contraindications: Do not use in pregnant or lactating animals. Do not use in dogs <12 months of age (<18 months for giant breeds) or cats <6 weeks of age due to potential adverse effects on cartilage. Do not use in animals with persistent cartilage lesions. Do not use in dogs or cats with neurological disease especially epilepsy.

Adverse reactions: Most common is mild gastrointestinal upset.

Drug interactions: Decreased bioavailability if administered with agents containing metal cations (sucralfate, certain antacids, multivitamins). Combination with NSAIDs in animals with epilepsy may lower the seizure threshold. Fluoroquinolones may increase plasma levels of theophylline and digoxin.

DOSES
See Appendix for guidelines on responsible antibacterial use.
Dogs: 3 mg/kg p.o. q24h.
Cats: 3 mg/kg p.o. q24h (tablet), 5.0 mg/kg p.o. q24h (suspension).
Small mammals, Birds, Reptiles: No information available.

Pralidoxime
(Pralidoxime*) **POM**

Formulations: Powder for reconstitution: 1 g vial which produces 200 mg/ml solution.

Action: Reactivates the cholinesterase enzyme damaged by organophosphate (OP) and allows the destruction of accumulated acetylcholine at the synapse to be resumed. In addition, pralidoxime detoxifies certain OPs by direct chemical inactivation and retards the 'ageing' of phosphorylated cholinesterase to a non-reactive form.

Use: Management of OP toxicity. Most effective if given within 24 hours. Pralidoxime does not appreciably enter the CNS, thus CNS toxicity is not reversed. If given within 24 hours of exposure, treatment is usually only required for 24–36 hours. Respiratory support may be necessary. Treatment of OP toxicity should also include atropine. Use at a reduced dose with renal failure.

Safety and handling: Normal precautions should be observed.

Contraindications: Do not use for poisoning due to carbamate or OP compounds without anticholinesterase activity.

Adverse reactions: Nausea, tachycardia, hyperventilation, and muscular weakness are reported in humans.

Drug interactions: Aminophylline, morphine, phenothiazines or theophylline should be avoided in these patients.

DOSES
Dogs: Dilute to a 20 mg/ml solution and administer 20–50 mg/kg slowly i.v. (over 2 minutes at least – 500 mg/min max.) i.m., s.c. Repeat after 1h if still severe signs then q8–12h.
Cats: Dilute to a 20 mg/ml solution and administer 20–50 mg/kg slowly i.v. (over 2 minutes at least – 500 mg/min max.) i.m., s.c. Repeat after 1h if still severe signs then q8–12h.
Small mammals: No information available.
Birds: 10–100 mg/kg i.m., i.v. q24h prn.
Reptiles: No information available.

Praziquantel

(Bob Martin 2 in 1 Dewormer, Bob Martin 3 in 1
Dewormer, Bob Martin Spot-on Dewormer, Cazitel Plus,
Cestem Flavoured, Dolpac, Droncit, Droncit Spot-on,
Drontal cat, Drontal plus, Endoguard, Milbemax for cats,
Milbemax for dogs, Plerion, Prazitel, Profender Spot-on)
POM-V, NFA-VPS, AVM-GSL

Formulations: Oral: 50 mg and 175 mg praziquantel with pyrantel
and febantel tablets (Bob Martin 3 in 1 Dewormer, Cazitel Plus, Cestem
Flavoured, Drontal plus, Endoguard, Prazitel); 10 mg, 25 mg, 50 mg
and 125 mg praziquantel with oxantel and pyrantel tablets (Dolpac,
Plerion); 20 mg and 30 mg praziquantel with pyrantel tablets (Bob
Martin 2 in 1 Dewormer, Drontal cat); 25 mg and 125 mg praziquantel
with milbemycin tablets (Milbemax for dogs); 10 mg and 40 mg
praziquantel with milbemycin tablets (Milbemax for cats); 50 mg
praziquantel (Droncit). Topical: 20 mg, 30 mg, 60 mg, 96 mg in spot-on
pipette (Bob Martin Spot-on Dewormer, Droncit Spot-on); 85.8 mg/ml
praziquantel with emodepside in spot-on pipettes (Profendor Spot-on).

Action: Cestocide that increases cell membrane permeability of
susceptible worms, resulting in loss of intracellular calcium and
paralysis. This allows the parasites to be phagocytosed or digested.

Use: Treatment of *Dipylidium caninum*, *Taenia*, *Echinococcus
granulosus* and *Mesocestoides* in dogs and cats. Because it kills all
intestinal forms of *Echinococcus*, it is the preferred drug in most
Echinococcus control programmes. The PETS travel scheme requires
animals to be treated with praziquantel prior to entry into the UK. The
inclusion of pyrantel and febantel in some preparations increases the
spectrum of efficacy. Drontal plus can be used from 2 weeks of age.
Drontal cat tablets can be used from 6 weeks of age. Retreatment is
usually unnecessary unless reinfection takes place.

Safety and handling: Normal precautions should be observed.
Solutions containing emodepside should not be handled by women
of child-bearing age.

Contraindications: Do not use in unweaned puppies or kittens, as
they are unlikely to be affected by tapeworms. Do not use the spot-on
preparation in animals <1 kg. Avoid the i.m. route in reptiles.

Adverse reactions: Injection may cause localized tissue sensitivity,
particularly in cats. Can cause transient hypersalivation if a cat licks
the site of spot-on application. Oral administration can occasionally
result in anorexia, vomiting, lethargy and diarrhoea. Injections in
reptiles may cause bruising and tissue necrosis at the site.

Drug interactions: No information available.

DOSES

Dogs: 3.5–7.5 mg/kg i.m., s.c.; 5 mg/kg p.o.; 8 mg/kg spot-on.

Cats: 3.5–7.5 mg/kg i.m., s.c.; 5 mg/kg p.o.; 8 mg/kg spot-on.
Small mammals: Ferrets: 5–10 mg/kg p.o., s.c., i.m. repeated in
10–14d; Rabbits: 5–10 mg/kg p.o., s.c., i.m. repeated in 10 days;
Gerbils, Rats, Mice: 30 mg/kg p.o. q14d (for 3 treatments).
Birds: Pigeons: 10–20 mg/kg p.o. or 7.5 mg/kg s.c.; Other birds:
10 mg/kg i.m., repeat after 7–10d.
Reptiles: 5–8 mg/kg p.o., repeat after 2 weeks in most species.

Prazosin
(Hypovase*, Prazosin*) **POM**

CIL

Formulations: Oral: 0.5 mg, 1 mg, 2 mg, 5 mg tablets.

Action: Prazosin is a post-synaptic alpha-1 blocking agent causing
arterial and venous vasodilation. This leads to reduction in blood
pressure and systemic vascular resistance.

Use: Adjunctive therapy of congestive heart failure secondary to
mitral regurgitation in cases that are refractory to standard therapy.
May be useful in promoting urine flow in patients with functional
urethral obstruction and in the management of systemic or pulmonary
hypertension. Efficacy may decline over time. Not often used.

Safety and handling: Normal precautions should be observed.

Contraindications: Hypotension, renal failure.

Adverse reactions: Hypotension, syncope, drowsiness, weakness,
GI upsets.

Drug interactions: Concomitant use of beta-blockers (e.g.
propranolol) or diuretics (e.g. furosemide) may increase the risk of a
first dose hypotensive effect. Calcium-channel blockers may cause
additive hypotension. Prazosin is highly protein-bound and so may be
displaced by, or displace, other highly protein-bound drugs (e.g.
sulphonamide) from plasma proteins.

DOSES
Dogs: 1 mg/dog p.o. q8–12h (dogs up to 15 kg); 2 mg/dog p.o. q8–12h
(dogs >15 kg). Monitor efficacy by measuring blood pressure and
clinical response.
Cats: 0.25–1 mg/cat p.o. q8–12h.
Small mammals, Birds, Reptiles: No information available.

Prednisolone
(PLT, Prednicare, Prednidale, Pred-forte*) **POM-V**

Formulations: Ophthalmic: Prednisolone acetate 0.5%, 1%
suspensions in 5 ml, 10 ml bottles (Pred-forte). Topical: Prednisolone
is a component of many topical dermatological, otic and ophthalmic
preparations. Injectable: Prednisolone sodium succinate 10 mg/ml

solution; 7.5 mg/ml suspension plus 2.5 mg/ml dexamethasone. Oral: 1 mg, 5 mg, 25 mg tablets. PLT is a compound preparation containing cinchophen.

Action: Binds to specific cytoplasmic receptors which then enter the nucleus and alter the transcription of DNA, leading to alterations in cellular metabolism which result in anti-inflammatory, immunosuppressive and antifibrotic effects. Also has glucocorticoid activity and acts in dogs as an ADH antagonist.

Use: Management of chronic allergic/inflammatory conditions (e.g. atopy, inflammatory bowel disease), immune-mediated conditions, hypoadrenocorticism, and lymphoproliferative and other neoplasms. In combination with cinchophen (PLT) it is used in the management of osteoarthritis. Prednisolone has approximately 4 times the anti-inflammatory potency and half the relative mineralocorticoid potency of hydrocortisone. It, like methylprednisolone, is considered to have an intermediate duration of activity and is suitable for alternate-day use. Animals on chronic therapy should be tapered off their steroids when discontinuing the drug. There are no studies comparing protocols for tapering immunosuppressive or anti-inflammatory therapy; it is appropriate to adjust the therapy according to laboratory or clinical parameters. For example, cases with immune-mediated haemolytic anaemia should have their therapy adjusted following monitoring of their haematocrit. There is no evidence that long-term low doses of glucocorticoids do, or do not, prevent relapse of immune-mediated conditions. Impaired wound healing and delayed recovery from infections may be seen. Use glucocorticoids with care in rabbits as they are sensitive to these drugs. If using in birds must make sure bird is genuinely pruritic and underlying infectious disease, e.g. aspergillosis, chlamydophilosis, has been excluded before use. The use of steroids in most cases of shock and spinal cord injury is of no benefit and may be detrimental.

Safety and handling: Shake suspension before use.

Contraindications: Do not use in pregnant animals. Systemic corticosteroids are generally contraindicated in patients with renal disease and diabetes mellitus. Topical corticosteroids are contraindicated in ulcerative keratitis.

Adverse reactions: Prolonged use of glucocorticoids suppresses the hypothalamic-pituitary axis (HPA), causing adrenal atrophy, and may cause significant proteinuria and glomerular changes in the dog. Catabolic effects of glucocorticoids leads to weight loss and cutaneous atrophy. Iatrogenic hyperadrenocorticism may develop with chronic use. Vomiting, diarrhoea and GI ulceration may develop; the latter may be more severe when corticosteroids are used in animals with neurological injury. Hyperglycaemia and decreased serum T4 values may be seen in patients receiving prednisolone. Even small single doses can cause severe adverse reactions in rabbits. In birds there is a high risk of immunosuppression and side effects, such as hepatopathy and a diabetes mellitus-like syndrome.

Drug interactions: There is an increased risk of GI ulceration if used concurrently with NSAIDs. Hypokalaemia may develop if acetazolamide, amphotericin B or potassium-depleting diuretics (e.g. furosemide, thiazides) are administered concomitantly with corticosteroids. Glucocorticoids may antagonize the effect of insulin. The metabolism of corticosteroids may be enhanced by phenytoin or phenobarbital and decreased by antifungals (e.g. itraconazole).

DOSES
See Appendix for chemotherapy and immunosuppression protocols.
Dogs:
- Ophthalmic: Dosage frequency and duration of therapy is dependent upon type of lesion and response to therapy. Usually 1 drop in affected eye(s) q4–24h tapering in response to therapy.
- Hypoadrenocorticism: 0.2–0.3 mg/kg with fludrocortisone. The use of prednisolone may be discontinued in most cases once the animal is stable.
- Allergy: 0.5–1.0 mg/kg p.o. q12h initially, tapering to lowest q48h dose.
- Anti-inflammatory: 0.5 mg/kg p.o. q12–24h; taper to 0.25–0.5 mg/kg q48h.
- Immunosuppression: 1.0–2.0 mg/kg p.o. q24h, tapering slowly to 0.5 mg/kg q48h (for many conditions this will take 6 months).
- Lymphoma: see Appendix.

Cats:
- Ophthalmic, Hypoadrenocorticism, Allergy: Doses as for dogs.
- Anti-inflammatory: 0.5–1.0 mg/kg p.o. q12–24h; taper to 0.5 mg/kg q48h.
- Immunosuppression: 1.0–2.0 mg/kg p.o. q12–24h, tapering slowly to 0.5-1.0 mg/kg q48h (for many conditions this will take 6 months).
- Lymphoma: see Appendix.

Small mammals: Ferrets: lymphoma (see Appendix), anti-inflammatory: 1–2 mg/kg p.o. q24h; postoperative management of adrenalectomy: 0.25–0.5 mg/kg p.o. q12h, taper to q48h; Rabbits: anti-inflammatory: 0.25–0.5 mg/kg p.o. q12h for 3 days, then q24h for 3 days, then q48h; Others: anti-inflammatory: 1.25–2.5 mg/kg p.o. q24h.

Birds: Pruritus: 1 mg/kg p.o. q12h, reduced to minimum effective dose as quickly as possible.

Reptiles: Analgesic, Anti-inflammatory: 2–5 mg/kg p.o. q 24–48h; Lymphoma: 40 mg/m^2 q48h with chlorambucil 2 mg/m^2 q24h q30d.

Pregabalin
(Lyrica) **POM**

Formulations: Oral: 25 mg, 50 mg, 75 mg, 100 mg, 150 mg, 200 mg, 225 mg, 300 mg capsules; 20 mg/ml solution.

Action: Similar mechanism of action to gabapentin and is considered the next generation gabapentin, binding to voltage-dependent calcium channel in the CNS reducing calcium influx. Pregabalin also decreases release of excitatory neurotransmitters (including glutamate and noradrenaline) and increases neuronal GABA levels. The mode of action of its analgesic effect is unknown.

Use: Adjunctive therapy in the treatment of epileptic seizures refractory to conventional treatment. Treatment of neuropathic pain. Use with care in patients with renal impairment.

Safety and handling: Normal precautions should be observed.

Contraindications: Avoid use in pregnant animals as toxicity has been demonstrated in experimental studies. Do not discontinue abruptly.

Adverse reactions: Many dogs develop sedation or ataxia, though not usually severe enough to warrant cessation of the therapy. Mild increases in hepatic enzymes may also occur following prolonged therapy.

Drug interactions: No information available.

DOSES
Dogs: 3–4 mg/kg p.o. q8h, starting at 2 mg/kg and gradually increasing.
Cats: No information available, but a similar dose to dogs has been suggested.
Small mammals, Birds, Reptiles: No information available.

Prochlorperazine
(Buccastem*, Prochlorperazine*, Stemetil*) **POM**

Formulations: Injectable: 12.5 mg/ml solution in 1 ml ampoule. Oral: 3 mg, 5 mg tablets; 5 mg/ml syrup.

Action: Blocks dopamine, muscarinic acetylcholine and 5-HT3 receptors in chemoreceptor trigger zone and vomiting centre.

Use: Predominantly to control motion sickness and emesis associated with vestibular disease. Maropitant and metoclopramide are authorized as antiemetics in dogs and so in this species prochlorperazine is not a first choice.

Safety and handling: Normal precautions should be observed.

Contraindications: No information available.

Adverse reactions: Sedation, depression, hypotension and extrapyramidal reactions (rigidity, tremors, weakness, restlessness, etc.).

Drug interactions: CNS depressant agents (e.g. anaesthetics, narcotic analgesics) may cause additive CNS depression if used with prochlorperazine. Antacids or antidiarrhoeal preparations (e.g. bismuth subsalicylate or kaolin/pectin mixtures) may reduce GI absorption of oral phenothiazines. Increased blood levels of both drugs may result if propranolol is administered with phenothiazines. Phenothiazines block alpha-adrenergic receptors, which may lead to unopposed beta activity causing vasodilation and increased cardiac rate if adrenaline is given.

DOSES
Dogs, Cats: 0.1–0.5 mg/kg i.v., i.m., s.c. q6–8h; 0.5–1 mg/kg p.o. q8–12h.
Small mammals: Rabbits: 0.2–0.5 mg/kg p.o. q8h.
Birds, Reptiles: No information available.

Progesterone
(Progesterone*) **POM**

Formulations: Injectable: 25 mg/ml oily solution.

Action: Binds to specific cytoplasmic receptors, which then enter the nucleus and alter the transcription of DNA leading to alterations in cellular metabolism.

Use: Threatened or habitual abortion, induction of parturition and postponement of oestrus. Doses of 2 mg/kg i.m. q48h will maintain plasma progesterone values >2 ng/ml, the level required to maintain pregnancy. Parturition can be expected 72 hours after the last injection. Parturition should be planned for day 57 after the onset of cytological dioestrus in the bitch or 64 days after mating in the queen. Other medications are authorized for the postponement of oestrus.

Safety and handling: Normal precautions should be observed.

Contraindications: Do not use in animals with diabetes mellitus.

Adverse reactions: Reversible masculinization of the external genitalia may occur in female puppies born to bitches treated during pregnancy. Prolonged therapy may result in pathological uterine changes in bitches.

Drug interactions: No information available.

DOSES
Dogs: 1–3 mg/kg i.m., s.c.
Cats: 0.2–2 mg/kg i.m., s.c.
Small mammals, Birds, Reptiles: No information available.

Proligestone
(Delvosteron) **POM-V**

Formulations: Injectable: 100 mg/ml suspension.

Action: Alters the transcription of DNA, leading to alterations in cellular metabolism which mimic those caused by progesterone.

Use: Postponement of oestrus in the bitch, queen and jill ferret, treatment and prevention of false pregnancy in the bitch and rabbit, and control of miliary dermatitis in the cat. It has also been used to increase hair growth in dogs with pituitary dwarfism. Miliary dermatitis can also be treated with glucocorticoids which may have fewer side effects. As coat colour changes may occasionally occur, injection into the medial side of the flank fold is recommended for thin-skinned or show animals.

Safety and handling: Normal precautions should be observed.

Contraindications: Best avoided in diabetic animals, as insulin requirements are likely to change unpredictably. Do not give to bitches before or at first oestrus.

Adverse reactions: Proligestone does not appear to be associated with as many or as serious adverse effects as other progestogens (e.g. megestrol acetate, medroxyprogesterone acetate). However, adverse effects associated with long-term progestogen use, e.g. temperament changes (listlessness and depression), increased thirst or appetite, cystic endometrial hyperplasia/pyometra, diabetes mellitus, acromegaly, adrenocortical suppression, mammary enlargement/neoplasia and lactation, may be expected. Irritation at site of injection may occur and calcinosis circumscripta at the injection site has been reported.

Drug interactions: No information available.

DOSES
Dogs: 10–33 mg/kg depending on body weight:

Body weight (kg)	Dose (mg)
<5	100–150
5–10	150–250
10–20	250–350
20–30	350–450
30–45	450–550
45–60	550–600
thereafter	10 mg/kg

This dose should be given once for the suppression of oestrus and prevention/treatment of false pregnancy. If permanent postponement of oestrus is required, dose is given during pro-oestrus, a second dose 3 months later, a third dose 4 months after the second, and subsequent doses given every 5 months thereafter. Once dosing ceases bitches may come into oestrus, on average 6–7 months later. Doses for treatment of acromegaly are as above, given monthly by injection until signs of hair growth are evident.
Cats:
- Oestrus postponement: 100 mg/cat s.c.

- Miliary dermatitis: 33–50 mg/kg s.c. repeated once after 14 days if the response is inadequate.

Small mammals: Ferrets: 50 mg/ferret s.c., if no response give 25 mg/ferret after 7 days, repeat at further 7 days; Rabbits: 30 mg/kg for pseudopregnancy.

Birds, Reptiles: No information available.

Promethazine
(Phenergan*) **POM**

Formulations: Oral: 10 mg, 25 mg tablets; 1 mg/ml syrup. Injectable: 25 mg/ml solution.

Action: Binds to H1 histamine receptors and prevents histamine from binding.

Use: Management of allergic disease and early treatment of anaphylaxis. Specific doses for dogs and cats have not been determined by pharmokinetic studies. Not widely used. Use with caution in cases with urinary retention, angle-closure glaucoma and pyloroduodenal obstruction.

Safety and handling: Normal precautions should be observed.

Contraindications: No information available.

Adverse reactions: May cause mild sedation. May reduce seizure threshold.

Drug interactions: No information available.

DOSES
Dogs, Cats: 0.2–0.4 mg/kg i.v., i.m. q6–8h, 12.5–25 mg/dog p.o. q24h.
Small mammals, Birds, Reptiles: No information available.

Propantheline
(Pro-Banthine*) **POM**

Formulations: Oral: 15 mg tablet.

Action: Quarternary antimuscarinic agent.

Use: Treatment of anticholinergic-responsive bradycardia, incontinence caused by detrusor hyper-reflexia, as a peripherally acting antiemetic and as an adjunctive therapy to treat GI disorders associated with smooth muscle spasm.

Safety and handling: Normal precautions should be observed.

Contraindications: No information available.

Adverse reactions: Antimuscarinics may cause constipation and paralytic ileus with resultant bacterial overgrowth. Other adverse effects include sinus tachycardia, ectopic complexes, mydriasis, photophobia, cycloplegia, increased intraocular pressure, vomiting, abdominal distension, urinary retention and drying of bronchial secretions.

Drug interactions: Antihistamines and phenothiazines may enhance the activity of propantheline and its derivatives. Chronic corticosteroid use (may increase intraocular pressure) may potentiate the adverse effects of propantheline and its derivatives. Propantheline and its derivatives may enhance the actions of sympathomimetics and thiazide diuretics. Propantheline and its derivatives may antagonize the actions of metoclopramide.

DOSES
Dogs:
- Bradycardia: 0.2–0.5 mg/kg p.o. q8–12h.
- Incontinence: 0.2 mg/kg p.o. q6–8h.
- GI indications: 0.25 mg/kg p.o. q8–12h (round dose to nearest 3.75 mg).

Cats:
- Incontinence: 7.5 mg/cat p.o. q3d.
- GI indications: Doses as for dogs.

Small mammals, Birds, Reptiles: No information available.

Proparacaine see **Proxymetacaine**

Propentofylline
(Propentofylline, Vitofyllin, Vivitonin) **POM-V**

Formulations: Oral: 50 mg, 100 mg tablets.

Action: Propentofylline is a xanthine derivative that increases blood flow to the heart, muscle and CNS via inhibition of phosphodiesterase. It also has an antiarrhythmic action, bronchodilator effects, positive inotropic and chronotropic effects on the heart, inhibitory effects on platelet aggregation and reduces peripheral vascular resistance.

Use: Relief of bronchospasm. Improvement of demeanour in animals. Treatment of age-related behaviour problems, in particular in combination with selegiline and dietary management for canine cognitive dysfunction. Use with care in patients with cardiac disease.

Safety and handling: Normal precautions should be observed.

Contraindications: Do not administer to pregnant bitches or breeding animals, as it has not yet been evaluated in this class of animal.

Adverse reactions: May increase myocardial oxygen demand.

Drug interactions: No information available.

DOSES
Dogs: 2.5–5 mg/kg p.o. q12h. Administer 30 min prior to food.
Birds: 5 mg/kg p.o. q12h.
Cats, Small mammals, Reptiles: No information available.

Propofol
(Norofol, Procare, PropoFlo Plus, PropoFol, Rapinovet)
POM-V

Formulations: Injectable: 10 mg/ml solution: lipid emulsion available both without a preservative or antibacterial or with a preservative (benzyl alcohol), 20 ml, 50 ml and 100 ml glass bottles. The solution containing a preservative can be used for up to 28 days after the vial is first broached.

Action: The mechanism of action is not fully understood but it is thought to involve modulation of the inhibitory activity of GABA at GABA receptors.

Use: Induction of anaesthesia and maintenance of anaesthesia using intermittent boluses or a continuous rate infusion. The solution containing benzyl alcohol preservative should not be used for maintenance of anaesthesia by continuous rate infusion due to the risk of toxicity caused by prolonged administration. Injection i.v. produces a rapid loss of consciousness as the CNS takes up the highly lipophilic drug. Over the next few minutes propofol distributes to peripheral tissues and the concentration in the CNS falls such that, in the absence of further doses, the patient wakes up. In dogs propofol is rapidly metabolized in the liver and other extrahepatic sites, although the clinical relevance of extrahepatic metabolism in animals is not established and may be species-dependent: in cats recovery is less rapid due to the phenolic nature of the compound. Propofol does not have analgesic properties, therefore it is better used in combination with other drugs to maintain anaesthesia; for example, a continuous rate infusion of a potent opioid. Considerable care must be taken with administration in hypovolaemic animals and those with diminished cardiopulmonary, hepatic and renal reserves.

Safety and handling: Shake the lipid emulsion well before use and do not mix with other therapeutic agents or therapeutic fluids prior to administration. If using a preparation that contains no bacteriostat, opened bottles should be stored in a refrigerator and used within 8 hours or discarded. Once broached, the lipid preparation with a preservative has a shelf-life of 28 days.

Contraindications: No information available.

Adverse reactions: The rapid injection of large doses causes apnoea, cyanosis, bradycardia and severe hypotension. Problems are less likely when injection is made over 30–60 seconds. Muscle rigidity, paradoxical muscle movements and tremors can sometimes occur in dogs immediately after i.v. administration. The muscle movements are unresponsive to management with diazepam, and further doses of propofol compound the problem. The tremors and movements wane with time without treatment. One study has shown that repeated daily administration (for 5 days) of the lipid preparation was associated with Heinz body anaemia in cats, although more recent studies have found conflicting results. Propofol is not irritant to tissues but a pain reaction is commonly evident during i.v. injection; the underlying mechanism causing pain is unknown.

Drug interactions: No information available.

DOSES

Dogs: Unpremedicated: 6–7 mg/kg i.v.; premedicated 1–4 mg/kg i.v. Continuous rate infusion for sedation or maintenance of anaesthesia: 0.1–0.4 mg/kg/minute. Lower doses are required when propofol is combined with other drugs for maintenance of anaesthesia.

Cats: Unpremedicated: 8 mg/kg i.v.; premedicated 2–5 mg/kg i.v. Continuous rate infusion for maintenance of anaesthesia is likely to result in a prolonged recovery in cats, doses of 0.1–0.4 mg/kg/minute are appropriate depending on other agents given in combination.

Small mammals: Ferrets: 2–8 mg/kg i.v.; Rabbits: unpremedicated 10 mg/kg i.v.; premedicated 2–6 mg/kg i.v.; Rats 7.5–10 mg/kg i.v.; Mice: 12–26 mg/kg i.v.

Birds: 10 mg/kg i.v. by slow infusion to effect: supplemental doses up to 3 mg/kg.

Reptiles: 5–10 mg/kg i.v., intraosseously.

Propranolol   CIL

(Inderal*, Propranolol*) **POM**

Formulations: Injectable: 1 mg/ml solution. Oral: 10 mg, 40 mg, 80 mg, 160 mg tablets.

Action: Non-selective beta-blocker. Blocks the chronotropic and inotropic effects of beta-1 adrenergic stimulation on the heart, thereby reducing myocardial oxygen demand. Blocks the dilatory effects of beta-2 adrenergic stimulation on the vasculature and bronchial smooth muscle. The antihypertensive effects are mediated through reducing cardiac output, altering the baroreceptor reflex sensitivity and blocking peripheral adrenoceptors.

Use: Management of cardiac arrhythmias (sinus tachycardia, atrial fibrillation or flutter, supraventricular tachycardia, ventricular arrhythmias), hypertrophic cardiomyopathy or obstructive heart disease. Potential efficacy as an additional antihypertensive drug and can be used in phaeochromocytoma if combined with an alpha-blocker. Used to reverse some of the clinical features of thyrotoxicosis prior to surgery in patients with hyperthyroidism. May be used in behavioural therapy to reduce somatic signs of anxiety and is therefore useful in the management of situational anxieties and behavioural problems where contextual anxiety is a component. Some authors suggest using propranolol in combination with phenobarbital for the management of fear- and phobia-related behaviour problems. There is a significant difference between i.v. and oral doses. This is a consequence of propranolol's lower bioavailability when administered orally as a result of decreased absorption and a high first pass effect. Wean off slowly when using chronic therapy.

Safety and handling: Normal precautions should be observed.

Contraindications: Do not use in patients with bradyarrhythmias, acute or decompensated congestive heart failure. Relatively contraindicated in animals with medically controlled congestive heart failure as is poorly tolerated. Do not administer concurrently with alpha-adrenergic agonists (e.g. adrenaline).

Adverse reactions: Bradycardia, AV block, myocardial depression, heart failure, syncope, hypotension, hypoglycaemia, bronchospasm, diarrhoea and peripheral vasoconstriction. Depression and lethargy are occasionally seen as a result of CNS penetration. Propranolol may exacerbate any pre-existing renal impairment. Sudden withdrawal of propranolol may result in exacerbation of arrhythmias or the development of hypertension.

Drug interactions: The hypotensive effect of propranolol is enhanced by many agents that depress myocardial activity including anaesthetic agents, phenothiazines, antihypertensive drugs, diuretics and diazepam. There is an increased risk of bradycardia, severe hypotension, heart failure and AV block if propranolol is used concurrently with calcium-channel blockers. Concurrent digoxin administration potentiates bradycardia. The metabolism of propranolol is accelerated by thyroid hormones, thus reducing its effect. The dose of propranolol may need to be decreased when initiating carbimazole therapy. Oral aluminium hydroxide preparations reduce propranolol absorption. Cimetidine may decrease the metabolism of propranolol, thereby increasing its blood levels. Propranolol enhances the effects of muscle relaxants (e.g. suxamethonium, tubocurarine). Hepatic enzyme induction by phenobarbital or phenytoin may increase the rate of metabolism of propranolol. There is an increased risk of lidocaine toxicity if administered with propranolol due to a reduction in lidocaine clearance. The bronchodilatory effects of theophylline may be blocked by propranolol. Although the use of propranolol is not contraindicated in patients with diabetes mellitus, insulin requirements should be monitored as propranolol may enhance the hypoglycaemic effect of insulin.

DOSES
Dogs:
- Cardiac indications: 0.02–0.08 mg/kg i.v. slowly over 5 min q8h; 0.1–1.5 mg/kg p.o. q8h. Start at the lower doses if myocardial function is poor.
- Phaeochromocytoma: 0.15–0.5 mg/kg p.o. q8h in conjunction with an alpha-blocker.
- Behavioural modification: 0.5–3.0 mg/kg p.o. as required up to q12h.

Cats:
- Cardiac indications: 0.02–0.06 mg/kg i.v. slowly (i.e. dilute 0.25 mg in 1 ml of saline and administer 0.2 ml boluses i.v. to effect); 2.5–5 mg/cat p.o. q8h.
- Behavioural modification: 0.2–1.0 mg/kg p.o. as required up to q8h.

Small mammals: Ferrets: 0.2–2 mg/kg p.o., s.c. q12–24h for hypertrophic cardiomyopathy.
Birds: Supraventricular tachycardia: 0.04 mg/kg slow i.v.
Reptiles: No information available.

Prostaglandin E2 see **Dinoprostone**
Prostaglandin F2 see **Dinoprost tromethamine**

Protamine sulphate
(Protamine sulphate*) **POM**

Formulations: Injectable: 10 mg/ml solution.

Action: An anticoagulant that, when administered in the presence of heparin, forms a stable salt, causing the loss of anticoagulant activity of both compounds.

Use: Heparin overdosage. The effects of heparin are neutralized within 5 minutes of protamine administration, with the effect persisting for approximately 2 hours.

Safety and handling: Do not store diluted solutions.

Contraindications: No information available.

Adverse reactions: Anaphylaxis, hypotension, bradycardia, nausea, vomiting, pulmonary hypertension and lassitude are seen in humans.

Drug interactions: No information available.

DOSES
Dogs, Cats: 1 mg of protamine inactivates 80–100 IU of heparin. Heparin disappears rapidly from the circulation. Decrease the dose of protamine by half for each 30-minute period since the heparin was administered. Give protamine i.v. very slowly over 1–3 min. Do not exceed 50 mg in any 10-minute period. Dilute protamine in 5% dextrose or normal saline.
Small mammals, Birds, Reptiles: No information available.

Proxymetacaine (Proparacaine)

(Proxymetacaine*) **POM**

Formulations: Ophthalmic: 0.5% (± fluorescein 0.25%), 1.0% solution (single-use vials).

Action: Local anaesthetic action is dependent on reversible blockade of the sodium channel, preventing propagation of an action potential along the nerve fibre. Sensory nerve fibres are blocked before motor nerve fibres, allowing a selective sensory blockade at low doses.

Use: Proxymetacaine is used on the ocular surface (cornea and conjunctival sac), the external auditory meatus and the nares. It acts rapidly (within 10 seconds) and provides anaesthesia for 25–55 minutes in the conjunctival sac depending on the species. Serial application increases duration and depth of anaesthesia. Topical anaesthetics block reflex tear production and should not be applied before a Schirmer tear test.

Safety and handling: Store in refrigerator and in the dark; reduced efficacy if stored at room temperature for >2 weeks.

Contraindications: Do not use for therapeutic purposes.

Adverse reactions: Conjunctival hyperaemia is common; local irritation manifested by chemosis may occasionally occur for several hours after administration (less likely than with tetracaine). All topical anaesthetics are toxic to the corneal epithelium and delay healing of ulcers.

Drug interactions: No information available.

DOSES

Dogs: Ophthalmic: 1–2 drops/eye; maximal effect at 15–25 min, duration 45–55 min. Aural/nasal: 5–10 drops/ear or nose every 5–10 min (maximum 3 doses if used intranasally).
Cats: Ophthalmic: 1–2 drops/eye; duration 25 min.
Small mammals: Ophthalmic: 1–2 drops/eye; duration 1 h in rabbits.
Birds, Reptiles: No information available.

Pyrantel

(Bob Martin 2 in 1 Dewormer, Bob Martin 3 in 1 Dewormer, Cazitel Plus, Cestem Flavoured, Dolpac, Drontal cat, Drontal plus, Drontal puppy, Endoguard Flavour/Plus, Plerion, Prazitel) **POM-V**

Formulations: Oral: Pyrantel with praziquantel and febantel (50 mg, 50 mg, 150 mg; 175 mg, 175 mg, 525 mg) tablets (Bob Martin 3 in 1 Dewormer, Cazitel Plus, Cestem Flavoured, Drontal plus, Endoguard, Prazitel); pyrantel with praziquantel and oxantel (10 mg, 10 mg, 40 mg; 25 mg, 25 mg, 100 mg; 50 mg, 50 mg, 200 mg; 125 mg, 125 mg,

500 mg) tablets (Dolpac, Plerion); pyrantel embonate with praziquantel (230 mg, 20 mg; 345 mg, 30 mg) tablets (Bob Martin 2 in 1 Dewormer, Drontal cat); 14.4 mg/ml pyrantel embonate with 15 mg/ml febantel suspension (Drontal puppy). Note: some formulations and doses give content of pyrantel (febantel, oxantel) in terms of pyrantel embonate/pamonate (50 mg pyrantel is equivalent to 144 mg pyrantel embonate/pamonate).

Action: A cholinergic agonist which interferes with neuronal transmission in parasites and thereby kills them. Febantel and oxantel are derivatives of pyrantel with increased activity against whipworms.

Use: Control of *Toxocara canis*, *Toxascaris leonina*, *Trichuris vulpis*, *Uncinaria stenocephala*, *Ancylostoma caninum* and *A. braziliensis*.

Safety and handling: Normal precautions should be observed.

Contraindications: Do not use in puppies <2 months or <1 kg. Safety has not been established in pregnant or lactating animals and therefore its use is not recommended.

Adverse reactions: Vomiting and diarrhoea may be observed.

Drug interactions: The addition of febantel or oxantel has a synergistic effect. Do not use with levamisole, piperazine or cholinesterase inhibitors.

DOSES
Dogs: 5 mg/kg pyrantel + 15 mg/kg febantel or 20 mg/kg oxantel p.o., repeat as required.
Cats: 57.5 mg/kg pyrantel embonate.
Small mammals: Ferrets: 4.4 mg/kg (pyrantel embonate) p.o., repeat in 14 days; Rabbits: 5–10 mg/kg (pyrantel embonate) p.o., repeat in 14 days; Rodents: 50 mg/kg (pyrantel embonate) p.o., repeat as required.
Birds: No information available.
Reptiles: 5 mg/kg p.o., repeat in 14 days.

Pyridostigmine
(Mestinon*) **POM**

Formulations: Oral: 60 mg tablets.

Action: Reversible inhibitor of cholinesterase activity, with a similar mechanism of action to neostigmine, but with a slower onset of activity and longer duration of action. It inhibits the enzymic hydrolysis of acetylcholine by acetylcholinesterase and other cholinesterases, thereby prolonging and intensifying the physiological actions of acetylcholine. It may also have direct effects on skeletal muscle.

Use: Treatment of myasthenia gravis. It can also be used to reverse the neuromuscular blockade produced by competitive neuromuscular blockers, but in general is less effective than neostigmine. It may also have a role in treatment of paralytic ileus. It is specifically used to increase the activity of acetylcholine at nicotinic receptors and thereby stimulate skeletal muscle, the autonomic ganglia, and the adrenal medulla. However, it also prolongs the effect of acetylcholine released from postganglionic parasympathetic nerves and also from some postganglionic sympathetic nerves to produce peripheral actions which correspond to those of muscarine. The muscarinic actions primarily comprise vasodilation, cardiac depression, stimulation of the vagus and parasympathetic nervous system, and increases in lacrimal, salivary and other secretions. The dosage should be reduced by 25% if muscarinic adverse effects appear. Treat muscarinic adverse effects with atropine. Animals with megaoesophagus should receive injectable therapy until able to swallow liquid or tablets.

Safety and handling: Normal precautions should be observed.

Contraindications: Do not use in patients with mechanical GI or urinary tract obstructions or peritonitis. Use with caution in patients with bronchial disease (especially feline asthma), bradycardia (and other arrhythmias), hypotension, renal impairment or epilepsy.

Adverse reactions: Vomiting, increased salivation, diarrhoea and abdominal cramps. Clinical signs of overdosage are related to muscarinic adverse effects and are generally less severe for pyridostigmine than for other parasympathomimetics (particularly neostigmine), but may include bronchoconstriction, increased bronchial secretions, lacrimation, involuntary defecation and micturition, miosis, nystagmus, bradycardia, heart block, arrhythmias, hypotension, agitation and weakness eventually leading to fasciculation and paralysis.

Drug interactions: Aminoglycosides, clindamycin, lincomycin and propranolol may antagonize the effect of pyridostigmine. Pyridostigmine may enhance the effect of depolarizing muscle relaxants (e.g. suxamethonium) but antagonize the effect of non-depolarizing muscle relaxants (e.g. pancuronium and vecuronium).

DOSES
Dogs: 0.2–5 mg/kg p.o. q8–12h.
Cats: 0.25 mg/kg p.o. q8–12h.
Small mammals, Birds, Reptiles: No information available.

Pyrimethamine
(Daraprim*, Fansidar*) **P**

Formulations: Oral: 25 mg tablet. Fansidar also contains sulfadoxine.

Action: Interference with folate metabolism of the parasite and thereby prevents purine synthesis (and therefore DNA synthesis).

Use: Infections caused by *Toxoplasma gondii* and *Neospora caninum*. Should not be used in pregnant or lactating animals without adequate folate supplementation. Used in birds to treat atoxoplasmosis, sarcocystosis and leucocytozoonosis.

Safety and handling: Normal precautions should be observed.

Contraindications: No information available.

Adverse reactions: Depression, anorexia and reversible bone marrow suppression (within 6 days of the start of therapy). Folate supplementation (5 mg/day) may prevent bone marrow suppression.

Drug interactions: Increased antifolate effect if given with phenytoin or sulphonamides. Folate supplementation for the host will reduce the efficacy of the drug if given concomitantly and should thus be given a few hours before pyrimethamine.

DOSES
Dogs, Cats: 1 mg/kg p.o. q24h for 4 weeks, alongside sulphonamides.
Small mammals: No information available.
Birds: 0.5–1 mg/kg p.o. q12h for 28 days.
Reptiles: No information available.

Pyriprole
(Prac-tic) **POM-V**

Formulations: Topical: 125 mg/ml spot-on pipettes of various sizes.

Action: Interaction with ligand-gated (GABA) chloride channels, blocking pre- and post-synaptic transfer of chloride ions, leads to death of parasites.

Use: Treatment and prevention of flea infestations (*Ctenocephalides canis, C. felis*) and tick prevention in dogs >8 weeks and >2 kg. For treatment of flea infestations the additional use of an approved insect growth regulator is recommended. For large dogs, the 5 ml dose should be applied in 2–3 spots. Bathing is not recommended for 48 hours prior to and 24 hours after application.

Safety and handling: Normal precautions should be observed.

Contraindications: Safety has not been established in pregnant and lactating females. Do not use on cats or rabbits.

Adverse reactions: Local pruritus or alopecia may occur at the site of application. May be harmful to aquatic organisms.

Drug interactions: No information available.

DOSES
Dogs: Minimum dose 12.5 mg/kg topically q4wk.
Cats: Do not use.
Small mammals: Rabbits: Do not use.
Birds, Reptiles: No information available.

Pyriproxyfen
(Indorex household spray) **AVM-GSL**

Formulations: Environmental spray.

Action: Juvenile hormone analogue. Arrests the development of flea larvae in the environment.

Use: Use as part of a comprehensive flea control programme in conjunction with on-animal adulticide products.

Safety and handling: Normal precautions should be observed. The product should not enter watercourses as this may be dangerous for fish and other organisms.

Contraindications: Do not use directly on animals.

Adverse reactions: None reported.

Drug interactions: None reported.

DOSES
Dogs, Cats: Use in the environment as directed.
Small mammals, Birds, Reptiles: No information available.

Quinalbarbitone/Cinchocaine see **Secobarbital**

Quinidine
(Kinidin Durules*, Quinidine sulphate*) **POM**

Formulations: Oral: 200 mg tablets; 250 mg sustained release tablets (Kinidin).

Action: An antiarrhythmic drug (class Ia with some class III actions) which decreases myocardial excitability and contractility, slows conduction velocity and prolongs refractory period in the atria, ventricles and His-Purkinje system. It is also an alpha-adrenoreceptor antagonist and may therefore also cause hypotension and peripheral vasodilation.

Use: Rarely used. Management of rapid or haemodynamically significant ventricular arrhythmias such as frequent, complex ventricular premature complexes or ventricular tachycardia. May be useful for some supraventricular arrhythmias, such as bypass tract-mediated supraventricular tachycardia and for cardioversion of acute atrial fibrillation in dogs. Patients exhibiting signs of toxicity or a lack of response should have their serum levels measured. Serum therapeutic levels are 0.0025–0.005 mg/ml in dogs. Toxic effects are not usually evident when serum levels are <0.01 mg/ml. Use with caution in patients with CHF, sinus node dysfunction, renal or hepatic insufficiency.

Safety and handling: Normal precautions should be observed.

Contraindications: Bradycardia, AV block, digitalis intoxication. Myasthenia gravis.

Adverse reactions: Weakness, anorexia, vomiting, diarrhoea, hypotension (especially with too rapid i.v. administration), myocardial depression, AV block, widening of QRS and QT intervals and ventricular proarrhythmia. Adverse effects are usually dose-related.

Drug interactions: Digoxin levels may be increased by quinidine. It is recommended that the dose of digoxin be decreased by half when adding quinidine and that serum drug levels of both quinidine and digoxin be assessed. The effect of neuromuscular blockers may be enhanced by quinidine. Drugs that alkalinize urine reduce the excretion of quinidine, thus prolonging its half-life. The half-life of quinidine may be reduced by as much as 50% as a consequence of hepatic enzyme induction by phenobarbital or phenytoin. Cimetidine inhibits the metabolism of quinidine by inhibiting hepatic microsomal enzymes, thereby increasing its effect. Additive cardiac depressant effects and an increased risk of ventricular arrhythmias may result if quinidine is used with other antiarrhythmic drugs. There is an increased risk of hypotension if quinidine is used with verapamil.

DOSES
Dogs: 6–11 mg/kg i.m., 6–20 mg/kg p.o. q6–8h.
Cats, Small mammals, Birds, Reptiles: No information available.

Ramipril
(Vasotop) **POM-V**

Formulations: Oral: 0.625 mg, 1.25 mg, 2.5 mg, 5 mg tablets.

Action: Angiotensin converting enzyme (ACE) inhibitor. It inhibits conversion of angiotensin I to angiotensin II and inhibits the breakdown of bradykinin. Overall effect is a reduction in preload and afterload via venodilation and arteriodilation, decreased salt and water retention via reduced aldosterone production and inhibition of the angiotensin-aldosterone-mediated cardiac and vascular remodelling. Efferent arteriolar dilation in the kidney can reduce intraglomerular pressure and therefore glomerular filtration. This may decrease proteinuria.

Use: Treatment of congestive heart failure in dogs. Often used in conjunction with diuretics when heart failure is present as most effective when used in these cases. Can be used in combination with other drugs to treat heart failure (e.g. pimobendan, spironolactone, digoxin). May be beneficial in cases of chronic renal insufficiency, particularly protein-losing nephropathies. May reduce blood pressure in hypertension. ACE inhibitors are more likely to cause or exacerbate prerenal azotaemia in hypotensive animals and those with poor renal perfusion (e.g. acute, oliguric renal failure). Use cautiously if hypotension, hyponatraemia or outflow tract obstruction are present. Regular monitoring of blood pressure, serum creatinine, urea and electrolytes is strongly recommended with ACE inhibitor treatment. The use of ACE inhibitors in cats with cardiac disease stems from extrapolation from theoretical benefits and studies showing a benefit in other species with heart failure and different cardiac diseases (mainly dogs and humans).

Safety and handling: Normal precautions should be observed.

Contraindications: Do not use in cases of haemodynamically relevant outflow tract obstruction (e.g. valvular stenosis, obstructive hypertrophic cardiomyopathy).

Adverse reactions: Potential adverse effects include hypotension, hyperkalaemia and azotaemia. Monitor blood pressure, serum creatinine and electrolytes when used in cases of heart failure. Dosage should be reduced if there are signs of hypotension (weakness, disorientation). Anorexia, vomiting and diarrhoea are rare. It is not recommended for breeding, pregnant or lactating bitches, as safety has not been established.

Drug interactions: Concomitant use of potassium-sparing diuretics (e.g. spironolactone) or potassium supplements could result in hyperkalaemia. However, in practice, spironolactone and ACE inhibitors appear safe to use concurrently. There may be an increased risk of nephrotoxicity and decreased clinical efficacy when used with NSAIDs. There is a risk of hypotension with concomitant administration of diuretics, vasodilators (anaesthetic agents, antihypertensive agents) or negative inotropes (beta-blockers).

DOSES

Dogs: 0.125 mg/kg p.o. q24h increasing to 0.25 mg/kg p.o. q24h after 2 weeks depending on the severity of pulmonary congestion.

Cats, Small mammals, Birds, Reptiles: No information available.

Ranitidine

(Ranitidine*, Zantac*) **POM**

CIL

Formulations: Injectable: 25 mg/ml solution Oral: 75 mg, 150 mg, 300 mg tablets; 15 mg/ml syrup.

Action: Ranitidine is a histamine (H2) receptor antagonist blocking histamine-induced gastric acid secretion. It is more potent than cimetidine but has lower bioavailability (50%) and undergoes hepatic metabolism. It also has some prokinetic effect through stimulation of local muscarinic acetylcholine receptors, which may be of benefit when gastric motility is impaired by gastritis or ulceration, and in feline idiopathic megacolon.

Use: Management of gastric and duodenal ulcers, idiopathic, uraemic or drug-related erosive gastritis, oesophagitis, and hypersecretory conditions secondary to gastrinoma, mast cell neoplasia or short bowel syndrome. Studies show minimal increases in gastric pH in dogs given ranitidine suggesting that it is of limited benefit in preventing GI ulcers in dogs. If used for the treatment of ulceration then treatment should continue for 2 weeks after remission of clinical signs which means typically a 1 month course. Absorption is not clinically significantly affected by food intake, anticholinergic agents, or antacids. Currently cimetidine is the only antiulcer drug with a veterinary market authorization. However, in situations where a GI prokinetic effect is desired, use of ranitidine may be justified under the cascade.

Safety and handling: Normal precautions should be observed.

Contraindications: No information available.

Adverse reactions: Rarely reported but include cardiac arrhythmias and hypotension, particularly if administered rapidly i.v.

Drug interactions: It is advisable, though not essential, that sucralfate is administered 2 hours before H2 blockers. Stagger oral doses of ranitidine when used with other antacids, digoxin or metoclopramide by 2 hours as it may reduce their absorption or effect.

DOSES

Dogs: 2 mg/kg slow i.v., s.c., p.o. q8–12h.

Cats: 2 mg/kg/day constant i.v. infusion, 2.5 mg/kg i.v. slowly q12h, 3.5 mg/kg p.o. q12h.

Small mammals: Ferrets: 3.5 mg/kg p.o. q12h; Rabbits: 4–6 mg/kg p.o., s.c. q8–24h; Chinchillas, Guinea pigs: 5 mg/kg p.o. q12h as a prokinetic.

Birds, Reptiles: No information available.

Retinol see **Vitamin A**

Rifampin (Rifampicin)

(Rifadin*, Rifampicin*, Rimactane*) **POM**

Formulations: Oral: 150 mg, 300 mg capsules; 20 mg/ml syrup.

Action: Bactericidal drug binding to the beta subunit of RNA polymerase and causing abortive initiation of RNA synthesis.

Use: Wide spectrum of antimicrobial activity including bacteria (particularly Gram-positives), *Chlamydophila*, *Rickettsia*, some protozoans and poxviruses. Very active against *Staphylococcus aureus* and *Mycobacterium tuberculosis*. Gram-negative aerobic bacteria are usually innately resistant. Obligate anaerobes (Gram-positive or -negative) are usually susceptible. Exact indications for small animal veterinary practice remain to be fully established. It has been suggested as part of the combination of treatments for atypical mycobacterial infections and for lesions in cats associated with *Rhodococcus equi*. It may also have a place in the management of chlamydophilosis, erhlichiosis and bartonellosis. Chromosomal mutations readily lead to resistance, therefore rifampin should be used in combination with other antimicrobial drugs to prevent the emergence of resistant organisms. Various combinations of clarithromycin, enrofloxacin, clofaxamine and doxycycline have been used with rifampin in the management of mycobacteriosis, including in birds. Until controlled studies are conducted to investigate the value of rifampin in these infections, recommendations remain empirical.

Safety and handling: Women of child-bearing age should not handle crushed or broken tablets or the syrup without the use of gloves.

Contraindications: Rifampin may be teratogenic at high doses and should not be administered to pregnant animals. It should not be administered to animals with liver disease.

Adverse reactions: In dogs, increases in serum levels of hepatic enzymes are commonly seen and this can progress to clinical hepatitis. Rifampin metabolites may colour urine, saliva and faeces orange-red.

Drug interactions: Rifampin is a potent hepatic enzyme inducer and increases the rate of metabolism of other drugs in humans, including barbiturates, theophylline and itraconazole. Increased dosages of these drugs may be required if used in combination with rifampin.

DOSES
See Appendix for guidelines on responsible antibacterial use.
Dogs, Cats: 10–15 mg/kg p.o. q24h.
Small mammals: No information available.
Birds: 10–20 mg/kg p.o. q12–24h.
Reptiles: No information available.

Robenacoxib

(Onsior) **POM-V**

Formulations: Oral: 5 mg, 10 mg, 20 mg, 40 mg flavoured tablets for dogs, 6 mg flavoured tablets for cats. Injectable: 20 mg/ml solution.

Action: Selectively inhibits COX-2 enzyme, thereby limiting the production of prostaglandins involved in inflammation. Robenacoxib is tissue selective, defined as being preferentially distributed and concentrated at sites of inflammation combined with having a short half-life in plasma (approximately 2 hours). This may confer advantages in terms of reducing exposure of target side effect organs (e.g. liver and kidneys) to robenacoxib in a 24-hour dose interval, although there are currently no clinical data to support this contention.

Use: Alleviation of inflammation and pain in both acute and chronic musculoskeletal disorders, and the reduction of postoperative pain and inflammation following orthopaedic and soft tissue surgery in dogs. Treatment of acute pain and inflammation in cats. Administer injectable preparation s.c. approximately 30 minutes before the start of surgery in order to provide perioperative analgesia. One injection provides pain control for up to 24 hours. All NSAIDs should be administered cautiously in the perioperative period as they may adversely affect renal perfusion during periods of hypotension. If hypotension during anaesthesia is anticipated, delay robenacoxib administration until the animal is fully recovered and normotensive. The oral dose may be administered directly into the mouth or for cats mixed with a small amount of food. It is recommended not to administer to dogs with food as this has been shown to reduce efficacy. In the cat, due to the longer half-life and narrower therapeutic index of NSAIDs, particular care should be taken to ensure the accuracy of dosing and not to exceed the recommended dose. The tablets are very palatable to cats and many cats will eat spontaneously facilitating dosing. In dogs, treatment with the oral preparation should be discontinued after 10 days if no clinical improvement is apparent.

Safety and handling: Normal precautions should be observed.

Contraindications: Do not give to dehydrated, hypovolaemic or hypotensive patients, or those with GI disease or blood clotting problems. Administration of robenacoxib to animals with renal disease must be carefully evaluated and is not advisable in the perioperative period. Do not give to pregnant animals or animals <12 weeks (dogs), <16 weeks (cats) or <2.5 kg body weight (cats and dogs).

Adverse reactions: GI signs are commonly reported, but most cases are mild and recover without treatment. Stop therapy if signs persists beyond 1–2 days. Some animals develop signs with one NSAID and not another. A 1–2-week wash-out period should be allowed before starting therapy with another NSAID. Stop therapy immediately if GI bleeding is suspected. There is a small risk that NSAIDs may precipitate cardiac failure in animals with cardiovascular disease. Liver disease will prolong the metabolism of robenacoxib, leading to the potential for drug accumulation and overdose with repeated dosing.

Drug interactions: Do not administer concurrently or within 24 hours of other NSAIDs and glucocorticoids. Do not administer with other potentially nephrotoxic agents, e.g. aminoglycosides.

DOSES
Dogs, Cats: 2 mg/kg s.c. q24h for a maximum of 2 doses; 1–2 mg/kg p.o. q24h (in cats for up to 6 days).
Small mammals, Birds, Reptiles: No information available.

Rocuronium
(Esmeron*) **POM**

Formulations: Injectable: 10 mg/ml solution.

Action: Inhibits the actions of acetylcholine at the neuromuscular junction by binding competitively to the nicotinic acetylcholine receptor on the post-junctional membrane.

Use: Provision of neuromuscular blockade during anaesthesia. This may be to improve surgical access through muscle relaxation, facilitate positive pressure ventilation or intraocular surgery. Rocuronium is very similar to vecuronium but it has a more rapid onset of action and shorter duration to spontaneous recovery in dogs. Its availability in aqueous solution and longer shelf-life increase convenience. Monitoring (using a nerve stimulator) and reversal of the neuromuscular blockade is recommended to ensure complete recovery before the end of anaesthesia. The neuromuscular blockade caused by rocuronium can be rapidly reversed using sugammadex (a cyclodextrin developed to reverse aminosteroidal neuromuscular blocking agents) at a dose of 8 mg/kg i.v. in dogs. Hypothermia, acidosis and hypokalaemia will prolong the duration of action of neuromuscular blockade. Hepatic disease may prolong duration of action of rocuronium; atracurium is preferred in this group of patients. The effects of renal disease on duration of action of rocuronium require further investigation; in an experimental study in cats, recovery from rocuronium was found to be independent of renal perfusion.

Safety and handling: Normal precautions should be observed.

Contraindications: Do not administer unless the animal is adequately anaesthetized and facilities to provide positive pressure ventilation are available.

Adverse reactions: Causes an increase in heart rate and a mild hypertension when used at high doses.

Drug interactions: Neuromuscular blockade is more prolonged when rocuronium is given in combination with volatile anaesthetics, aminoglycosides, clindamycin and lincomycin.

DOSES

Dogs: 0.4 mg/kg i.v. followed, when required, by a maintenance dose of 0.16 mg/kg i.v. prn or continuous rate infusion of 0.2 mg/kg/h.

Cats: Doses of 0.5–0.6 mg/kg i.v. have been evaluated in cats. This dose had a rapid onset and short duration of action (20 min). Rocuronium has been evaluated to improve conditions for endotracheal intubation in cats at a dose of 0.6 mg/kg; however, this strategy requires prompt successful intubation and ventilation until the effects of the neuromuscular blockade wane (or the effects are reversed) and spontaneous respiration resumes.

Small mammals, Birds, Reptiles: No information available.

S-Adenosylmethionine (SAMe)

(Denamarin, Denosyl, Doxion, Hepatosyl Plus, Samylin, Zentonil Advanced, Zentonil Plus) **GSL**

Formulations: Oral: 90 mg, 100 mg, 200 mg, 225 mg, 400 mg, 425 mg tablets; 50 mg, 100 mg, 200 mg capsules; 75 mg, 300 mg, 400 mg powder.

Action: S-Adenosylmethionine (SAMe) is an endogenous molecule synthesized by cells throughout the body and is a component of several biochemical pathways. SAMe is especially important in hepatocytes because of their central role in metabolism. Supplementation with SAMe may also improve signs of age-related mental decline in dogs. In humans, antidepressant effects of SAMe are also documented.

Use: Adjunctive treatment for liver disease, especially for acute hepatotoxin-induced liver disease. SAMe has been shown to increase hepatic glutathione levels; a potent antioxidant which protects hepatocytes from toxins and death. Can also be used in patients on long-term therapy with potentially hepatotoxic drugs. SAMe may improve bile flow in cats. May be used to improve cognitive function in aging dogs. The use as an antidepressant therapy in animals has yet to be established. The safety of exogenous SAMe has not been proven in pregnancy; therefore, it should be used with caution.

Safety and handling: Normal precautions should be observed.

Contraindications: No information available.

Adverse reactions: None reported. GI signs (nausea, vomiting, diarrhoea), dry mouth, headache, sweating and dizziness are occasionally reported in humans.

Drug interactions: Concurrent use of SAMe with tramadol, meperidine, pentazocine, MAOIs including selegiline, SSRIs such as fluoxetine, or other antidepressants (e.g. amitriptyline) could cause additive serotonergic effects. SAMe may increase the clearance of drugs that undergo hepatic glucuronidation, including paracetamol, diazepam and morphine.

DOSES
Dogs, Cats: 20 mg/kg p.o. q 24h.
Small mammals: Ferrets, Rodents: 20–100 mg/kg p.o. daily for liver support (anecdotal).
Birds, Reptiles: No information available.

Salbutamol

(Ventolin*) **POM** **CIL**

Formulations: Inhalational: 100 μg per metered inhalation (Evohaler).

Action: Selective beta-2 stimulation causes smooth muscle relaxation and bronchodilation.

Use: Treatment of bronchospasm in inflammatory airway disease and irritation in cats and dogs. Used in rats for mycoplasmosis-related chronic obstructive pulmonary disease (COPD).

Safety and handling: Normal precautions should be observed.

Contraindications: No information available.

Adverse reactions: In humans side effects of the beta-2 agonists include headache, muscle cramps and palpitation. Other side effects include tachycardia, arrhythmias, peripheral vasodilation, and disturbances of sleep and behaviour. Shivering and agitation is occasionally seen in dogs.

Drug interactions: In humans there is an increased risk of side effects if salbutamol is used by patients also taking diuretics, digoxin, theophylline or corticosteroids.

DOSES
Dogs: 100–300 µg (micrograms)/dog q4–6h or as needed for relief of bronchospasm.
Cats: 100 µg (micrograms)/cat q4–6h or as needed for relief of bronchospasm.
Small mammals: Rats: 100 µg (micrograms)/rat q4–6h (use a small chamber) or as needed for relief of bronchospasm.
Birds, Reptiles: No information available.

Secobarbital (Quinalbarbitone/ Cinchocaine)
(Somulose) POM-V CD SCHEDULE 2

Formulations: Injectable: 400 mg/ml secobarbital with 25 mg/ml cinchocaine solution.

Action: Rapidly and profoundly depresses the CNS, including the respiratory centres. Cinchocaine has marked cardiotoxic effects at high doses. When given in combination, the barbiturate produces rapid loss of consciousness and cessation of respiration while the cinchocaine depresses cardiac conduction, resulting in early cardiac arrest. Since cardiac arrest is not dependent on development of profound hypoxia, euthanasia with the secobarbital/cinchocaine combination is generally not accompanied by the gasping that may occur with other agents.

Use: For euthanasia of cats and dogs. Speed of injection is very important. An injection rate that is too slow may induce normal collapse but prolong the period until death. It is always advisable to have an alternative method of euthanasia available. Perivascular administration of secobarbital may delay the onset of effect and cause pain and result in excitement. Placement of a venous catheter is therefore recommended and care should be taken to ensure (by aspiration) that the injection is correctly placed in the vein.

Safety and handling: This is a potent drug which is rapidly and highly toxic to humans. Extreme care should be taken to avoid accidental self-administration. Use an i.v. catheter instead of a needle whenever possible. Only administer in the presence of an assistant/other individual. Wear suitable protective gloves when handling. Wash off splashes from skin and eyes immediately. In the event of accidental self-administration, by injection or skin absorption, do not leave the person unattended, seek urgent medical assistance advising medical service of barbiturate and local anaesthetic poisoning, and show the label advice to a doctor. Maintain airways in the injured person and give symptomatic and supportive treatment. Cinchocaine can cause hypersensitivity following skin contact; this can lead to contact dermatitis, which can become severe.

Contraindications: Somulose must not be used for anaesthesia as it is non-sterile and cardiotoxic.

Adverse reactions: No information available.

Drug interactions: No information available.

DOSES
Dogs, Cats: Euthanasia: 0.25 ml/kg i.v. over 10–15 seconds to minimize premature cardiac arrest.
Small mammals, Birds, Reptiles: No information available.

Selamectin
(Stronghold) **POM-V**

Formulations: Topical: Spot-on pipettes of various sizes containing 6% or 12% selamectin.

Action: Interacts with GABA and glutamate-gated channels leading to flaccid paralysis of parasite.

Use: Treatment and prevention of flea and ear mite infestations, sarcoptic acariasis, biting lice and adult roundworms (*Toxocara canis*), and prevention of heartworm disease (*Dirofilaria immitis*) in dogs. In cats it is used for treatment and prevention of flea and ear mite infestations, and for the treatment of adult roundworms (*Toxocara cati*), hookworm (*Ancylostoma tubaeforme*) and biting lice. Frequent shampooing may reduce the efficacy of the product. Can be used in lactation and pregnancy.

Safety and handling: Highly toxic to aquatic organisms; therefore, take care with disposal.

Contraindications: Not for use in cats and dogs <6 weeks.

Adverse reactions: Transient pruritus and erythema at the site of application may occur.

Drug interactions: No information available.

DOSES

Dogs: Minimum dose recommendation 6 mg/kg. For effective treatment of sarcoptic mange apply product on three occasions at 2-week intervals.

Cats: Minimum dose recommendation 6 mg/kg as required.

Small mammals: Ferrets, Rabbits, Rodents: 6–15 mg/kg monthly.

Birds, Reptiles: No information available.

Selegiline (L-Deprenyl)

(Selgian) **POM-V**

Formulations: Oral: 4 mg, 10 mg tablets.

Action: Selegiline modifies the concentration of monoaminergic neurotransmitters, especially phenylethylamine and dopamine, by selectively inhibiting the activity of type-B monoamine oxidase (which normally breaks down these chemicals). It also appears to have neuroprotective properties.

Use: Authorized for the treatment of behavioural disorders of purely emotional origin, such as depression and anxiety, and, in association with behaviour therapy, for the treatment of signs of emotional origin observed in behavioural conditions such as overactivity, separation problems, generalized phobia and unsocial behaviour. These emotional disorders are characterized by a modification of feeding, drinking, autostimulatory behaviour, sleep, exploratory behaviour, aggression related to fear and/or irritation, social behaviour and somatic disorders (tachycardia, emotional micturition). It may also enhance learning in certain contexts and is indicated for the treatment of canine cognitive dysfunction, especially when signs of anxiety and/or social withdrawal are associated with these problems. It may also be used to treat signs of cognitive decline in older cats. Treatment can be stopped suddenly without gradual dose reduction.

Safety and handling: Normal precautions should be observed.

Contraindications: Selegiline should not be used in animals with a known sensitivity to the drug or administered to lactating or pregnant bitches as it may act on prolactin secretion.

Adverse reactions: No information available.

Drug interactions: Selegiline should not be administered with alpha-2 antagonists (or within 24 hours before or after their use), pethidine, fluoxetine, tricyclic antidepressants (e.g. amitriptyline, doxepin, clomipramine), ephedrine, potential monoamine oxidase inhibitors (e.g. amitraz) or phenothiazines. The effect of morphine is potentiated when used simultaneously. Potential interactions with metronidazole, prednisolone and trimethoprim may exist.

DOSES
Dogs: 0.5–1 mg/kg p.o. q24h for a minimum of 2 months.
Cats: 1 mg/kg p.o. q24h.
Small mammals, Birds, Reptiles: No information available.

Sertraline
(Lustral*) **POM**

Formulations: Oral: 50 mg, 100 mg tablets.

Action: Blocks serotonin re-uptake in the brain, resulting in antidepressive activity and a raising in motor activity thresholds.

Use: Treatment of compulsive type behaviour including acral lick in dogs. The atypical tricyclic antidepressant clomipramine is authorized for use in dogs.

Safety and handling: Normal precautions should be observed.

Contraindications: Known sensitivity to sertraline or other SSRIs, history of seizures.

Adverse reactions: Possible reactions include lethargy, decreased appetite and vomiting. Trembling, restlessness, GI disturbance and an apparent paradoxical increase in anxiety may occur in some cases. Owners should be warned of a potential increase in aggression in response to medication.

Drug interactions: Sertraline should not be used within 2 weeks of treatment with an MAOI (e.g. selegiline) and an MAOI should not be used within 6 weeks of treatment with sertraline. Sertraline, like other SSRIs, antagonizes the effects of anticonvulsants and so is not recommended for use with epileptic patients or in association with other agents which lower seizure threshold, e.g. phenothiazines. Caution is warranted if sertraline is used concomitantly with aspirin or other anticoagulants since the risk of increased bleeding in the case of tissue trauma may be increased.

DOSES
Dogs: 1–3 mg/kg p.o. q24h.
Cats, Small mammals, Birds: No information available.
Reptiles: A dose of 10 mg/kg has been used to reduce inter-male aggression in one species of lizard (*Anolis carolinesis*).

Serum gonadotrophin (PMSG, Equine chorionic gonadotrophin)
(PMSG-Intervet*) **POM-V**

Formulations: Injectable: 5000 IU freeze-dried plug.

Action: Mimics action of FSH.

Use: Induction of oestrus by stimulation of ovarian follicle development. Increases spermatogenesis, though with low efficiency.

Safety and handling: Normal precautions should be observed.

Contraindications: No information available.

Adverse reactions: Anaphylactoid reactions may occur rarely.

Drug interactions: No information available.

DOSES
Dogs:
- Oestrus induction: 20 IU/kg s.c. q24h for 10 days, followed by 500 IU chorionic gonadotrophin i.m. on day 10.
- To stimulate spermatogenesis: 400–800 IU i.m. twice weekly for 4–8 weeks.

Cats: No information available.
Small mammals: Guinea pigs: 1000 IU/animal i.m., repeat in 7–10 days.
Birds, Reptiles: No information available.

Sevelamer hydrochloride
(Renagel) **POM**

Formulations: Oral: 800 mg tablets.

Action: Sevelamer is an organic ion exchange resin that binds intestinal phosphate.

Use: Reduction of serum phosphate in azotaemia. Hyperphosphataemia is implicated in the progression of chronic renal failure. Phosphate-binding agents are usually only used if low phosphate diets are unsuccessful. Monitor serum phosphate levels at 10–14 day intervals and adjust dosage accordingly if trying to normalize serum concentrations. May inhibit vitamin absorption including vitamin K; consider monitoring prothrombin time.

Safety and handling: Normal precautions should be observed.

Contraindications: GI obstruction.

Adverse reactions: Pills are hygroscopic and will expand. Constipation is possible.

Drug interactions: No information available.

DOSES
Dogs, Cats: 30–40 mg/kg p.o. q8h, titrated to the desired serum phosphate concentration. Should be given at least 1 hour before or 3 hours after other medications.
Small mammals, Birds, Reptiles: No information available.

Sevoflurane
(SevoFlo) **POM-V**

Formulations: Inhalational: 250 ml bottle.

Action: The mechanism of action of volatile anaesthetic agents is not fully understood.

Use: Induction and maintenance of anaesthesia. Sevoflurane is potent and highly volatile so should only be delivered from a suitable calibrated vaporizer. It is less soluble in blood than halothane and isoflurane; therefore induction and recovery from anaesthesia are quicker. Sevoflurane has a less pungent smell than isoflurane and induction of anaesthesia using chambers or masks is usually well tolerated in small dogs and cats. The concentration of sevoflurane required to maintain anaesthesia depends on the other drugs used in the anaesthesia protocol; the concentration should be adjusted according to clinical assessment of anaesthetic depth. The cessation of administration results in rapid recovery, which may occasionally be associated with signs of agitation. Sevoflurane does not sensitize the myocardium to catecholamines to the extent that halothane does. Not currently authorized for use in cats, although widespread clinical use in this species has not been associated with complications. Use with caution in guinea pigs.

Safety and handling: Measures should be adopted to prevent contamination of the environment.

Contraindications: No information available.

Adverse reactions: Causes a dose-dependent hypotension that does not wane with time. The effects of sevoflurane on respiration are dose-dependent and comparable to isoflurane, i.e. more depressant than halothane. Sevoflurane crosses the placental barrier and will affect neonates delivered by caesarean section. Sevoflurane is degraded by soda lime to compounds that are nephrotoxic in rats (principally Compound A). Conditions accelerating degradation (i.e. low gas flows, high absorbent temperatures and high sevoflurane concentrations) should be avoided in long operations, although no studies in dogs have demonstrated Compound A to accumulate in concentrations capable of causing renal toxicity.

Drug interactions: Opioid agonists, benzodiazepines and nitrous oxide reduce the concentration of sevoflurane required to achieve surgical anaesthesia. The effects of sevoflurane on the duration of action of non-depolarizing neuromuscular blocking agents are similar to those of isoflurane, i.e. greater potentiation compared with halothane.

DOSES

Dogs, Cats, Small mammals, Birds: The expired concentration required to maintain surgical anaesthesia in 50% of recipients is about 2.5% in animals (minimum alveolar concentration). Administration of other anaesthetic agents and opioid analgesics reduces the dose requirement of sevoflurane; therefore the dose should be adjusted according to individual requirement. 6–8% sevoflurane concentration is required to induce anaesthesia in unpremedicated patients.

Reptiles: Induction: 6–8% in 100% oxygen; Maintenance: 3–5% in 100% oxygen.

Sildenafil

(Viagra*) **POM**

CIL

Formulations: Oral: 25 mg, 50 mg, 100 mg tablets.

Action: Vasodilation, due to an increase in vascular levels of cGMP caused by inhibition of cGMP-specific phosphodiesterase type V.

Use: Indicated for the treatment of pulmonary arterial hypertension. Data from clinical studies suggest that while sildenafil therapy in dogs with pulmonary hypertension does not significantly reduce the echocardiographic measurements, patients receiving therapy may have improvements in quality of life.

Safety and handling: Normal precautions should be observed.

Contraindications: Systemic hypotension, significant hepatic or renal impairment or bleeding disorders.

Adverse reactions: Vomiting, dizziness and raised intraocular pressure.

Drug interactions: Cimetidine, erythromycin and itraconazole increase plasma sildenafil concentration. Avoid concomitant use of nitrates, which significantly enhance its hypotensive effect.

DOSES

Dogs: 0.5–2.7 mg/kg p.o. q8–24h; suggested median dose from clinical studies in dogs is 3 mg/kg/day.
Cats, Small mammals, Birds, Reptiles: No information available.

Silver sulfadiazine

(Flamazine*) **POM**

Formulations: Topical: 1% cream (water-soluble).

Action: Slowly releases silver in concentrations that are toxic to bacteria and yeasts. The sulfadiazine component also has anti-infective qualities.

Use: Topical antibacterial and antifungal drug particularly active against Gram-negative organisms such as *Pseudomonas aeruginosa*. Used in the management of second and third degree burns. Up to 10% may be absorbed, depending on the size of area treated.

Safety and handling: Use gloves.

Contraindications: Do not use in neonates or pregnant animals.

Adverse reactions: Patients hypersensitive to sulphonamides may react to silver sulfadiazine. It may accumulate in patients with impaired hepatic or renal function.

Drug interactions: No information available.

DOSES
See Appendix for guidelines on responsible antibacterial use.
Dogs, Cats:
- Burns/skin infection: Apply antiseptically to the affected area to a thickness of approximately 1.5 mm. Initially, apply as often as necessary to keep wound covered, then reduce as healing occurs to once a day applications. Dressings may be applied if necessary. Keep the affected area clean.
- Otitis (resistant *Pseudomonas*/refractory *Malassezia*): Dilute 1:1 with sterile water and apply topically.

Small mammals: Apply sparingly to wounds q12–24h.
Birds: Doses as for dogs and cats.
Reptiles: Apply topically to wounds q24–72h.

Silybin (Milk thistle, Silibinin, Silymarin)
(Denamarin, Doxion, Hepatosyl Plus, Marin, Samylin, Zentonil Advanced) **general sale**

Formulations: Oral: 9 mg, 24 mg, 25 mg, 35 mg, 40 mg, 50 mg, 70 mg, 100 mg tablets; 10 mg, 40 mg, 53 mg powder.

Action: Silybin is the active component of milk thistle or silymarin. It acts as an antioxidant and free radical scavenger, promotes hepatocyte protein synthesis, increases the level of glutathione, and stimulates biliary flow and the production of hepatoprotective bile acids. It also inhibits leucotriene production so reducing the inflammatory response.

Use: Adjunctive treatment for liver disease, especially for acute hepatotoxin-induced liver disease. Silybin has been shown to increase hepatic glutathione levels; a potent antioxidant which protects hepatocytes from toxic damage. Can also be used in patients on long-term therapy with potentially hepatotoxic drugs.

Safety and handling: Normal precautions should be observed.

Contraindications: No information available.

Adverse reactions: None reported. GI signs, pruritus and headaches have been recognized in primates.

Drug interactions: Silybin may inhibit microsomal cytochrome P450 isoenzyme 2C9 (CYP2C9). May increase plasma levels of beta-blockers (e.g. propranolol), calcium-channel blockers (e.g. verapamil), diazepam, lidocaine, metronidazole, pethidine and theophylline. Silymarin may increase the clearance of drugs that undergo hepatic glucuronidation, including paracetamol, diazepam and morphine. Clinical significance has not been determined for this interaction and the usefulness of silymarin for treating paracetamol toxicity has not been determined.

DOSES
Dogs, Cats: Therapeutic dosage is unknown, but suggested doses range from 50–250 mg/kg p.o. q 24h.
Small mammals: Ferrets: 50–250 mg/kg p.o. q24h. (Note: herbivorous rodents may denature active principles in the stomach.)
Birds: 50–75 mg/kg p.o. q12h.
Reptiles: No information available.

Sodium acetate/acetic acid
(Walpole's solution*) **POM-V**

Formulations: Urethral irrigation: 1.17% sodium acetate and glacial acetic acid.

Action: Acidity causes struvite to dissolve.

Use: Used to flush out struvite urethral calculi in cats and dogs.

Safety and handling: Normal precautions should be observed.

Contraindications: No information available.

Adverse reactions: May worsen any pre-existing urethral inflammation.

Drug interactions: No information available.

DOSES
Dogs, Cats: Flush the urethra with 1 ml of solution, repeating prn until the obstruction is breached.
Small mammals, Birds, Reptiles: No information available.

Sodium acid phosphate see Phosphate enema

Sodium bicarbonate
(Sodium bicarbonate*) **POM**

Formulations: Injectable: 1.26%, 4.2%, 8.4% solutions for i.v. infusion (8.4% solution = 1 mmol/ml). Oral: 300 mg, 500 mg, 600 mg tablets.

Action: Provision of bicarbonate ions.

Use: Management of severe metabolic acidosis, to alkalinize urine, and as an adjunctive therapy in the treatment of hypercalcaemic or hyperkalaemic crisis. Active correction of acid-base inbalance requires blood gas analysis. Do not attempt specific therapy unless this facility is immediately available. 1 g of sodium bicarbonate provides 11.9 mEq of Na^+ and 11.9 mEq of bicarbonate. In hypocalcaemic patients use sodium bicarbonate cautiously and administer slowly. As oral sodium bicarbonate (especially at higher doses) may contribute significant amounts of sodium, use with caution in patients on salt-restricted intakes, e.g. those with congestive heart failure.

Safety and handling: Normal precautions should be observed.

Contraindications: Should not be used in animals that are unable to effectively expel carbon dioxide (e.g. hypoventilating, hypercapnoeic patients).

Adverse reactions: Excessive use of sodium bicarbonate i.v. can lead to metabolic alkalosis, hypernatraemia, congestive heart failure, a shift in the oxygen dissociation curve causing decreased tissue oxygenation, and paradoxical CNS acidosis leading to respiratory arrest.

Drug interactions: Sodium bicarbonate is incompatible with many drugs and calcium salts: do not mix unless checked beforehand. Alkalinization of the urine by sodium bicarbonate decreases the excretion of quinidine and sympathomimetic drugs, and increases the excretion of aspirin, phenobarbital and tetracyclines (especially doxycycline).

DOSES
Dogs, Cats:
- Severe metabolic acidosis: mmol $NaHCO_3$ required = base deficit x 0.5 x body weight (kg) (0.3 is recommended instead of 0.5 in some references). Give half the dose slowly over 3–4 hours, recheck blood gases and clinically re-evaluate the patient. Avoid over-alkalinization.
- Acutely critical situations (e.g. cardiac arrest): 1 mmol/kg i.v. over 1–2 min followed by 0.5 mmol/kg at intervals of 10 min during the arrest.
- Adjunctive therapy of hypercalcaemia: 0.5–1 mmol/kg i.v. over 30 min.
- Adjunctive therapy of hyperkalaemia: 2–3 mmol/kg i.v. over 30 min.
- Metabolic acidosis secondary to renal failure or to alkalinize the urine: Initial dose 8–12 mg/kg p.o q8h and then adjust dose to maintain total CO_2 concentrations at 18–24 mEq/l. The dose may be increased to 50 mg/kg to adjust urine pH in patients with normal renal, hepatic and cardiac function.

Small mammals, Birds, Reptiles: No information available.

Sodium chloride

(Aqupharm, Hypertonic saline, Sodium chloride, Vetivex)
POM-V

Formulations: Injectable: 0.45% to 7% NaCl solutions; 0.18% NaCl with 4% glucose and 0.9% NaCl with 5% glucose solutions. Oral: 300 mg, 600 mg tablets. Ophthalmic: 5% ointment (compounded by an ocular pharmacy).

Action: Expands plasma volume and replaces lost extracellular fluid.

Use: When used for fluid replacement NaCl (0.45% and 0.9%) will expand the plasma volume compartment. Compared with colloids, 2.5 to 3.0 times as much fluid must be given because the crystalloid is distributed to other sites. Normal saline is also the treatment of choice for patients with hypercalcaemia or hyperchloraemic alkalosis. Sodium chloride solutions are often used as a drug diluent. Hypertonic saline is used to expand the circulating blood volume rapidly in animals with shock, particularly during the preoperative period. The hypertonic ophthalmic ointment is used in the management of corneal oedema. Hypertonic saline solutions have very high sodium concentrations and it is important to monitor serum sodium concentrations before and after their administration; maintenance with an isotonic crystalloid is usually required after administration to correct electrolyte and fluid disturbances created by the administration of the hypertonic solution. Oral sodium supplementation is recommended by some authors in the long-term management of hypoadrenocorticism.

Safety and handling: Hypertonic saline solutions should be regarded as drugs and not as intravenous fluids and should be stored separately to prevent confusion.

Contraindications: No information available.

Adverse reactions: Peripheral oedema is more likely to occur after crystalloids because muscle and subcutaneous capillaries are less permeable to protein. Normal saline contains higher amounts of chloride than plasma, which will increase the risk of acidosis. The degree of acidosis is not likely to be a problem in a healthy patient but acidosis may be exacerbated in a compromised patient. Hypertonic saline administered at fluid rates >1 ml/kg/min can cause a vagally mediated bradycardia, therefore the rate of fluid administration must be carefully controlled. Enteric-coated products for oral use may not be adequately absorbed by dogs and therefore may be of unpredictable efficacy. The ophthalmic ointment may cause a stinging sensation.

Drug interactions: No information available.

DOSES
Dogs, Cats:
- Fluid therapy: fluid requirements depend on the degree of dehydration and ongoing losses. In uncomplicated cases

0.45–3% solutions should be administered at a dose of 50–60 ml/kg/day i.v., p.o. Higher doses are required if the animal is dehydrated. Solutions containing 0.9% to 3% NaCl are suitable for replacing deficits. Solutions containing 0.45% NaCl (with added potassium) are indicated for longer term maintenance.

- Hypotension/shock: 5% to 7.5% NaCl solutions (hypertonic saline) at doses of 3–8 ml/kg i.v. Solutions of this concentration are hypertonic, therefore they should be used with caution and with other appropriate fluid replacement strategies. Hypertonic NaCl may be combined with colloid solutions to stabilize the increase in vascular volume provided by the hypertonic solution.
- Salt-wasting syndromes (hypoadrenocorticism): 1–5 g p.o. q24h.
- Corneal oedema: apply a small amount of ointment q4–24h.

Small mammals, Birds, Reptiles: No information available.

Sodium chromoglycate see Sodium cromoglicate

Sodium citrate
(Micolette*, Micralax*, Relaxit*) **P**

Formulations: Rectal: micro-enemas containing 450 ml sodium citrate with 45 mg sodium alkylsulphoacetate (Micralax) or 45 mg sodium lauryl sulphoacetate (Micolette) or 75 mg sodium lauryl sulphate (Relaxit).

Action: An osmotic laxative that causes water to be retained within the lumen of the GI tract. It is formulated with a stool softener that augments its action.

Use: Low volume enema used to treat constipation and to prepare the lower GI tract for proctoscopy and radiography.

Safety and handling: Normal precautions should be observed.

Contraindications: Not recommended for use in cases with inflammatory bowel disease.

Adverse reactions: Uncommon. Largely due to water and electrolyte disturbances.

Drug interactions: No information available.

DOSES
Dogs, Cats: 1 enema inserted per rectum to full length of nozzle.
Small mammals, Birds, Reptiles: No information available.

Sodium cromoglicate (Sodium chromoglycate)

(Haycrom*, Opticrom*, Rynacrom*, Sodium cromoglicate*, Vividrin*) **P, POM**

Formulations: Topical: 2% ocular drops; 2%, 4% nasal spray.

Action: Stabilizes mast cell membranes, preventing degranulation.

Use: Management of allergic conjunctivitis and rhinitis. Action is localized to the site of application.

Safety and handling: Normal precautions should be observed.

Contraindications: No information available.

Adverse reactions: May cause local irritation.

Drug interactions: No information available.

DOSES
Dogs, Cats: 1–2 drops in eye or nose q6h.
Small mammals, Birds, Reptiles: No information available.

Sodium stibogluconate

(Pentostam*) **POM**

Formulations: Injectable: 100 mg/ml solution.

Action: Active against the amastigote stages of *Leishmania*; exact mode of action unknown.

Use: Treatment of leishmaniosis in dogs. Animals may be clinically normal after treatment but remain carriers, and follow-on treatment with allopurinol may be beneficial. Seek expert advice before treating leishmaniosis. Use with caution in patients with hepatic impairment.

Safety and handling: Normal precautions should be observed.

Contraindications: Significant renal impairment; lactating animals.

Adverse reactions: Pain and inflammation at the injection site, anorexia and vomiting, and myalgia. Meglumine antimonate is said to be less toxic.

Drug interactions: No information available.

DOSES
Dogs: 30–50 mg/kg i.v., s.c. q24h for 3–4 weeks. If giving i.v., administer slowly (over at least 5 min) to avoid cardiac toxicity.
Cats, Small mammals, Birds, Reptiles: No information available.

Somatotropin (Growth hormone)
(Genotropin*, Humatrope*, Norditropin*) **POM**

Formulations: Injectable: 2–16 IU vials for reconstitution.

Action: Recombinant human growth hormone that mimics growth hormone action in other species.

Use: Treatment of growth hormone deficiency. Serum IGF-1 measurements may be helpful to monitor therapy. Antibody formation may limit its effectiveness in the long term.

Safety and handling: Normal precautions should be observed.

Contraindications: No information available.

Adverse reactions: Growth hormone is diabetogenic; monitor blood glucose. Local reactions may be seen; rotate injection sites.

Drug interactions: No information available.

DOSES
Dogs, Cats: 0.3–0.7 IU/kg weekly divided into 3–5 doses s.c., i.m. (painful). Continue for at least 6 weeks to evaluate response.
Small mammals, Birds, Reptiles: No information available.

Sotalol `CIL`
(Beta Cardone*, Sotacor*, Sotalol*) **POM**

Formulations: Oral: 40 mg, 80 mg, 160 mg, 200 mg tablets. Injectable: 10 mg/ml solution.

Action: Produces a prolongation of action potential duration and refractory period, via selective inhibition of potassium channels. Non-selective beta-adrenergic blocker.

Use: Treatment of supraventricular or ventricular arrhythmias. The beta-blocking activity is about one-third that of propranolol. Used most commonly in dogs with ventricular arrhythmias secondary to myocardial disease. Preferable to assess efficacy with repeated Holter ECG monitoring. Use with caution in patients with renal failure or medically controlled CHF.

Safety and handling: Normal precautions should be observed.

Contraindications: Asthma, sinus bradycardia, AV block or decompensated CHF.

Adverse reactions: The non-selective beta-blocking effects can decrease heart rate, stroke volume and cardiac output in dogs and may precipitate congestive heart failure. The drug is eliminated in urine and faeces and elimination half-life may increase with renal insufficiency, leading to accumulation at standard doses. Adverse effects include hypotension, bradyarrhythmias, bronchospasm, depression, nausea, vomiting and diarrhoea. The drug is potentially pro-arrhythmic and can cause torsades de pointes, especially if hypokalaemia is present.

Drug interactions: Sympathomimetics (e.g. terbutaline, phenylpropanolamine, adrenaline) may have their actions blocked by sotalol and they may, in turn, reduce the efficacy of sotalol. Additive myocardial depression may occur with the concurrent use of sotalol and other beta-blockers or myocardial depressant anaesthetic agents. Hypotensive effects may be enhanced by phenothiazines, furosemide, hydralazine and other vasodilators. Sotalol may prolong the hypoglycaemic effects of insulin therapy. Concurrent use of negative inotropics (e.g. calcium-channel blockers) should be done with caution, particularly in patients with pre-existing systolic dysfunction or CHF.

DOSES
Dogs: 0.5–3 mg/kg p.o. q12h. Start with lower doses if myocardial function is reduced. No data available on i.v. doses.
Cats: 10–20 mg/cat p.o. q12h.
Small mammals, Birds, Reptiles: No information available.

Spinosad
(Comfortis) **POM-V**

Formulations: Oral: 90 mg, 140 mg, 270 mg, 425 mg, 665 mg, 1040 mg, 1620 mg chewable tablets.

Action: Activation of nicotinic acetylcholine receptors.

Use: Treatment and prevention of flea infestations. As it acts on larvae and adults, there will be a short lag phase after administration due to the emergence of adult fleas from pupae already in the environment. If used as part of a treatment programme for flea allergy dermatitis, then combine with an insect growth regulator.

Safety and handling: Normal precautions should be observed.

Contraindications: Avoid in dogs and cats weighing <1.2 kg or <14 weeks of age.

Adverse reactions: Vomiting occurs occasionally. Rare side effects include lethargy, diarrhoea, anorexia, ataxia and seizures.

Drug interactions: This is a P-glycoprotein substrate, therefore, use with caution if combining with other substrate drugs (e.g. digoxin, doxorubicin).

DOSES
Dogs: 45–70 mg/kg p.o. q28d with or immediately after food.
Cats: 50–75 mg/kg p.o. q28d with or immediately after food.
Small mammmals, Birds, Reptiles: No information available.

Spiramycin see **Metronidazole**

Spironolactone

(Cardalis, Prilactone, Tempora, Aldactone*,
Spironolactone*) **POM-V, POM**

Formulations: Oral: 10 mg, 25 mg, 40 mg, 50 mg, 80 mg, 100 mg
tablets; 1 mg/ml, 2 mg/ml, 5 mg/ml, 10 mg/ml, 20 mg/ml syrups;
spironolactone with benazepril (2.5 mg benazepril/20 mg
spironolactone; 5 mg benazepril/40 mg spironolactone; 10 mg
benazepril/80 mg spironolactone).

Action: Aldosterone receptor antagonist that acts on the kidneys as
a weak potassium-sparing diuretic (preventing sodium resorption in
the distal tubule) and acts on the myocardium and vasculature to
inhibit aldosterone-mediated fibrosis and remodelling.

Use: Treatment of congestive heart failure. Authorized for use in
combination with standard therapy for treatment of CHF caused by
valvular regurgitation in dogs. Used in the management of ascites
secondary to hepatic failure (when hypokalaemia can exacerbate
hepatic encephalopathy) and in treatment of hyperaldosteronism
due to adrenal tumours. Spironolactone is a weak diuretic and does
not have a diuretic effect in healthy dogs. Its beneficial effects in
heart failure appear to be related to inhibition of myocardial fibrosis,
vascular remodelling and endothelial dysfunction. It is particularly
useful for hypokalaemic patients with heart failure. Use with caution
in patients with renal or hepatic dysfunction.

Safety and handling: Normal precautions should be observed.

Contraindications: Do not use in animals with
hypoadrenocorticism, hyperkalaemia or hyponatraemia. Do not give
in conjunction with NSAIDs to animals with renal insufficiency.
Do not use during pregnancy, lactation, or in animals intended
for breeding.

Adverse reactions: Hyponatraemia and hyperkalaemia may
develop. Discontinue if hyperkalaemia occurs. Reversible prostatic
atrophy may occur in entire male dogs. Severe ulcerative facial
dermatitis has been reported in Maine Coon cats. Hepatotoxicity is
reported in humans.

Drug interactions: Potentiates thiazide and loop diuretics.
Hyperkalaemia may result if ACE inhibitors, NSAIDs, ciclosporin or
potassium supplements are administered in conjunction with
spironolactone. However, in practice, spironolactone and ACE
inhibitors appear safe to use concurrently. Monitor renal function
and serum potassium levels in animals receiving spironolactone and
ACE inhibitors. There is an increased risk of nephrotoxicity if
spironolactone is administered with NSAIDs. The plasma
concentration of digoxin may be increased by spironolactone.

DOSES

Dogs, Cats: 2–4 mg/kg p.o. q24h.

Small mammals, Birds, Reptiles: No information available.

Sterculia
(Peridale, Normacol*) **AVM-GSL, GSL**

Formulations: Oral: 98% granules (Peridale); 118 mg capsules (Normacol).

Action: Bulk-forming agent that increases faecal mass and stimulates peristalsis.

Use: Management of impacted anal sacs, diarrhoea and constipation, and the control of stool consistency after surgery. Sterculia is inert and not absorbed. During treatment, fluid should be provided or a moist diet given. As the preparations swell in contact with water, they should be administered with plenty of water available.

Safety and handling: Normal precautions should be observed.

Contraindications: Do not use in cases of intestinal obstruction or where enterotomy or enterectomy is to be performed.

Adverse reactions: No information available.

Drug interactions: No information available.

DOSES

Dogs: 1.5 g p.o. q24h (dogs <5 kg); 3 g p.o. q12–24h (5–15 kg); 4 g p.o. q12–24h (>15 kg). Sprinkle over feed or place on tongue.

Cats: Kittens: 1 capsule q24h; Adults: 1 capsule q12h.

Small mammals, Birds, Reptiles: No information available.

Streptomycin
(Devomycin) **POM-V**

Formulations: Injectable: Streptomycin (250 mg/ml); Streptomycin (150 mg/ml) with dihydrostreptomycin (150 mg/ml) (Devomycin D).

Action: Inhibits bacterial protein synthesis, resulting in a bactericidal effect that is concentration-dependent.

Use: Active against a range of Gram-negative and some Gram-positive pathogens although resistance is quite widespread and it is less active than other aminoglycosides. It is specifically indicated in the treatment of infections caused by *Leptospira* and *Mycobacterium tuberculosis* (in combination with other drugs). Aminoglycosides require an oxygen-rich environment to be effective, thus they are ineffective in sites of low oxygen tension (abscesses, exudates) and all obligate anaerobes are resistant. Use of streptomycin is limited and if an aminoglycoside is indicated other members of the family are more commonly employed, e.g. gentamicin. There is a marked post-antibiotic effect, allowing the use of pulse-dosing regimens which may limit toxicity. Dosing 2–3 times a week is used to treat mycobacteriosis in humans.

Safety and handling: Normal precautions should be observed.

Contraindications: Do not use in guinea pigs, hamsters, gerbils and mice.

Adverse reactions: Streptomycin is one of the more ototoxic aminoglycosides, interfering with balance and hearing, which can be permanent. Cats are especially sensitive to ototoxicity. Nephrotoxicosis may be a problem but is less likely than with other aminoglycosides. Toxic to birds, especially raptors.

Drug interactions: Increased risk of nephrotoxicity when used with cephalosporins (notably cefalotin) and cytotoxic drugs. Ototoxicity is increased with loop diuretics. The effects of neostigmine and pyridostigmine may be antagonized by aminoglycosides. The effect of non-depolarizing muscle relaxants, e.g. pancuronium, may be enhanced. Penicillin and streptomycin act synergistically. Aminoglycosides may be chemically inactivated by beta-lactam antibiotics (e.g. penicillins, cephalosporins) or heparin when mixed *in vitro* .

DOSES
See Appendix for guidelines on responsible antibacterial use.
Dogs: 25 mg/kg i.m. q24h.
Cats: 25 mg/kg i.m. q24h.
Small mammals: Rabbits: 50 mg/kg streptomycin in combination with 40 mg/kg penicillin s.c. q24h.
Birds: 10–30 mg/kg i.m. q8–12h.
Reptiles: No information available.

Succinylcholine see Suxamethonium

Sucralfate
(Antepsin*, Antepsin suspension*, Carafate*) **POM** `CIL`

Formulations: Oral: 1 g tablet; 0.2 g/ml suspension.

Action: In an acidic medium an aluminium ion detaches from the compound, leaving a very polar, relatively non-absorbable ion. This ion then binds to proteinaceous exudates in the upper GI tract, forming a chemical diffusion barrier over ulcer sites, preventing further erosion from acid, pepsin and bile salts. However, its major action appears to relate to stimulation of mucosal defences and repair mechanisms (stimulation of bicarbonate and PGE production and binding of epidermal growth factor). These effects are seen at neutral pH.

Use: Treatment of oesophageal, gastric and duodenal ulceration, used with an H2 receptor antagonist or proton pump inhibitor but given separately. The efficacy of sucralfate as a phosphate binder in renal failure is uncertain.

Safety and handling: Normal precautions should be observed.

Contraindications: Perforated ulcer.

Adverse reactions: Minimal; constipation is the main problem in humans. Bezoar formation and hypophosphataemia are also reported in humans.

Drug interactions: Sucralfate may decrease the bioavailability of H2 antagonists, phenytoin and tetracycline. Although there is little evidence to suggest that this is of clinical importance, it may be a wise precaution to administer sucralfate at least 2 hours before these drugs. Sucralfate interferes significantly with the absorption of fluoroquinolones and digoxin.

DOSES
Dogs: 500 mg/dog p.o. q6–8h (dogs up to 20 kg); 1–2 g/dog p.o. q6–8h (>20 kg).
Cats: 250 mg/cat p.o. q8–12h.
Small mammals: Ferrets: 25–125 mg/kg q6–12h; Rabbits: 25 mg/kg p.o. q8–12h; Rodents: 25–50 mg/kg p.o. q6–8h.
Birds: 25 mg/kg p.o. q8h.
Reptiles: 500–1000 mg/kg p.o. q6–8h.

Sulfadimethoxine
(Coxi Plus) **POM-V**

Formulations: Oral: 1000 mg/4 g sachet.

Action: Competitively inhibits bacterial and protozoal synthesis of folic acid.

Use: Coccidiosis in ferrets, rabbits, birds and reptiles; atoxoplasmosis in passerine birds. Use with care in reptiles with reduced renal function, renal failure or dehydration.

Safety and handling: Normal precautions should be observed.

Contraindications: No information available.

Adverse reactions: No information available.

Drug interactions: No information available.

DOSES
Dogs, Cats: No information available.
Small mammals: Ferrets: 50 mg/kg p.o., then 25 mg/kg q24h for 5–10 days; Rabbits: 50 mg/kg p.o., then 25 mg/kg q24h for 10–20 days; Others: 10–15 mg/kg p.o. q12h.

Birds: 1 g/l of drinking water daily for 2 days, then 3 days off and 2 days on.
Reptiles: 90 mg/kg p.o. once; then 45 mg/kg p.o. q24h for 5–7 days.

Sulfasalazine

CIL

(Salazopyrin*, Sulphasalazine*) **POM**

Formulations: Oral: 500 mg tablet; 250 mg/ml oral suspension.

Action: Sulfasalazine is a pro-drug: a diazo bond binding sulfapyridine to 5-ASA is cleaved by colonic bacteria to release free 5-ASA, which acts locally in high concentrations in the colon as an anti-inflammatory.

Use: Used in the management of colitis. There is a significant risk of keratoconjunctivitis sicca and periodic Schirmer tear tests should be performed.

Safety and handling: Normal precautions should be observed.

Contraindications: No information available.

Adverse reactions: Uncommon but include keratoconjunctivitis sicca (KCS), vomiting, allergic dermatitis and cholestatic jaundice. Owners should be made aware of the seriousness of KCS and what signs to monitor. The cause of the KCS is not clear. Historically sulfapyridine has been blamed. Olsalazine has been recommended as the incidence of KCS is less with its use, though not completely abolished. It is possible that 5-ASA may sometimes be responsible.

Drug interactions: The absorption of digoxin may be inhibited by sulfasalazine, and the measurement of serum folate concentration may be interfered with. Sulfasalazine may cause a reduction in serum thyroxine concentrations.

DOSES
Dogs: 15–30 mg/kg p.o. q8–12h, maximum 6 g/day.
Cats: 10–20 mg/kg p.o. q8–12h.
Small mammals, Birds, Reptiles: No information available.

Sulphonamide see **Trimethoprim/sulphonamide**

Suxamethonium (Succinylcholine)

(Suxamethonium*) **POM**

Formulations: Injectable: 50 mg/ml solution.

Action: Competitively binds to the nicotinic acetylcholine receptor. The persistent depolarization prevents the transmission of further action potentials, resulting in muscle relaxation.

Use: Used to facilitate intubation in cats and primates. There are no indications for suxamethonium in dogs. Suxamethonium has a very rapid onset of action (5–15 s) and short duration of action (3–5 min). However, use of neuromuscular blockade to facilitate intubation is rarely required in small animals and suxamethonium has been largely replaced by non-depolarizing drugs. Use with caution in patients with hepatic disease.

Safety and handling: Store in refrigerator.

Contraindications: Do not administer unless the animal is adequately anaesthetized and facilities to provide positive pressure ventilation are available. Do not use in animals exposed to organophosphate compounds.

Adverse reactions: Can cause arrhythmias (sinus bradycardia, ventricular arrhythmias) via stimulation of muscarinic receptors in the sinus node. A small rise in potassium concentration is expected after suxamethonium; patients with burns and neuromuscular disorders are at severe risk of hyperkalaemia.

Drug interactions: The actions of suxamethonium may be enhanced by beta-adrenergic blockers (e.g. propranolol), furosemide, isoflurane, lidocaine, magnesium salts and phenothiazines. Diazepam may reduce the duration of action of suxamethonium. Neostigmine and pyridostigmine should not be administered with suxamethonium as they inhibit pseudocholinesterases, thereby enhancing suxamethonium's effect.

DOSES

Dogs: Do not use.

Cats: 1.0 mg/kg i.v. A total dose of 3.5 mg is satisfactory in cats >3.5 kg.

Small mammals, Birds: No information available.

Reptiles: Giant chelonians: 0.25–1 mg/kg i.m. for immobilization only. IPPV required, as paralysis of respiratory muscles will occur.

T3 see **Liothyronine**
T4 see **Levothyroxdine**

Tacrolimus (FK 506)
(Protopic*) **POM**

Formulations: Topical: 0.03%, 0.1% ointments. Oral: Various preparations – avoid switching between brands.

Action: T lymphocyte inhibition.

Use: Recently described for topical ophthalmic use as the aqueous formulation to treat canine keratoconjunctivitis sicca that is unresponsive to topical ciclosporin. In laboratory animals, ciclosporin may affect circulating levels of insulin and cause an increase in glycaemia; in the presence of suggestive signs of diabetes mellitus, the effect of treatment on glycaemia must be monitored. Has also been used for localized autoimmune dermatoses and localized lesions of atopic dermatitis. Long-term effects, potential adverse effects and toxicities are as yet unknown and tacrolimus must be reserved for special cases only. Although the limited studies to date have used aqueous formulations, there are anecdotal reports that the skin (0.1%) formulation (dissolved in hypromellose) has been used successfully and without adverse effects. Systemic (oral) administration has been used for a limited number of cases.

Safety and handling: Use gloves.

Contraindications: No information available.

Adverse reactions: Discomfort on application (blepharospasm).

Drug interactions: No information available.

DOSES
See Appendix for immunosuppression protocols.
Dogs: Apply small amount of ointment to the affected eye q12h.
Cats, Small mammals, Birds, Reptiles: No information available.

Telmisartan
(Semintra) **POM-V**

Formulations: Oral: 4 mg/ml solution.

Action: Angiotensin II receptor (type AT1) antagonist which acts to inhibit the effects of angiotensin (i.e. vasoconstriction, increased aldosterone synthesis, sodium and water retention and renal, vascular and cardiac remodelling). In the kidney, angiotensin II may result in glomerular capillary hypertension and increased protein in the glomerular filtrate, which could trigger or potentiate interstitial fibrosis.

Use: Authorized for the reduction of proteinuria associated with chronic kidney disease in cats. The effects on the long term prognosis of feline kidney disease are currently not established. In the one study published to date, telmisartan would appear to be as effective as benazepril at delaying deterioration in proteinuria over 6 months in cats with chronic kidney disease (IRIS stages IIa to IV, urine specific gravity <1.035 and no co-morbid conditions). Reduction in proteinuria was reported within 7 days of starting treatment in this study. Monitoring of blood pressure is recommended in cats that develop clinical signs referable to hypotension or cats undergoing general anaesthesia. The oral solution was accepted well by most cats in a separate palatability study.

Safety and handling: Normal precautions should be observed.

Contraindications: The safety of telmisartan has not been established in breeding, pregnant or lactating cats or cats <6 months of age.

Adverse reactions: Rare during the clinical study but included mild and transient GI signs (regurgitation, vomiting, diarrhoea) and increased ALT activity that resolved within a few days of stopping therapy. Healthy cats administered five times the recommended dose for 6 months experienced decreases in blood pressure and RBC count and increases in BUN. These were not observed in the clinical study.

Drug interactions: Cats that received concomitant therapy with amlodipine at the recommended dose did not experience clinical evidence of hypotension.

DOSES
Cats: 1 mg/kg p.o. q24h.
Dogs, Small mammals, Birds, Reptiles: No information available.

Tepoxalin
(Zubrin) **POM-V**

Formulations: Oral: 50 mg, 100 mg, 200 mg tablets.

Action: Reduction in both prostaglandin and leukotriene synthesis, leading to anti-inflammatory, analgesic and antipyretic effects. 5-Lipoxygenase enzyme inhibition may be associated with an improved GI safety profile compared to some other NSAIDs.

Use: Control of musculoskeletal pain and inflammation in dogs, particularly that associated with osteoarthritis. Tepoxalin is not COX-2 selective and is not authorized for preoperative administration to dogs. After placing the tablet in the dog's mouth, keep the mouth closed for approximately 4 seconds to ensure that the drug is fully dispersed. Administer the tablets within 1–2 hours of feeding. The tablets can also be placed in moist food or treat and offered to the dog immediately. Long-term treatment to manage chronic conditions should be accompanied by regular examination of the animal for signs of adverse effects. Liver disease will prolong the metabolism of tepoxalin, leading to the potential for drug accumulation and overdose with repeated dosing. Administration to animals with renal disease must be carefully evaluated.

Safety and handling: The tablets are lyophilisates designed to dissolve rapidly in water. Ensure that they are handled with dry hands to prevent dissolution during administration.

Contraindications: Do not give to dehydrated, hypovolaemic or hypotensive patients or those with GI disease or blood clotting problems. Do not administer perioperatively until the animal is fully recovered from anaesthesia and normotensive. Do not give to pregnant or very young animals, as tepoxalin has not been evaluated in animals <6 months.

Adverse reactions: GI signs may occur in all animals after NSAID administration. Stop therapy if this persists beyond 1–2 days. Some animals develop signs with one NSAID and not another. A 1–2-week wash-out period should be allowed before starting another NSAID after cessation of therapy. Stop therapy immediately if GI bleeding is suspected. There is a small risk that NSAIDs may precipitate cardiac failure in animals with cardiovascular disease.

Drug interactions: Do not administer concurrently with, or within 24 hours of, other NSAIDs and glucocorticoids. Do not administer with other potentially nephrotoxic agents, e.g. aminoglycosides.

DOSES
Dogs: 10 mg/kg p.o. q24h with food.
Cats: No published data. Do not use.
Small mammals, Birds, Reptiles: No information available.

Terbinafine
(Lamisil*) **POM**

Formulations: Oral: 250 mg tablets. Topical: 1% cream.

Action: Inhibits ergosterol synthesis by inhibiting squalene epoxidase, an enzyme that is part of the fungal cell wall synthesis pathway.

Use: Management of dermatophytosis, *Malassezia* dermatitis, subcutaneous and systemic fungal infections in cats and dogs, and aspergillosis in birds. Optimal therapeutic regimes are still under investigation. Pre-treatment and monitoring CBC, renal and liver function tests are advised.

Safety and handling: Normal precautions should be observed.

Contraindications: No information available.

Adverse reactions: Vomiting, diarrhoea, increased liver enzymes, pruritus (cats).

Drug interactions: No information available.

DOSES

Dogs, Cats: 20–40 mg/kg p.o. q24h; can use week-on, week-off schedule.
Small mammals: Rodents: 10–30 mg/kg p.o. q24h for 4–6 weeks.
Birds: 10–15 mg/kg p.o. q12h, or nebulization of 1 mg/ml for 20 min q8h.
Reptiles: No information available.

Terbutaline

(Bricanyl*, Monovent*) **POM**

Formulations: Injectable: 0.5 mg/ml solution. Oral: 5 mg tablets; 1.5 mg/5 ml syrup.

Action: Selective beta-2 adrenergic agonist that directly stimulates bronchodilation.

Use: Bronchodilation. Maintenance of heart rate in animals with sick sinus syndrome. Use with caution in patients with diabetes mellitus, hyperthyroidism, hypertension or seizure disorders.

Safety and handling: Normal precautions should be observed.

Contraindications: No information available.

Adverse reactions: Fine tremor, tachycardia, hypokalaemia, hypotension and hypersensitivity reactions. Administration i.m. may be painful.

Drug interactions: There is an increased risk of hypokalaemia if theophylline or high doses of corticosteroids are given with high doses of terbutaline. Use with digitalis glycosides or inhalational anaesthetics may increase the risk of cardiac arrhythmias. Beta-blockers may antagonize its effects. Other sympathomimetic amines may increase the risk of adverse cardiovascular effects.

DOSES

Dogs: 1.25–5 mg/dog p.o. q8–12h, 0.01 mg/kg i.m., s.c., i.v. q4h.
Cats: 0.312–1.25 mg/cat p.o. q8–12h, 0.01 mg/kg i.m., s.c., i.v. q4h.
Small mammals: Rats: 5 mg/kg p.o. q12h.
Birds, Reptiles: No information available.

Testosterone

(Durateston) **POM-V**

Formulations: Injectable: 50 mg/ml comprising 6 mg/ml testosterone propionate, 12 mg/ml testosterone phenylpropionate, 12 mg/ml testosterone isocaproate and 20 mg/ml testosterone decanoate.

Action: Male androgenic steroid.

Use: Management of feminization associated with oestrogen-producing testicular tumours and testosterone-responsive incontinence and alopecia in male dogs. Can be used to suppress oestrus in the bitch and for false pregnancy but other medications are generally preferred and the use of this drug in racing greyhounds is discouraged.

Safety and handling: Normal precautions should be observed.

Contraindications: Include prostatic enlargement, perineal hernia, recurrence or exacerbation of perianal adenomas, cardiac insufficiency, liver or renal disease. Do not use in pregnant animals.

Adverse reactions: Use of testosterone in male cats may cause spraying. Administration of androgens to prepubertal animals may result in early closure of epiphyseal growth plates. Undesirable signs of virilization (low grade vaginitis, clitoral enlargement) may occur in certain individuals.

Drug interactions: Insulin requirements may be decreased in diabetic patients receiving androgenic therapy at normal doses. At higher doses insulin resistance may be encountered.

DOSES
Dogs: 2.5–10 mg/kg (0.05–0.2 ml) i.m., s.c. monthly.
Cats: 2.5–5 mg/kg (0.05–0.1 ml) i.m., s.c. monthly.
Small mammals, Birds, Reptiles: No information available.

Tetanus antitoxin
(Tetanus antitoxin behring) **POM-V**

Formulations: Injectable: 500–1500 IU/ml solution.

Action: Antibody binds to tetanus toxin.

Use: Preventive measure in animals at risk of developing tetanus from wounds. In established tetanus cases it is less effective as it does not displace bound toxin. Best used in developing cases of tetanus (i.e. immediately clinical signs are seen or when contamination of wound is severe and progression to a severe form of tetanus is possible). Risk of tetanus in dogs and cats is very low and therefore routine prophylaxis is not warranted.

Safety and handling: Normal precautions should be observed.

Contraindications: Avoid in cats (cannot metabolize phenol preservative).

Adverse reactions: All antisera have the potential to produce anaphylactoid reactions, particularly if the patient has previously received products containing horse protein. Repeated doses may lead to hypersensitivity reactions. Adrenaline or antihistamines may be used to manage these adverse effects.

Drug interactions: No information available.

DOSES

Dogs: Prophylactic: 80 IU/kg (maximum of 2500 IU/dog) i.m., s.c. once. Therapy of developing tetanus: 100–500 IU/kg s.c. once, maximum 20,000 IU/animal.
Cats: Not required.
Small mammals, Birds, Reptiles: No information available.

Tetracaine (Amethocaine)
(Amethocaine hydrochloride*) **POM**

Formulations: Ophthalmic: 0.5%, 1% solution (single-use vials).

Action: Local anaesthetic action is dependent on reversible blockade of the sodium channel, preventing propagation of an action potential along the nerve fibre. Sensory nerve fibres are blocked before motor nerve fibres, allowing a selective sensory blockade at low doses.

Use: Local anaesthesia of the ocular surface (cornea and conjunctival sac). Although effective, it is rarely used in veterinary practice. An alternative topical ophthalmic anaesthetic such as proxymetacaine is advised. Duration of action has not been reported in companion animal species. Topical anaesthetics block reflex tear production and should not be applied before a Schirmer tear test.

Safety and handling: Store in refrigerator.

Contraindications: Do not use for therapeutic purposes.

Adverse reactions: Tetracaine often causes marked conjunctival irritation, chemosis and pain on application. All topical anaesthetics are toxic to the corneal epithelium and delay healing of ulcers.

Drug interactions: No information available.

DOSES

Dogs, Cats, Small mammals: Ophthalmic: 1 drop per eye, single application.
Birds, Reptiles: No information available.

Tetracosactide (Tetracosactrin, ACTH)
(Synacthen*) **POM**

Formulations: Injectable: 0.25 mg/ml solution for intravenous use. In the event of availability problems, an alternative lyophilized formulation (0.25 mg/ml) for intramuscular use may be imported on a named patient basis.

Action: ACTH analogue that binds to specific receptors on the cell membrane of adrenocortical cells and induces the production of steroids from cholesterol.

Use: To stimulate cortisol production in the diagnosis of hyperadrenocorticism (Cushing's syndrome) and hypoadrenocorticism (Addison's disease). See *BSAVA Manual of Canine and Feline Endocrinology* for advice on performance and interpretation of ACTH stimulation test. Used in ferrets for the diagnosis of hypo- (but not hyper-) adrenocorticism. Availability problems at time of writing. It is recommended to use lower doses than previously published and reserve for diagnosis of hypoadrenocorticism. The effect on cortisol production in cats is less dramatic than in dogs, so the same reference ranges cannot be used.

Safety and handling: Normal precautions should be observed. Small aliquots of the intravenous and intramuscular preparations may be frozen and thawed once without undue loss of activity.

Contraindications: No information available.

Adverse reactions: None reported.

Drug interactions: None reported.

DOSES
Dogs: 0.125 mg/dog i.v. (dogs up to 5 kg body weight) or 0.25 mg/dog (dogs >5 kg body weight). Doses as low as 5 µg (micrograms)/kg produce maximal stimulation in healthy animals so doses higher than this are not necessary. The same doses may be used for the lyophilized product but must be administered intramuscularly.
Cats: Same doses as dogs.
Small mammals: Ferrets: 1 µg (micrograms)/kg i.m. for diagnosis of hypoadrenocorticism.
Birds, Reptiles: No information available.

2,2,2-Tetramine see **Trientine**

Theophylline
(Corvental-D) **POM-V**

Formulations: Oral: 100 mg, 200 mg, 500 mg sustained release capsules.

Action: Causes inhibition of phosphodiesterase, alteration of intracellular calcium, release of catecholamine, and antagonism of adenosine and prostaglandin, leading to bronchodilation and other effects.

Use: Spasmolytic agent and has a mild diuretic action. It has been used in the treatment of small airway disease. Beneficial effects include bronchodilation, enhanced mucociliary clearance stimulation of respiratory centre, increased sensitivity to P_aCO_2, increased diaphragmatic contractility, stabilization of mast cells and a mild inotropic effect. Theophylline has a low therapeutic index and should be dosed on a lean body weight basis. Administer with caution in patients with severe cardiac disease, gastric ulcers, hyperthyroidism, renal or hepatic disease, severe hypoxia or severe hypertension. Therapeutic plasma theophylline values are 5–20 µg/ml.

Safety and handling: Normal precautions should be observed.

Contraindications: Patients with a known history of arrhythmias or seizures.

Adverse reactions: Vomiting, diarrhoea, polydipsia, polyuria, reduced appetite, tachycardia, arrhythmias, nausea, twitching, restlessness, agitation, excitement and convulsions. Hyperaesthesia is seen in cats. Most adverse effects are related to the serum level and may be symptomatic of toxic serum concentrations. The severity of these effects may be decreased by the use of modified-release preparations. They are more likely to be seen with more frequent administration.

Drug interactions: Agents that may increase the serum levels of theophylline include cimetidine, diltiazem, erythromycin, fluoroquinolones and allopurinol. Phenobarbital may decrease the serum concentration of theophylline. Theophylline may decrease the effects of pancuronium. Theophylline and beta-adrenergic blockers (e.g. propranolol) may antagonize each others effects. Theophylline administration with halothane may cause an increased incidence of cardiac dysrhythmias and with ketamine an increased incidence of seizures.

DOSES

Dogs: 20 mg/kg p.o. q24h or 10 mg/kg p.o. q12h which may be increased to 15 mg/kg p.o. q12h if no side effects on lower dose. Note: Manufacturer only recommends q24h dosing. Some texts indicate q12h dosing of the sustained release preparation is required to maintain therapeutic serum levels.

Cats: 10 mg/kg p.o. q24h (sustained release preparation).

Small mammals: Ferrets: 4.25–10 mg/kg p.o. q8–12h; Guinea pigs, Rats: 10–20 mg/kg p.o. q8–12h.

Birds, Reptiles: No information available.

Thiabendazole see Tiabendazole
Thiamazole see Methimazole
Thiamine see Vitamin B1

Thyroid stimulating hormone
(Thyrotropin alfa, TSH)
(Thyrogen*) **POM**

Formulations: Injectable: 1.1 mg vial; after reconstitution with 1.2 ml sterile water the TSH concentration is 0.9 mg/ml.

Action: Binds to specific receptors on thyroid follicular cell membranes and in so doing stimulates the proteolytic degradation of thyroglobulin and the release of thyroxine (T4) and smaller quantities of tri-iodothyronine (T3).

Use: Stimulation of thyroid hormone production in the diagnosis of canine hypothyroidism. The diagnostic value in cats has not been fully assessed.

Safety and handling: Normal precautions should be observed.

Contraindications: Repeated administration is not advisable.

Adverse reactions: Chemical grade TSH may be associated with anaphylactic responses; do not use.

Drug interactions: Anabolic or androgenic steroids, carbimazole, barbiturates, corticosteroids, diazepam, heparin, mitotane (o,p'-DDD), phenylbutazone, phenytoin and salicylates may all decrease serum T4 levels. Fluorouracil, insulin, oestrogens, propranolol and prostaglandins may cause T4 levels to be increased. All these drugs will make the TSH stimulation test hard to interpret.

DOSES
Dogs: 50–100 µg (micrograms)/dog.
Cats: 25 µg (micrograms)/cat.
Small mammals, Birds, Reptiles: No information available.

Thyrotropin alfa see **Thyroid stimulating hormone**
L-Thyroxine see **Levothyroxine**

Tiabendazole (Thiabendazole)
(Auroto ear drops) **POM-V**

Formulations: Topical (aural): 4% solution combined with neomycin 0.5% and tetracaine hydrochloride.

Action: Fungicidal effect is due to the effect on the mitochondrial electron transport chain. The acaricidal effect is not understood.

Use: Management of *Malassezia* otitis externa and *Otodectes cynotis* infestations (additional topical acaricidal treatment on the hair coat advised).

Safety and handling: Normal precautions should be observed.

Contraindications: Do not use if tympanum is ruptured.

Adverse reactions: Ataxia, nystagmus and deafness may occur if used when the tympanum is ruptured.

Drug interactions: No information available.

DOSES

Dogs, Cats: 3–5 drops in affected ear(s) for 7 days. For ear mites the regimen should continue or be repeated within a 3-week period.
Small mammals, Birds, Reptiles: No information available.

Ticarcillin

(Timentin*) **POM**

Formulations: Injectable: 3 g ticarcillin and 200 mg clavulanic acid powder for reconstitution.

Action: Beta-lactam antibiotics bind penicillin-binding proteins involved in cell wall synthesis, decreasing bacterial cell wall strength and rigidity, and affecting cell division, growth and septum formation. The effect is bactericidal and killing occurs in a time-dependent fashion. Clavulanic acid acts as a non-competitive 'suicide' inhibitor for beta-lactamase enzymes.

Use: A carboxypenicillin that, like piperacillin, is indicated for the treatment of serious (usually but not exclusively life-threatening) infections caused by *Pseudomonas aeruginosa*, although it also has activity against certain other Gram-negative bacilli including *Proteus* spp. and *Bacteroides fragilis*. For *Pseudomonas* septicaemias antipseudomonal penicillins are often given with an aminoglycoside (e.g. gentamicin) as there is a synergistic effect. As ticarcillin kills bacteria by a time-dependent mechanism, dosing regimens should be designed to maintain tissue concentration above the MIC throughout the interdosing interval. Pharmacokinetic information on the ticarcillin/clavulanic acid combination is limited in veterinary species. After reconstitution it is stable for 48–72 hours.

Safety and handling: Normal precautions should be observed.

Contraindications: Do not administer penicillins to hamsters, gerbils, guinea pigs, chinchillas or rabbits.

Adverse reactions: Nausea, diarrhoea and skin rashes may be seen.

Drug interactions: Do not mix with aminoglycosides in the same syringe because there is mutual inactivation. There is synergism *in vivo* between the beta-lactams and the aminoglycosides.

DOSES

See Appendix for guidelines on responsible antibacterial use.
Dogs, Cats: 40–100 mg/kg i.v., i.m. q4–6h.
Small mammals: Rabbits, Chinchillas, Guinea pigs, Hamsters, Gerbils: Do not use.
Birds: 150–200 mg/kg i.v., i.m. q8–12h.
Reptiles: 50–100 mg/kg i.m. q24h.

Timolol maleate

(Azarga*, CoSopt*, Timolol*, Timoptol*) **POM**

Formulations: Ophthalmic: 0.25%, 0.5% solutions (5 ml bottle, single-use vials; 0.5% solution most commonly used); 1% brinzolamide with 0.5% timolol (Azarga); 2% dorzolamide with 0.5% timolol (CoSopt) (5 ml bottle, single-use vials).

Action: A topical non-selective beta-blocker that decreases aqueous humour production via beta-adrenoreceptor blockade in the ciliary body. See also Brinzolamide, Dorzolamide.

Use: Management of canine and feline glaucoma. It can be used alone or in combination with other topical glaucoma drugs, such as a topical carbonic anhydrase inhibitor. Dorzolamide/timolol or brinzolamide/timolol can be used in the control of most types of glaucoma in dogs; dorzolamide/timolol can be used in cats. The combination may be more effective than either drug alone. The combination causes miosis and is therefore not the drug of choice in uveitis or anterior lens luxation. Although no specific guidelines are available, it may be appropriate to use 0.25% in cats and small dogs <10 kg.

Safety and handling: Normal precautions should be observed.

Contraindications: Avoid in uncontrolled heart failure and asthma.

Adverse reactions: Ocular adverse effects include miosis, conjunctival hyperaemia and local irritation. Systemic absorption may occur following topical application causing bradycardia and reduced blood pressure.

Drug interactions: Additive adverse effects may develop if given concurrently with oral beta-blockers. Concomitant administration of timolol with verapamil may cause a bradycardia and asystole. Prolonged AV conduction times may result if used with calcium antagonists or digoxin.

DOSES

Dogs: One drop per affected eye q8–12h.
Cats: One drop per affected eye q12h.
Small mammals: Rabbits: 1 drop per eye q12h.
Birds, Reptiles: No information available.

Tobramycin

(Nebcin*, Tobramycin*) **POM**

Formulations: Injectable: 40 mg/ml solution.

Action: Aminoglycosides inhibit bacterial protein synthesis. They are bactericidal and their mechanism of killing is concentration-dependent, leading to a marked post-antibiotic effect, allowing pulse-dosing regimens which may limit toxicity.

Use: Treatment of Gram-negative infections. It is less active against most Gram-negative organisms than gentamicin, but appears to be more active against *Pseudomonas aeruginosa*. Aminoglycosides are ineffective at sites of low oxygen tension (e.g. abscesses) and all obligate anaerobic bacteria are resistant. More pharmacokinetic work is necessary to be sure of the dose rate, particularly in cats. The doses below are for general guidance only, and should be assessed according to the clinical response. Cellular casts found in the urine sediment are an early sign of nephrotoxicity. Monitor renal function during use. If giving i.v., administer slowly. Geriatric animals or those with decreased renal function should only be given this drug systemically when absolutely necessary and then q12h or less frequently.

Safety and handling: Normal precautions should be observed.

Contraindications: Do not use ophthalmic product where corneal ulceration is present.

Adverse reactions: Tobramycin is considered to be less nephrotoxic than gentamicin.

Drug interactions: Avoid concurrent use of other nephrotoxic, ototoxic or neurotoxic agents (e.g. amphotericin B, furosemide). Increase monitoring and adjust dosages when these drugs must be used together. Aminoglycosides may be chemically inactivated by beta-lactam antibiotics (e.g. penicillins, cephalosporins) or heparin when mixed *in vitro*. The effect of non-depolarizing muscle relaxants (e.g. pancuronium) may be enhanced by aminoglycosides. Synergism may occur when aminoglycosides are used with penicillins or cephalosporins.

DOSES
See Appendix for guidelines on responsible antibacterial use.
Dogs, Cats: Systemic: 2–4 mg/kg slow i.v., i.m., s.c. q8–24h. Pulse dosing (q24h) may be more effective (as for gentamicin).
Small mammals: No information available.
Birds: 2.5–5 mg/kg i.m. q8–12h.
Reptiles: 2.5 mg/kg i.m. q24–72h.

Toceranib
(Palladia) **POM-V**

Formulations: Oral: 10 mg, 15 mg, 50 mg film-coated tablets.

Action: Selective protein tyrosine kinase inhibitor with particular effects on the split kinase TK family, which may also have an effect on angiogenesis.

Use: Treatment of non-resectable grade 2 or 3 recurrent cutaneous mast cell tumours. Phase I trials have also demonstrated some efficacy in other canine malignancies (including mammary gland carcinomas, soft tissue sarcomas, multiple myelomas, melanomas and other carcinomas). Dogs should be monitored closely during treatment. As a guideline urinalysis, haematology and biochemistry should be undertaken before starting therapy, and then at least once a month (some clinicians may also check these parameters 1 week after drug initiation). Full coagulation profiles and faecal occult blood tests should be undertaken if adverse clinical signs are witnessed. It is good practice to contact owners once a week for the first 6 weeks of therapy to check for potential side effects, so that prompt action can be taken if these occur. Use with caution in dogs with pre-existing liver disease.

Safety and handling: Cytotoxic drug; see Appendix and specialist texts for further advice on chemotherapeutic agents.

Contraindications: Do not use in pregnant or lactating bitches, in dogs <2 years old, in dogs <3 kg, if there are any signs of GI haemorrhage, or if the patient has shown previous hypersensitivity to toceranib.

Adverse reactions: Weight loss, GI signs (diarrhoea, haemorrhage, anorexia, vomiting), lethargy, myelosuppression, lameness/musculoskeletal disorders, dermatitis and pruritus. Can also cause anaemia, increase in ALT activity, coagulation derangements (including pulmonary thromboembolism) and decrease in albumin. Uncommon events that may be related to toceranib administration include seizures, epistaxis, circulatory shock and death.

Drug interactions: No information available, but use with caution when combining with chemotherapeutic agents and drugs that have the potential to cause GI toxicity (i.e. steroids, NSAIDs) until further information is available.

DOSES
See Appendix for chemotherapy protocols.
Dogs: 2.5–3.25 mg/kg p.o. q48h.
Cats, Small mammals, Birds, Reptiles: No information available.

Toldimphos see Phosphate

Tolfenamic acid
(Tolfedine) **POM-V**

Formulations: Injectable: 40 mg/ml solution. Oral: 6 mg, 20 mg, 60 mg tablets.

Action: Inhibition of cyclo-oxygenase but uncertain if preferentially inhibits COX-2 over COX-1. COX inhibition limits the production of prostaglandins involved in inflammation. Also reported to have a direct antagonistic action on prostaglandin receptors.

Use: Alleviation of inflammation and pain in dogs and cats. Also used in the management of chronic locomotor disease in dogs and for the management of fever and the treatment of upper respiratory tract disorders, in combination with antibiotics, in cats. Injectable is authorized for preoperative administration to cats and dogs. Liver disease will prolong the metabolism of tolfenamic acid leading to the potential for drug accumulation and overdose with repeated dosing. In the cat, due to the longer half-life and narrower therapeutic index, particular care should be taken not to exceed the recommended dose and the use of a 1 ml graduated syringe is recommended to measure the dose accurately. Use with caution in renal diseases and in the perioperative period, as may adversely affect renal perfusion during periods of hypotension. There is emerging evidence, using *in vitro* models and dog tumour cell lines, that tolfenamic acid may have anticancer activity against some tumour types.

Safety and handling: Normal precautions should be observed.

Contraindications: Do not give to dehydrated, hypovolaemic or hypotensive patients or those with GI disease or blood clotting problems. Do not give to pregnant animals or animals <6 weeks old. Do not give i.m. to cats.

Adverse reactions: GI signs may occur in all animals after NSAID administration. Stop therapy if this persists beyond 1–2 days. Some animals develop signs with one NSAID drug and not another. A 1–2-week wash-out period should be allowed before starting another NSAID after cessation of therapy. Stop therapy immediately if GI bleeding is suspected. There is a small risk that NSAIDs may precipitate cardiac failure in animals with cardiovascular disease.

Drug interactions: Do not administer concurrently with, or within 24 hours of, other NSAIDs and glucocorticoids. Do not administer with other potentially nephrotoxic agents, e.g. aminoglycosides.

DOSES
Dogs: 4 mg/kg i.m., s.c., may be repeated once after 24h; 4 mg/kg p.o. for 3 days. Treatment starts with a single injection on day 1. The oral dosage regimen may be repeated once a week (i.e. 4 days of treatment with 3 days rest).
Cats: 4 mg/kg s.c., may be repeated once after 24h; 4 mg/kg p.o. for 3 days. Treatment starts with a single injection on day 1. Repeated dosing on a weekly basis is not recommended in cats.
Small mammals: Guinea pigs: 2 mg/kg s.c. q24h.
Birds, Reptiles: No information available.

Topiramate
(Topamax) **POM**

Formulations: Oral: 25 mg, 50 mg, 100 mg, 200 mg tablets; 15 mg, 25 mg, 50 mg sprinkle capsules.

Action: The exact antiepileptic mode of action is unknown, but may involve inhibition of voltage-dependent sodium channels and enhancement of GABA activity at GABA$_A$ receptors.

Use: As an adjunctive therapy in animals refractory to standard anticonvulsant therapies and where other adjunctive therapies have been unsuccessful. Use with care in patients with hepatic impairment.

Safety and handling: Normal precautions should be observed.

Contraindications: Avoid rapid withdrawal. Do not use in patients with severe hepatic disease.

Adverse reactions: Nausea and anorexia.

Drug interactions: No information available.

DOSES
Dogs: 2–20 mg/kg p.o. q8–12h. Experimentally, daily doses of 10–150 mg/kg p.o. q24h have been used with no evidence of serum accumulation.
Cats: Experimental single dose of 30 mg/kg p.o. has been described. No further information is available.
Small mammals, Birds, Reptiles: No information available.

Torasemide (Torsemide)
(Torem*) **POM**

Formulations: Oral: 5 mg, 10 mg tablets.

Action: Loop diuretic inhibiting the $Na^+/K^+/Cl^-$ co-transporter in the thick ascending limb of the loop of Henle. The net effect is a loss of sodium, potassium, chloride and water in the urine. Potassium excretion is less than with an equivalent dose of furosemide. Torasemide also increases excretion of calcium, magnesium and hydrogen, as well as renal blood flow and glomerular filtration rate. It has an anti-aldosteronergic effect, which is the result of dose-dependent inhibition of receptor-bound aldosterone. The diuretic effect of torasemide is equivalent to 10 times the effect of furosemide (mg for mg).

Use: Torasemide is not authorized for veterinary species and thus should not be used as a first-line loop diuretic. However, it can be effective for managing congestive heart failure in dogs and cats that is refractory to standard therapy including furosemide, by replacing the furosemide with torasemide. Compared with furosemide at an equivalent dose, torasemide has a higher bioavailability, a longer duration of action (12h with a peak effect of 2h in dogs and 4h in cats) and results in less kaliuresis and calciuresis. Dogs receiving torasemide for 14 days experienced less diuretic resistance and had greater increases in BUN compared with dogs receiving furosemide for 14 days. Has been used to treat oedema associated with hepatic cirrhosis and renal failure in humans. Use with caution in patients with severe electrolyte depletion, hepatic failure, renal failure and diabetes mellitus.

Safety and handling: Normal precautions should be observed.

Contraindications: Dehydration and anuria.

Adverse reactions: Hypokalaemia, hypochloraemia, hypocalcaemia, hypomagnesaemia, hyponatraemia, dehydration, polyuria/polydipsia and prerenal azotaemia occur readily. A marked reduction in cardiac output can occur in animals with diseases in which cardiac output is already impaired, such as severe pulmonary hypertension, low-output heart failure, hypertrophic cardiomyopathy, pericardial or myocardial disorders and cardiac tamponade. Other adverse effects reported in humans include ototoxicity, blurred vision, GI disturbances, leucopenia, anaemia, weakness and dermatological reactions.

Drug interactions: No information available.

DOSES
Dogs, Cats: Replace furosemide p.o. with torasemide p.o. at a daily dose that is $1/10^{th}$ to $1/13^{th}$ of the total daily furosemide dose divided q12–24h. Doses up to 0.3 mg/kg p.o. q12h have been reported in dogs and cats, but higher doses may be tolerated.
Small mammals, Birds, Reptiles: No information available.

Tramadol

CIL

(Tramadol ER*, Ultracet*, Ultram*, Zamadol*) **POM CD Schedule 3**

Formulations: Oral: 50 mg tablets; 100 mg, 200 mg, 300 mg extended release tablets; smaller tablet sizes (10 mg, 25 mg) are available from some veterinary wholesalers; 5 mg/ml oral liquid. Injectable: 50 mg/ml solution (may be difficult to source in the UK).

Action: Some metabolites of tramadol are agonists at all opioid receptors, particularly mu receptors. The parent compound also inhibits the re-uptake of noradrenaline and 5-HT, and stimulates presynaptic 5-HT release, which provides an alternative pathway for analgesia involving the descending inhibitory pathways within the spinal cord. In people, good and poor metabolizers of tramadol are described, with good metabolizers developing more opioid-like effects following drug administration and improved analgesia. Whether similar individual differences in metabolism of tramadol occur in cats and dogs is currently unknown.

Use: Management of mild to moderate acute pain and as an adjunctive analgesic in the management of chronic pain resulting from osteoarthritis or neoplasia. Increasing body of literature describing pharmacokinetics (PK) and pharmacodynamics (PD) in dogs and cats, although not authorized for use in these species. The recommended dose range is currently largely empirical due to a lack of combined PK/PD studies. When used for management of osteoarthritis in dogs, recent evidence suggests that doses around 4 mg/kg three times daily are required to produce analgesia; similar studies in cats to support dose recommendations are not available. Perioperatively, injectable tramadol is used instead of opioids to provide analgesia for acute pain, although the injectable preparation can be difficult to obtain in the UK. One study has shown tramadol 2 mg/kg to provide equivalent analgesia to morphine 0.2 mg/kg i.v. after ovariohysterectomy in dogs, and there are a number of studies that show tramadol 2 mg/kg to be efficacious for the management of acute pain in cats and dogs with dosing 3–4 times daily. Injectable tramadol has also been administered epidurally in dogs but does not appear to confer advantages over systemic administration. Tramadol has similar actions to morphine but causes less respiratory depression, sedation and GI side effects. It is attractive as an adjunct to manage chronic pain because it can be given orally and is not subject to controlled drug regulations; however, a larger body of evidence to support dose recommendations is needed. Cats seem to be more susceptible to the dysphoric effects of tramadol, although both dogs and cats can develop nausea and behavioural changes or sedation following repeated dosing. The oral preparations are unpalatable to cats and therefore difficult to administer, even when reformulated in gelatin capsules.

Safety and handling: Normal precautions should be observed.

Contraindications: No information available.

Adverse reactions: Sedation can occur after administration of high doses to dogs. Dysphoria is more likely in cats. Contraindicated in humans with epilepsy. Owners should be informed that there may be a slightly increased risk of seizures in treated animals.

Drug interactions: Tramadol can be given in combination with other classes of analgesic drugs such as NSAIDs, amantadine and gabapentin. It has the potential to interact with drugs that inhibit central 5-HT and noradrenaline re-uptake such as tricyclic antidepressants (e.g. amitriptyline), monoamine oxidase inhibitors (e.g. selegiline), selective serotonin re-uptake inhibitors and some opioids (e.g. fentanyl, pethidine and buprenorphine), causing serotonin syndrome that can result in seizures and death. Should signs of serotonin syndrome develop (manifest in mild form as hyperthermia, elevated blood pressure and CNS disturbances such as hypervigilance and excitation) these must be managed symptomatically and contributing drug treatments stopped.

DOSES
Dogs: 2–5 mg/kg p.o. q8h, 2 mg/kg i.v.
Cats: 2–4 mg/kg p.o. q8h, 1–2 mg/kg i.v., s.c.
Small mammals: Rabbits: 3–10 mg/kg p.o. q8–12h; Rats: 10–20 mg/kg p.o., s.c. q8–12h.
Birds: Bald eagles: 5 mg/kg p.o. q12h; Hispaniolan Amazons: 30 mg/kg p.o. q6h to achieve human therapeutic levels. Reduced thermal withdrawal response for 6 hours post-dosing; Red-tailed hawks: 15 mg/kg p.o. q12h to achieve human therapeutic levels.
Reptiles: 10 mg/kg i.m., p.o. q24–48h.

Travoprost
(Travatan*) **POM**

Formulations: Ophthalmic: 40 μg/ml (0.004%) solution in 2.5 ml bottle.

Action: Agonist for receptors specific for prostaglandin F. It reduces intraocular pressure by increasing uveoscleral outflow and may have a profound effect on intraocular pressure in the dog.

Use: Its main indication is in the management of primary canine glaucoma and it is useful in the emergency management of acute primary glaucoma (superseding mannitol and acetazolamide). There is little published data on its use in the cat but other tested topical prostaglandin analogues have been ineffective in this species. Often used in conjunction with other topical antiglaucoma drugs such as carbonic anhydrase inhibitors. It may be useful in the management of lens subluxation despite being contraindicated in anterior lens luxation. Travoprost has comparable activity to latanoprost.

Safety and handling: Normal precautions should be observed.

Contraindications: Uveitis and anterior lens luxation.

Adverse reactions: Miosis in dogs; conjunctival hyperaemia and mild irritation may develop. Increased iridal pigmentation has been noted in humans but not in dogs.

Drug interactions: Do not use in conjunction with thiomersal-containing preparations.

DOSES
Dogs: 1 drop per eye once daily (evening), or q8–12h.
Cats: No information available.
Small mammals: Rabbits: 1 drop/eye q12h.
Birds, Reptiles: No information available.

Trazodone
(Molipaxin*, Trazodone*) **POM**

Formulations: Oral: 50 mg, 100 mg, 150 mg tablets/capsules; 10 mg/ml liquid.

Action: Trazodone is an atypical antidepressant with mixed serotonergic agonistic and antagonistic actions. Its mode of action in alleviating anxiety is not fully understood.

Use: Chronic anxiety-related problems in dogs that are unresponsive to other pharmacological interventions. Should be used in conjunction with a behaviour modification plan. Use with caution and carefully monitor patients with renal disease. Less risk in patients with cardiac disease than tricyclic antidepressants such as amitriptyline.

Safety and handling: Normal precautions should be observed.

Contraindications: Glaucoma, history of seizures or urinary retention and severe liver disease.

Adverse reactions: Sedation, vomiting, excitability and dry mouth.

Drug interactions: Should not be used with monoamine oxidase inhibitors or drugs metabolized by cytochrome P450 2D6 (e.g. chlorphenamine, cimetidine). There is a risk of serotonin syndrome if combined with other serotonergic substances, but adjunctive therapy is sometimes used (see below). Ketoconazole will inhibit the breakdown of trazodone, leading to increased blood levels, while carbamazepine will have the opposite effect; itraconazole may be similar, although there is no clinical evidence of this.

DOSES
Dogs: 5–10 kg, 25 mg p.o. q24h; 11–20 kg, 50 mg p.o. q24h; >21 kg, 100 mg p.o. q24h. Doses may be titrated upwards every 10 to 14 days to a maximum of double the recommended dose. Doses for dogs >40 kg may be titrated to a maximum of 300 mg p.o. q24h. Dose may need to be increased if used long term as tolerance over time is common. Lower end doses may be used adjunctively with SSRIs (e.g. fluoxetine) but not MAOIs, but the risk of serotonin syndrome should be recognized.
Cats, Small mammals, Birds, Reptiles: No information available.

Tretinoin see **Vitamin A**

Triamcinolone
(Kenalog*) **POM**

Formulations: Injectable: 40 mg/ml suspension for deep i.m., intra-articular or intralesional use.

Action: Alters the transcription of DNA, leading to alterations in cellular metabolism which reduces inflammatory response.

Use: Management of inflammatory arthritides and dermatoses. Unsuitable for alternate-day use because of its duration of activity. Has 1.25 times the anti-inflammatory potency of prednisolone. On a dose basis, 0.8 mg triamcinolone is equivalent to 1 mg prednisolone. It has negligible mineralocorticoid activity. Animals on chronic therapy should be tapered off their steroids when discontinuing the drug.

Safety and handling: Normal precautions should be observed.

Contraindications: Do not use in pregnant animals. Systemic corticosteroids are generally contraindicated in patients with renal disease and diabetes mellitus. Do not use in birds.

Adverse reactions: Prolonged use of glucocorticoids suppresses the hypothalamic-pituitary axis (HPA) and cause adrenal atrophy.

Catabolic effects of glucocorticoids lead to weight loss and cutaneous atrophy. Iatrogenic hyperadrenocorticism may develop with chronic use. Vomiting and diarrhoea may be seen in some patients. GI ulceration may develop. Glucocorticoids may increase urine glucose levels and decrease serum T3 and T4 values. Impaired wound healing and delayed recovery from infections may be seen.

Drug interactions: There is an increased risk of GI ulceration if systemic glucocorticoids are used concurrently with NSAIDs. Hypokalaemia may develop if potassium-depleting diuretics (e.g. furosemide, thiazides) are administered with corticosteroids. Insulin requirements may increase in patients taking glucocorticoids. Metabolism of corticosteroids may be enhanced by phenobarbital or phenytoin and decreased by antifungals (e.g. itraconazole).

DOSES
Dogs: Systemic: 0.1–0.2 mg/kg i.m. initially then 0.02–0.04 mg/kg maintenance. A single i.m. dose of the long-acting preparations is effective for 3–4 weeks. Intralesional: 1.2–1.8 mg (total dose) injected intralesionally. Maximum 0.6 mg at any one site; separate injections by 0.5–2.5 cm.
Cats: Systemic, Intralesional: as for dogs. Intra-articular: 1–3 mg.
Birds: Do not use.
Small mammals, Reptiles: No information available.

Trientine (2,2,2-Tetramine)
(Trientine*) **POM**

Formulations: Oral: 300 mg capsule.

Action: Trientine is a copper chelator used in the management of copper toxicosis and acts primarily to increase the urinary elimination of copper.

Use: Treatment of dogs with copper hepatotoxicosis, especially those intolerant of penicillamine. Compared to penicillamine, it has greater affinity for plasma copper but reduced affinity for tissue copper.

Safety and handling: Normal precautions should be observed.

Contraindications: No information available.

Adverse reactions: Nausea, vomiting, abdominal pain, melaena and weakness. Chronic therapy can, rarely, lead to copper deficiency.

Drug interactions: Inhibits the absorption of iron, zinc and other minerals; separate doses by a minimum of 2 hours.

DOSES
Dogs: 10–15 mg/kg p.o. q12h. Vomiting may be reduced by giving in divided doses with food.
Cats, Small mammals, Birds, Reptiles: No information available.

Trifluorothymidine (Trifluridine, F3T)
(Viroptic* (USA)) **POM**

Formulations: Ophthalmic: 1% solution in 10 ml bottle (with/without preservative depending on availability from compounding pharmacy).

Action: Inhibits viral replication (viral DNA polymerase); does not depend on viral thymidine kinase for phosphorylation.

Use: A topical antiviral that is effective against feline herpesvirus-1 (FHV-1) *in vitro*; its efficacy *in vivo* has not been demonstrated. Usually reserved for corneal ulceration caused by herpetic disease. It is available in the UK if compounded by an ophthalmic pharmacy (e.g. Moorfields Eye Hospital, London). It has a short shelf-life of 12 weeks from the manufacturer, even unopened, and is expensive. Trifluorothymidine is virostatic and is unable to eradicate latent viral infection. In refractory and severe cases, combined therapy including topical antiviral medication, topical interferon and oral lysine, can be used. Treatment should not be continued for more than 3 weeks. Rarely used now in the UK as it has been superseded by oral famciclovir.

Safety and handling: Normal precautions should be observed.

Contraindications: No information available.

Adverse reactions: Ocular irritation may occur; frequency of application should be reduced if this develops.

Drug interactions: No information available.

DOSES
Cats: 1 drop per eye q4–6h for a maximum of 3 weeks. More frequent application q1–2h for acute infection is safe if tolerated.
Dogs, Small mammals, Birds, Reptiles: No information available.

L-Tri-iodothyronine see **Liothyronine**

Trilostane
(Vetoryl) **POM-V**

Formulations: Oral: 10 mg, 30 mg, 60 mg, 120 mg capsules.

Action: Blocks adrenal synthesis of glucocorticoids. Effects on mineralocortioids are relatively minor.

Use: Treatment of canine pituitary- and adrenal-dependent hyperadrenocorticism. It has been reported to be useful in the treatment of feline hyperadrenocorticism and canine 'alopecia X' syndrome. It is not considered to be useful in treating ferrets with hyperadrenocorticism. Perform ACTH stimulation tests (start test 3–5h post-dosing) 10 days, 4 weeks, 12 weeks and then every

3 months. The aim is for a post-ACTH cortisol of 40–120 nmol/l. In cases where clinical signs persist or polydipsia appears within the 24-hour period, ACTH stimulation tests performed later in the day and/or sequential cortisol determinations may be needed for dose adjustment (either mg/kg or frequency). Dosage adjustments may be necessary even after prolonged periods of stability.

Safety and handling: Normal precautions should be observed.

Contraindications: Do not use in patients with renal or hepatic insufficiency.

Adverse reactions: In humans, idiosyncratic reactions include diarrhoea, colic, muscle pain, nausea, hypersalivation and rare cases of skin changes (rash or pigmentation). Reported adverse effects in dogs include mild increases in serum potassium, bilirubin and calcium. Clinical hypoadrenocorticism can be seen. Adrenal necrosis has been reported. Adrenal hyperplasia has been noted with prolonged treatment but the effects of this are unknown. Prolonged adrenal suppression after drug withdrawal has been noted in some cases.

Drug interactions: Trilostane should not be administered concurrently with other drugs that suppress adrenal function, e.g. mitotane, itraconazole.

DOSES
Dogs: 2–5 mg/kg p.o. q24h. Start at the low end of the range and increase gradually. Twice-daily dosing is needed in some cases when clinical signs persist despite suppression of the cortisol response to ACTH stimulation. The total daily dose should be increased but not as much as doubled when switching from once to twice daily dosing.
Cats: 30 mg/cat p.o. q24h, adjusting dose according to clinical signs and post-treatment ACTH stimulation tests.
Small mammals, Birds, Reptiles: No information available.

Trimethoprim/Sulphonamide (Potentiated sulphonamides)
(Co-Trimazine, Duphatrim, Norodine, Tribrissen, Trimacare, Trimedoxine, Trinacol, Septrin*) **POM-V**

Formulations: Trimethoprim and sulphonamide are formulated in a ratio of 1:5. Injectable: trimethoprim 40 mg/ml and sulfadiazine 200 mg/ml (240 mg/ml total) suspension. Each 5 ml of paediatric suspension contains 200 mg sulfamethoxazole and 40 mg trimethoprim = 48 mg/ml suspension. Oral: trimethoprim and sulfadiazine in a variety of tablet sizes designated by the amount of trimethoprim e.g. 20 mg, 80 mg.

Action: Trimethoprim and sulphonamides block sequential steps in the synthesis of tetrahydrofolate, a cofactor required for the synthesis of many molecules, including nucleic acids. Sulphonamides block the synthesis of dihydropteroic acid by competing with para-aminobenzoic acid, and trimethoprim inhibits the enzyme dihydrofolate reductase, preventing the reduction of dihydrofolic acid to tetrahydrofolic acid. This two-step mechanism ensures that bacterial resistance develops more slowly than to either agent alone. In addition the effect of the combination tends to be bactericidal as against a bacteriostatic effect of either agent alone.

Use: Many organisms are susceptible, including *Nocardia*, *Brucella*, Gram-negative bacilli, some Gram-positive organisms (*Streptococcus*), plus *Pneumocystis carinii*, *Toxoplasma gondii* and other coccidians. *Pseudomonas* and *Leptospira* are usually resistant. Trimethoprim/sulphonamide is useful in the management of urinary, respiratory tract and prostatic infections, but ineffective in the presence of necrotic tissue. Trimethoprim alone may be used for urinary, prostatic, systemic salmonellosis and respiratory tract infections. Fewer adverse effects are seen with trimethoprim alone. Trimethoprim is a weak base which becomes ion-trapped in fluids that are more acidic than plasma (e.g. prostatic fluid and milk). Monitor tear production particularly during long-term use and in breeds susceptible to keratoconjunctivitis sicca. Ensure patients receiving sulphonamides are well hydrated and are not receiving urinary acidifying agents.

Safety and handling: Normal precautions should be observed.

Contraindications: Avoid use in animals with keratoconjunctivitis sicca (KCS) or previous history of adverse reaction to sulphonamides such as KCS or polyarthritis. Beware use in reptiles where renal disease is suspected.

Adverse reactions: Drowsiness, anorexia, leucopenia, anaemia and hypersalivation may be seen in cats. Acute hepatitis, vomiting, cholestasis, immune-mediated thrombocytopenia and an immune-mediated polyarthritis may be seen in dogs. Dobermanns would seem to be more susceptible to the development of immune-mediated systemic adverse effects. Acute hypersensitivity reactions are possible with sulphonamide products; they may manifest as a type III hypersensitivity reaction. Haematological effects (anaemias, agranulocytosis) are possible but rare in dogs. Sulphonamides may reversibly suppress thyroid function. Dermatological reactions (e.g. toxic epidermal necrolysis) have been associated with the use of sulphonamides in some animals. KCS has been reported in dogs treated with sulfapyridine and other sulphonamides. Sulphonamide crystal formation can occur in the urinary tract, particularly in animals producing very concentrated acidic urine.

Drug interactions: Antacids may decrease the bioavailability of sulphonamides if administered concomitantly. Urinary acidifying agents will increase the tendency for sulphonamide crystals to form within the urinary tract. Concomitant use of drugs containing procaine may inhibit the action of sulphonamides since procaine is a precursor for para-amino benzoic acid. When using the Jaffe alkaline picrate reaction assay for creatinine determination, trimethoprim/ sulphonamide may cause an over-estimation of approximately 10%.

DOSES

See Appendix for guidelines on responsible antibacterial use.
Doses (mg) of total product (trimethoprim + sulphonamide).
Dogs, Cats: 15 mg/kg p.o. q12h.
Small mammals: Ferrets: trimethoprim/sulfamethoxazole 15–30 mg/kg p.o., s.c. q12h; Rabbits: trimethoprim/sulfadiazine 30 mg/kg p.o., s.c. q24h; trimethoprim/sulfamethoxazole 30 mg/kg p.o., s.c. q24h; Chinchillas, Guinea pigs, Hamsters: 15–30 mg/kg p.o. i.m., s.c. q12–24h; Gerbils, Rats, Mice: 50–100 mg/kg p.o. s.c. q24h.
Birds: 8–30 mg/kg i.m. q12h; 20–100 mg/kg p.o. q12h; Pigeons: 475–970 mg/l drinking water.
Reptiles: Coccidiosis: 25 mg/kg p.o. q24h for 7 days.

Tropicamide
(Mydriacyl*, Tropicamide*) **POM**

Formulations: Ophthalmic: 0.5%, 1% solution, single-use vials, 5 ml bottle.

Action: Inhibits acetylcholine at the iris sphincter and ciliary body muscles, causing mydriasis (pupil dilation) and cycloplegia (paralysis of the ciliary muscle).

Use: Synthetic, short-acting antimuscarinic used for mydriasis and cycloplegia. It is the mydriatic of choice for intraocular examination due to its rapid onset (20–30 min) and short duration of action (4–12 h). Tropicamide is more effective as a mydriatic than as a cycloplegic and is therefore less effective than atropine in relieving ciliary body muscle spasm associated with uveitis. Use with care in patients with lens luxation.

Safety and handling: Normal precautions should be observed.

Contraindications: Avoid in glaucoma.

Adverse reactions: May cause salivation in cats, but less marked than with atropine.

Drug interactions: No information available.

DOSES
Dogs, Cats: 1 drop per eye, repeat after 20–30 min if necessary.
Small mammals: Rabbits, Chinchillas, Hamsters, Rats: 1 drop per eye, repeat after 20–30 min if necessary.
Birds, Reptiles: Ineffective because of complex arrangement of musculature in iris and ciliary body.

TSH see Thyroid stimulating hormone

Tylosin
(Bilosin, Tylan, Tyluvet) **POM-V**

Formulations: Injectable: 200 mg/ml solutions (Bilosin, Tylan, Tyluvet). Oral: 100 g/bottle soluble powder (Tylan).

Action: A bacteriostatic macrolide antibiotic that binds to the 50S ribosomal subunit, suppressing bacterial protein synthesis.

Use: Tylosin has good activity against mycoplasmas and has the same antibacterial spectrum of activity as erythromycin but is generally less active against bacteria. Although rarely indicated in small animal medicine, it has been used for the treatment of antibiotic-responsive diarrhoea in dogs and for cryptosporidiosis. Administration is predominantly by the oral route in dogs and cats.

Safety and handling: Normal precautions should be observed.

Contraindications: Do not give to hamsters, guinea pigs or rabbits.

Adverse reactions: GI disturbances. The activity of tylosin is enhanced in an alkaline pH. Tylosin can cause pain at the site of injection.

Drug interactions: Not well documented in small animals. It does not appear to inhibit the same hepatic enzymes as erythromycin.

DOSES
See Appendix for guidelines on responsible antibacterial use.
Dogs, Cats: 2–10 mg/kg i.m. q24h, 7–11 mg/kg p.o. q6–8h. May need higher dosages for dogs with chronic colitis and in the treatment of cryptosporidiosis. Doses of up to 40 mg/kg q12h have been recommended by some authors.
Small mammals: Ferrets, Chinchillas, Rats, Mice: 10 mg/kg p.o., i.m., s.c. q12h; Not recommended for Rabbits, Hamsters or Guinea pigs.
Birds: 20–40 mg/kg i.m. q8–12h (not chickens), or by nebulization of 100 mg diluted in 5 ml DMSO and 10 ml saline; Passerines: 1 g/l drinking water for 7–10 days; Pigeons: 50 mg/kg p.o. q24h, 25 mg/kg i.m. q6–8h, or 800 mg/l drinking water.
Reptiles: 5 mg/kg i.m. q24h q10–60d.

Ursodeoxycholic acid (UDCA) | CIL

(Destolit*, Ursodeoxycholic acid*, Ursofalk*, Ursogal*)
POM

Formulations: Oral: 150 mg, 300 mg, 500 mg tablets; 250 mg capsule; 50 mg/ml suspension.

Action: A relatively hydrophilic bile acid with cytoprotective effects in the biliary system. It inhibits ileal absorption of hydrophobic bile acids, thereby reducing their concentration in the body pool; hydrophobic bile acids are toxic to hepatobiliary cell membranes and may potentiate cholestasis. It also has an immunomodulatory effect, and may modify apoptosis of hepatocytes.

Use: An adjunctive therapy for patients with liver disease, particularly where cholestasis is present. The administration of UDCA does not alter the bile acids tolerance test of normal healthy dogs but a small but significant increase has been demonstrated in cats.

Safety and handling: Normal precautions should be observed.

Contraindications: No information available.

Adverse reactions: Vomiting is a rare effect. Safety has not been demonstrated in dogs or cats but side effects appear to be rare. Serious hepatotoxicity has been recognized in rabbits and non-human primates, but not in dogs or cats. Some human patients have an inability to sulphate lithocholic acid (a naturally metabolite of UDCA), which is a known hepatotoxin; the veterinary significance of this is unclear.

Drug interactions: Aluminium-containing antacids may bind to UDCA, thereby reducing its efficacy.

DOSES
Dogs, Cats: 10–15 mg/kg p.o. q24h.
Small mammals, Birds, Reptiles: No information available.

Vasopressin (ADH)
(Pitressin*) **POM**

Formulations: Injectable, topical: 20 IU/ml of argipressin (synthetic vasopressin) in aqueous solution.

Action: Posterior pituitary hormone with vasopressive and antidiuretic properties.

Use: Diagnosis and treatment of central diabetes insipidus. Desmopressin is generally preferred and is better researched.

Safety and handling: Normal precautions should be observed.

Contraindications: Do not use if cardiac disease is present.

Adverse reactions: Nausea, muscle cramp, hypersensitivity reactions and constriction of myocardial arteries are seen in humans.

Drug interactions: No information available.

DOSES
Dogs, Cats: 0.5 IU/kg i.m., s.c. prn; maximum dose 5 IU/animal.
Small mammals, Birds, Reptiles: No information available.

Vecuronium
(Norcuron*) **POM**

Formulations: Injectable: 10 mg powder for reconstitution.

Action: Inhibits the actions of acetylcholine at the neuromuscular junction by binding competitively to the alpha subunit of the nicotinic acetylcholine receptor on the post-junctional membrane.

Use: Provision of neuromuscular blockade during anaesthesia. This may be to improve surgical access through muscle relaxation, to facilitate positive pressure ventilation or for intraocular surgery. Intermediate dose-dependent duration of action of approximately 20 min. Has no cardiovascular effects and does not cause histamine release. Monitoring (using a nerve stimulator) and reversal of the neuromuscular blockade are recommended to ensure complete recovery before the end of anaesthesia. Hypothermia, acidosis and hypokalaemia will prolong the duration of neuromuscular blockade. In healthy animals repeated doses are relatively non-cumulative and it can be given by infusion i.v. to maintain neuromuscular blockade. It is metabolized by the liver; therefore in animals with liver dysfunction atracurium is advised rather than vecuronium. The duration of action of vecuronium is shorter in diabetic dogs compared with non-diabetic animals, although the underlying reasons for this difference are unclear. This may be clinically relevant when using vecuronium to provide neuromuscular blockade in diabetic dogs undergoing ocular surgery. Sugammadex (a cyclodextrin) developed to reverse neuromuscular blockade induced by rocuronium can also be used to reverse neuromuscular blockade caused by vecuronium in dogs at a dose of 8 mg/kg i.v. Used topically as a mydriatic in birds; ensure solution does not contain surface-penetrating agent.

Safety and handling: Unstable in solution and so is presented as a freeze-dried powder. The prepared solution can be diluted further if required.

Contraindications: Do not administer unless the animal is adequately anaesthetized and facilities to provide positive pressure ventilation are available.

Adverse reactions: No information available.

Drug interactions: Neuromuscular blockade is more prolonged when vecuronium is given in combination with volatile anaesthetics, aminoglycosides, clindamycin and lincomycin.

DOSES
Dogs, Cats: 0.1 mg/kg initially produces neuromuscular blockade for 25–30 min. The block can be maintained by increments of 0.03 mg/kg or a constant rate infusion of 0.1–0.2 mg/kg/h. Lower loading doses of 0.05 mg/kg i.v. produce neuromuscular blockade of shorter duration (16–19 min).
Birds: 1 drop of 0.8 mg/ml solution in 0.9% saline applied topically to eye; repeat after 2 minutes.
Small mammals, Reptiles: No information available.

Verapamil
(Cordilox*, Securon*, Verapamil*) **POM**

Formulations: Injectable: 2.5 mg/ml solution. Oral: 40 mg, 80 mg, 120 mg, 160 mg tablets.

Action: Inhibits inward movement of calcium ions through slow (L-type) calcium channels in myocardial cells, cardiac condution tissue and vascular smooth muscle. Verapamil causes a reduction in myocardial contractility (negative inotrope), depressed electrical activity (slows AV conduction) and vasodilation (cardiac vessels and peripheral arteries and arterioles).

Use: Primarily used to control supraventricular tachyarrhythmias, such as accessory pathway-mediated SVT, atrial tachycardia and flutter. In rabbits can be used perioperatively to minimize formation of surgical adhesions. Verapamil is a second-choice calcium-channel blocker behind diltiazem as it has a more pronounced negative inotropic effect. Patients with severe hepatic disease may have a reduced ability to metabolize the drug; reduce the dose by 70%.

Safety and handling: Normal precautions should be observed.

Contraindications: Do not use in patients with 2nd or 3rd degree AV block, hypotension, sick sinus syndrome, left ventricular dysfunction or heart failure.

Adverse reactions: Can cause hypotension, bradycardia, dizziness, precipitation or exacerbation of congestive heart failure, nausea, constipation and fatigue in humans.

Drug interactions: Do not use concurrently with beta-blockers. Both drugs have a negative inotropic and chronotropic effect and the combined effect can be profound. Co-administration with sodium channel blockers may also lead to cardiovascular depression and hypotension. Verapamil activity may be adversely affected by vitamin D or calcium salts. Cimetidine may increase the effects of verapamil. Verapamil may increase the blood levels of digoxin, digitoxin or theophylline, leading to potentially toxic effects from these drugs. Calcium-channel blockers may increase intracellular vincristine. The neuromuscular blocking effects of non-depolarizing muscle relaxants may be enhanced by verapamil.

DOSES
Dogs: 0.5–3 mg/kg p.o. q8h or 0.05 mg/kg slowly i.v. over 5–10 min (with ECG monitoring). Up to 4 repeat i.v. administrations at a reduced dose of 0.025 mg/kg q5min if necessary.
Cats: 0.5–1 mg/kg p.o. q8h or 0.025 mg/kg slowly i.v. over 5 min (with ECG monitoring). Up to 8 repeat i.v. administrations q5min if necessary.
Small mammals: Rabbits: 0.2 mg/kg slow i.v., p.o. after surgery and repeated q8h for 9 doses or 2.5–25 µg (micrograms)/kg/h i.p., s.c.; Hamsters: 0.25–0.5 mg/kg s.c. q12h.
Birds, Reptiles: No information available.

Vetrabutine
(Monzaldon) **POM-V**

Formulations: Injectable: 100 mg/ml solution.

Action: A chemical derivative of papaverine, an opium alkaloid that has a different chemical structure and pharmacological action from the opiates and which is used as a spasmolytic agent.

Use: Dilation of the cervix and coordination of the uterine contractions to ease and shorten parturition. May be useful in dystocia where there is insufficient relaxation of the birth canal.

Safety and handling: Pregnant women should preferably not handle this drug; if they must do so, then great care must be exercised to avoid self-injection.

Contraindications: Do not use in cats.

Adverse reactions: No information available.

Drug interactions: No information available.

DOSES
Dogs: 2 mg/kg i.m. q30–60 min up to 3 times.
Cats: Do not use.
Small mammals, Birds, Reptiles: No information available.

Vinblastine
(Velbe*, Vinblastine*) **POM**

Formulations: Injectable: 1 mg/ml solution.

Action: Interferes with microtubule assembly, causing metaphase arrest and ultimately resulting in cell death.

Use: In veterinary medicine vinblastine is used less frequently than vincristine for treatment of lymphoproliferative disorders, but it has been used with prednisolone for treatment of canine mast cell tumours. Use with care in patients with abnormal liver function; dose reduction recommended. Potentially a neurotoxic substrate of P-glycoprotein, use with caution in herding breeds (e.g. collies) that may have the gene mutation that causes a non-functional glycoprotein. Drug is locally irritant and must be administered i.v. through a carefully pre-placed catheter.

Safety and handling: Cytotoxic drug; see Appendix and specialist texts for further advice on chemotherapeutic agents. Store under refrigeration.

Contraindications: Bone marrow suppression.

Adverse reactions: Main dose-limiting toxicity is myelosuppression with neutropenia. Mucositis, stomatitis, ileus and GI tract toxicity may also occur.

Drug interactions: Any drugs that inhibit metabolism via hepatic cytochrome P450 system may reduce metabolism and thus increase toxicity of vinblastine, e.g. calcium-channel blockers, cimetidine, ciclosporin, erythromycin, metoclopramide, itraconazole. Drugs that are inhibitors of P-glycoprotein (ciclosporin, verapamil, phenothiazines, itraconazole) may increase the toxicity.

DOSES
See Appendix for chemotherapy protocols and conversion of body weight to body surface area.
Dogs, Cats: 2.0–2.5 mg/m^2 q7–14d.
Small mammals, Birds, Reptiles: No information available.

Vincristine
(Oncovin*, Vincristine*) **POM**

Formulations: Injectable: 1 mg, 2 mg, 5 mg vials.

Action: Interferes with microtubule assembly, causing metaphase arrest and ultimately resulting in cell death.

Use: With other neoplastic agents in the treatment of canine and feline neoplastic diseases, particularly lymphoproliferative disorders. May be used in the management of thrombocytopenia to stimulate release of platelets. Use with caution in patients with hepatic disease, leucopenia, infection, or pre-existing neuromuscular disease. Potentially a neurotoxic substrate of P-glycoprotein, use with caution in herding breeds (e.g. collies) that may have the gene mutation that causes a non-functional glycoprotein. Solution is locally irritant and must be administered i.v. through a carefully pre-placed catheter.

Safety and handling: Cytotoxic drug; see Appendix and specialist texts for further advice on chemotherapeutic agents. Store under refrigeration.

Contraindications: No information available.

Adverse reactions: Include peripheral neuropathy, ileus, GI tract toxicity/constipation and severe local irritation if administered perivascularly. Potentially myelosuppressive.

Drug interactions: Concurrent administration of vincristine with drugs that inhibit cytochromes of the CYP3A family may result in decreased metabolism of vincristine and increased toxicity. If vincristine is used in combination with crisantaspase it should be given 12–24 hours before the enzyme. Administration of crisantaspase with or before vincristine may reduce clearance of vincristine and increase toxicity.

DOSES
See Appendix for chemotherapy protocols and conversion of body weight to body surface area.
Dogs, Cats:
- Transmissible venereal tumours: 0.025 mg/kg i.v. q7d for 4 weeks.
- Other neoplastic diseases: usual doses are 0.5–0.75 mg/m².
- To increase circulating platelet numbers: 0.01–0.025 mg/kg i.v. q7d prn.

Small mammals: Ferrets: 0.025 mg/kg i.v. as part of chemotherapy protocol for lymphoma.
Birds, Reptiles: No information available.

Vitamin A (Retinol, Isotretinoin, Tretinoin)
(Retin-A, Isotrex*, Roaccutane*) **POM-VPS, POM**

Formulations: Injectable: Vitamin A (retinol) 50,000 IU/ml. Oral: 10 mg, 20 mg isotretinoin capsules (Roaccutane). Topical: 0.05% isotretinoin gel (Isotrex); 0.025% tretinoin cream; 0.01% tretinoin gel (Retin-A).

Action: Nutritional fat-soluble hormone that regulates gene expression. Tretinoin (all-trans retinoic acid) is the acid form of vitamin A and isotretinoin (13-cis retinoic acid) is an isomer of tretinoin.

Use: Treatment of hypovitaminosis A. Also used in conjunction with other appropriate therapies for sebaceous adenitis or primary seborrhoea of Cocker Spaniels. Animals receiving oral dosing should be monitored for vitamin A toxicity. Avoid concurrent use of oral and topical preparations because of toxicity. Avoid using formulations of vitamins A, D3 and E that are authorized for farm animals as they are too concentrated for small animal use.

Safety and handling: Vitamin A is teratogenic; gloves should be worn when applying topical preparations. Avoid contact with eyes, mouth or mucous membranes. Minimize exposure of the drug to sunlight.

Contraindications: Do not use in pregnant animals.

Adverse reactions: Many adverse effects are reported in humans following the use of oral isotretinoin, predominantly involving the skin, haematological parameters, hepatotoxicity, nervous system and bone changes. Similar abnormalities are reported in dogs and cats receiving high doses. Teratogenic if administered in the first trimester or at high doses. Redness and skin pigmentation may be seen after several days. It changes the lipid content of tears, which can result in keratoconjunctivitis sicca (KCS). It may also cause hyperlipidaemia and can be hepatotoxic at high doses. Prolonged use of vitamin A can promote loss of calcium from bone and lead to hypercalcaemia. Do not use topical preparations simultaneously with other topical drugs.

Drug interactions: Numerous, depending on preparation and route given. Consult specialist tests before using with another drug. Oral vitamin A may alter ciclosporin levels, which should therefore be monitored closely.

DOSES
Dogs:
- Hypovitaminosis A: 10,000–100,000 IU/dog i.m. q3d, no more than two doses; 10,000 IU/dog p.o. q24h for 3 days.
- Dermatological: 10,000 IU/dog p.o. q24h or apply isotretinoin/ tretinoin gel/cream to clean skin q12h; 1 mg isotretinoin/kg p.o. q12h for 1 month, reducing the dosage to 1 mg/kg p.o. q24h if improvement is seen.

Cats: Hypovitaminosis A: 10,000–100,000 IU/cat i.m. q3d, no more than two doses; 10, 000 IU/cat p.o. q24h for 3 days.

Small mammals: Rabbits: 500–1000 IU/kg i.m. once; Guinea pigs: 50–500 IU/kg i.m. or 10 mg beta carotene/kg food; Hamsters: 50–500 IU/kg i.m. or 2 µg (micrograms) vitamin A palmitate/g food.

Birds: 1000–20,000 IU/bird i.m. once or p.o. q12h.

Reptiles: 1000–2000 IU/kg p.o. q7–14d.

Vitamin B complex
(Anivit 4BC, Duphafral Extravite, Dupharal, Multivitamin injection, Vitamin B tablets) **POM-VPS, general sale**

Formulations: Various preparations containing varying quantities of vitamins are available, authorized for farm animals only. Most are for parenteral use and all those are POM-VPS.

Action: Cofactors for enzymes of intermediary metabolism and biosynthesis.

Use: Multiple deficiencies of B vitamins may occur in patients with renal or hepatic disease or significant anorexia. Dosages and routes vary with individual products. Check manufacturer's recommendations prior to use. Most products are intended for large animal use and some may contain vitamin C and other vitamins or minerals.

Safety and handling: All B vitamins are photosensitive and must be protected from light. Multi-dose vials require aseptic technique for repeated use.

Contraindications: No information available.

Adverse reactions: Anaphylaxis may be seen when used i.v. and products should be given slowly and/or diluted with i.v. fluids. Use of large animal products which also contain fat-soluble vitamins (A, D, E, K) may lead to toxicity.

Drug interactions: None reported.

DOSES
Dogs: 1 ml/dog (dogs up to 15 kg), 2–4 ml/dog (dogs >15 kg) s.c., i.m., i.v. q24h.
Cats: 1 ml/cat s.c., i.m., i.v. q24h or as required.
Small mammals: Rabbits: 0.02–0.4 ml/rabbit s.c., i.m. q24h or as required; Rodents: 0.02–0.2 ml/kg s.c., i.m. q24h or as required.
Birds: 1–3 mg/kg i.m. once. Should aim to achieve 10–30 mg/kg thiamine. Care must be taken not to exceed 3 mg/kg pyridoxine HCl (vitamin B6) as toxicity (acute death in 24–48 hours) recorded in raptors and pigeons.
Reptiles: No information available.

Vitamin B1 (Thiamine)
(Vitamin B1) POM-V, general sale

Formulations: Injectable: 100 mg/ml solution (authorized for veterinary use, though only in farm animals). Oral: various.

Action: Cofactor for enzymes in carbohydrate metabolism, it forms a compound with ATP to form thiamine diphosphate/thiamine pyrophosphate employed in carbohydrate metabolism. It does not affect blood glucose.

Use: Thiamine supplementation is required in deficient animals. Although uncommon this may occur in animals fed raw fish diets or uncooked soy products. Thiamine may be beneficial in alleviating signs of lead poisoning and ethylene glycol intoxication. It is used in birds and reptiles for the treatment of cerebral cortical necrosis.

Safety and handling: Protect from air and light; multi-dose vials require aseptic technique for repeated use.

Contraindications: Do not use in pregnant animals unless absolutely necessary.

Adverse reactions: Anaphylaxis can be seen with i.v. use; dilute with fluids and/or give slowly if using i.v. Adverse effects in pregnant animals are documented.

Drug interactions: There are no specific clinical interactions reported, although thiamine may enhance the activity of neuromuscular blocking agents.

DOSES
Dogs:
- Vitamin B1 deficiency: 50–250 mg/dog i.m., s.c., p.o. q12–24h for several days until signs resolve.
- Lead poisoning: 2 mg/kg i.m., s.c. q12h.
- Ethylene glycol intoxication: 100 mg/dog i.m., s.c., p.o q24h.

Cats: Vitamin B1 deficiency: 10–25 mg/cat i.m., s.c. q12–24h for several days until signs resolve or 10–20 mg/kg i.m. until signs resolve then 10 mg/kg p.o. for 21 days.

Small mammals: Ferrets, Rabbits: 1–2 mg/kg s.c., i.m. q12–24h for several days until signs resolve.

Birds: 10–30 mg/kg i.m. q24h.

Reptiles: Thiamine deficiency: 25–35 mg/kg p.o., i.m., s.c. q24h; Diet high in thiaminases: 30 g/kg of food fed q24h.

Vitamin B3 see **Nicotinamide**

Vitamin B12 (Cyanocobalamin, Hydroxocobalamin)
(Anivit B12 250 and 1000, Neo-Cytamen (hydroxocobalamin) Vitbee 250 and 1000) **POM-VPS**

Formulations: Injectable: 0.25 mg/ml, 1 mg/ml solutions.

Action: Essential cofactor for enzymes involved in DNA and RNA synthesis and in carbohydrate metabolism.

Use: Cyanocobalamin is used to treat vitamin B12 deficiency. Such a deficiency may develop in patients with significant disease of the distal ileum, small intestinal bacterial overgrowth, and exocrine pancreatic insufficiency. In humans, hydroxocobalamin has almost completely replaced cyanocobalamin in the treatment of vitamin B12 deficiency.

Safety and handling: Must be protected from light.

Contraindications: Do not give i.v.

Adverse reactions: Hypersensitivity to the phenol preservative in the injectable solutions can occur; patients should be monitored after injections for rash, fever and urticaria.

Drug interactions: None reported.

DOSES

Dogs: 0.25–1 mg/dog s.c., i.m. q7d for 4 weeks, then as needed to maintain normal levels.

Cats: 0.125–0.25 mg/cat s.c., i.m. q7d for 4–6 weeks, then as needed to maintain normal levels.

Small mammals: Rabbits: 20–50 µg (micrograms)/kg monthly to continue as long as deficiency is present.

Birds: 0.25–5 mg/kg i.m. q7d.

Reptiles: 0.05 mg/kg i.m., s.c.

Vitamin C (Ascorbic acid)

(Numerous trade names.) **POM, general sale**

Formulations: Injectable: 100 mg/ml. Oral: Various strength tablets, capsules, powders and liquids.

Action: Water-soluble antioxidant, also critical for crosslinking collagen precursors (growth and repair of tissue) and is involved in protein, lipid and carbohydrate metabolism.

Use: Vitamin C is used to reduce methaemoglobinaemia associated with paracetamol toxicity. Supplemental vitamin C may be required in conditions of increased oxidative stress, in cachexic patients and in those requiring nutritional support. There is no evidence to support long-term or high-dose therapy in dogs and cats, as they are able to synthesize vitamin C *de novo* to meet their needs.

Safety and handling: Normal precautions should be observed.

Contraindications: Avoid use in patients with liver disease.

Adverse reactions: May cause anaphylaxis if given i.v. Vitamin C supplementation may increase liver damage by increasing iron accumulation. Prolonged use can increase the risk of urate, oxalate and cystine crystalluria and stone formation.

Drug interactions: Large doses (oral or injectable) will acidify the urine and may increase the renal excretion of some drugs (e.g. mexiletine) and reduce the effect of some antibacterial drugs in the genitourinary system (e.g. aminoglycosides).

DOSES

Dogs, Cats: Methaemoglobinaemia: 30–40 mg/kg s.c. q6h for 7 treatments.

Small mammals: Rabbits: 50–100 mg/kg q12h; Guinea pigs: maintenance: 10–30 mg/kg/day or 200–400 mg/l drinking water; hypovitaminosis C: 100–200 mg/kg p.o. q24h.

Birds: No information available.

Reptiles: 10–20 mg/kg i.m. q7d; has been used at 100–250 mg/kg p.o. q24h in cases of infectious stomatitis in association with antimicrobial therapy.

Vitamin D

CIL

(1,25-dihydroxycolecalciferol (active vitamin D3), colecalciferol (vitamin D3))

(Alfacalcidol*, AT 10*, Calcijex*, Calcitriol*, One-alpha*, Rocaltrol*) **POM-VPS, POM**

Formulations: Oral: Alfacalcidol 2 µg/ml solution (One-alpha), 0.25–1 µg capsules (Alfacalcidol; One-alpha), Calcitriol 0.25 µg capsules (Calcitriol; Rocaltrol), Dihydrotachysterol 0.25 mg/ml solution (AT 10). Injectable: Calcitriol 1 µg/ml solution (Calcijex). Vitamin D is a general term used to describe a range of hormones that influence calcium and phosphorus metabolism. They include vitamin D2 (ergocalciferol or calciferol), vitamin D3 (colecalciferol), dihydrotachysterol, alfacalcidol and calcitriol (1,25-dihydroxycolecalciferol, the active form of vitamin D3). These different drugs have differing rates of onset and durations of action.

Action: In conjunction with other hormones (calcitonin and parathormone) regulates calcium homeostasis through numerous complex mechanisms, including accretion of calcium to bone stores, absorption of calcium from dietary sources.

Use: Chronic management of hypocalcaemia when associated with low parathyroid hormone concentrations which are most commonly associated with iatrogenic hypoparathyroidism following thyroidectomy and immune-mediated hypoparathyroidism. Calcitriol has also been used in the management of renal secondary hyperparathyroidism; in this circumstance it reduces serum parathyroid hormone concentrations. Vitamin D2 (ergocalciferol) has a very slow onset of action and has limited use in dogs and cats. Dihydrotachysterol has an onset of action within 24 hours and raises serum calcium within 1–7 days, with a discontinuation time of 1–3 weeks for serum calcium levels to normalize. Calcitriol and alfacalcidol (1-alpha-hydroxycolecalciferol) have a rapid onset of action (1–2 days) and a short half-life (<1 day); they are the preferred forms for use. Vitamin D requires two hydroxylations (one in the liver and the other in the kidney) to become active. Thus, only the active form (calcitriol) should be used in patients with renal failure. Vitamin D has a very narrow therapeutic index and toxic doses are easily achieved. Serum calcium and preferably ionized calcium concentrations need to be monitored closely and frequently. Avoid using formulations of vitamins A, D3 and E that are authorized for farm animals as they are too concentrated for small animal use.

Safety and handling: Normal precautions should be observed.

Contraindications: Do not use in patients with hyperphosphataemia or malabsorption syndromes. Do not use in pregnant animals.

Adverse reactions: Hypercalcaemia, hyperphosphataemia.

Drug interactions: Corticosteroids may negate the effect of vitamin

D preparations. Sucralfate decreases absorption of vitamin D. Drugs that induce hepatic enzyme systems (e.g. barbiturates) will increase the metabolism of vitamin D and lower its effective dose. Magnesium or calcium containing antacids may cause hypermagnesaemia or hypercalcaemia when used with vitamin D. Thiazide diuretics may also cause hypercalcaemia with concurrent use. Hypercalcaemia may potentiate the toxic effects of verapamil or digoxin; monitor carefully.

DOSES
Dogs:
* Hypocalcaemia/vitamin D deficiency: dihydrotachysterol: 0.02–0.03 mg/kg p.o. q24h initially, then 0.01–0.02 mg/kg p.o. q24–48h for maintenance; calcitriol: 10–15 ng (nanograms)/kg p.o. q12h for 3–4 days, then decrease to 2.5–7.5 ng/kg p.o. q12h for 2–3 days then give q24h.
* Renal secondary hyperparathyroidism: calcitriol: 1.5–3.5 ng (nanograms)/kg p.o. q24h; some authors recommend higher doses of up to 6 ng (nanograms)/kg/day if there is refractory hyperparathyroidism and ionized serum calcium concentrations can be assessed. Assess serum calcium and phosphate levels serially and maintain total calcium x phosphate product below 4.2 (calcium and phosphate in mmol/l). Do not use if this is not possible.

Cats:
* Hypocalcaemia: dihydrotachysterol: 0.02–0.03 mg/kg p.o. q24h initially, then 0.01–0.02 mg/kg p.o. q24–48h for maintenance; calcitriol: 10–15 ng (nanograms)/kg/day p.o. q12h for 3–4 days, then decrease to 2.5–7.5 ng/kg p.o. q12h for 2–3 days then give q24h.
* Renal secondary hyperparathyroidism: calcitriol 2.5–3.5 ng (nanograms)/kg/day p.o.

Small mammals: No information available.
Birds: Hypovitaminosis D: 3300–6600 IU/kg i.m. once (calcitriol).
Reptiles: No information available.

Vitamin E (Alpha tocopheryl acetate)
(Multivitamin injection, Vitamin E suspension) **POM-VPS**

Formulations: Oral: 20 mg/ml, 100 mg/ml suspension.

Action: Lipid-soluble antioxidant also regulates gene expression and is involved in cellular metabolism of sulphur compounds.

Use: Vitamin E supplementation is very rarely required in small animals. Patients with exocrine pancreatic insufficiency and other severe malabsorptive diseases may be at risk of developing deficiency. Vitamin E has been shown to be an effective antioxidant in dogs with liver disease, especially in patients with copper storage disease. Its use has been suggested for numerous conditions, including discoid lupus, demodicosis and hepatic diseases including fibrosis. These are, however, only anecdotal suggestions and there may be some significant risks. Avoid using formulations of vitamins A, D3 and E that are authorized for farm animals as they are too concentrated for small animal use.

Safety and handling: Normal precautions should be observed.

Contraindications: Do not use in patients at high risk for thrombosis. Do not use in neonates.

Adverse reactions: Thrombosis. Anaphylactoid reactions have been reported.

Drug interactions: Vitamin E may enhance vitamin A absorption, utilization and storage. Vitamin E may alter ciclosporin pharmacokinetics and, if used concurrently, ciclosporin therapy should be monitored by checking levels.

DOSES

Dogs: 1.6–8.3 mg/kg p.o. q24h for the first 30 days, then as needed. An alternative dose is 100–400 IU/dog.

Cats: 1.6–8.3 mg/kg p.o. for the first 30 days, then as needed. An alternative dose is 30 IU/cat.

Small mammals: No information available.

Birds: 0.06 mg/kg i.m. q7d in psittacids for hypovitaminosis E; once only in raptors to prevent/treat capture myopathy.

Reptiles: 1 IU/kg i.m. q24h for 7–14 days.

Vitamin K1 (Phytomenadione)   CIL
(Vitamine K1 Laboratoire TVM, Konakion*) **POM-V, NFA-VPS**

Formulations: Injectable: 10 mg/ml. Oral: 50 mg tablets.

Action: Involved in the formation of active coagulation factors II, VII, IX and X by the liver.

Use: Toxicity due to coumarin and its derivatives. Before performing liver biopsy in patients with prolonged coagulation times. Deficient states may also occur in prolonged significant anorexia. Although vitamin K is a fat-soluble vitamin its biological behaviour is like that of a water-soluble vitamin; it has a relatively short half-life and there are no significant storage pools. It may still require 6–12 hours for effect. Oral absorption is increased 4–5-fold in dogs if given with tinned food, especially those with increased fat content. One-stage prothrombin time is the best method of monitoring therapy. Use a small gauge needle when injecting s.c. or i.m. in a patient with bleeding tendencies.

Safety and handling: Normal precautions should be observed.

Contraindications: Avoid giving i.v. if possible.

Adverse reactions: Anaphylactic reactions have been reported following i.v. administration. Safety not documented in pregnant animals. Haemolytic anaemia occurs in cats when overdosed.

Drug interactions: Many drugs will antagonize the effects of vitamin K, including aspirin, chloramphenicol, allopurinol, diazoxide, cimetidine, metronidazole, erythromycin, itraconazole, propranolol and thyroid drugs as well as coumarin-based anticoagulants. If the patient is on other long-term medications it is advisable to check specific literature. The absorption of oral vitamin K is reduced by mineral oil.

DOSES
Dogs:
- Known 1st generation coumarin toxicity or vitamin K1 deficiency: Initially 2.5 mg/kg s.c. in several sites, then 1–2.5 mg/kg in divided doses p.o. q8–12h for 5–7 days.
- Known 2nd generation coumarin (brodifacoum) toxicity: Initially 5 mg/kg s.c. in several sites, then 2.5 mg/kg p.o. q12h for 3 weeks, then re-evaluate coagulation status. The patient's activity should be restricted for 1 week following treatment. Evaluate the coagulation status 3 weeks after cessation of treatment.
- Known inandione (diphacinone) or unknown anticoagulant toxicity: Initially 2.5–5 mg/kg s.c. over several sites. Then 2.5 mg/kg p.o. divided q8–12h for 3–4 weeks. Re-evaluate coagulation status 2 days after stopping therapy. If the PT time is elevated, continue therapy for 2 additional weeks. If not elevated repeat PT in 2 days. If normal, the animal should be rested for 1 week, if abnormal then continue therapy for an additional week and re-check PT times as above.
- Liver disease (pre-biopsy): 0.5–1.0 mg/kg s.c. q12h. After 2 days, re-evaluate coagulation status; postpone biopsy and continue supplementation if PT remains prolonged.

Cats:
- Coumarin rodenticide toxicity: doses as for dogs.
- Liver disease (pre-biopsy): 1.0 mg/kg s.c. q12h. After 2 days, re-evaluate coagulation status: postpone biopsy and continue supplementation if PT remains prolonged.

Small mammals: Ferrets: coumarin toxicity: doses as for dogs; Rabbits, Rodents: 1–10 mg/kg i.m. as needed depending upon clinical signs/clotting times.

Birds: 0.2–2.5 mg/kg i.m., p.o. q6–12h until stable, then q24h.

Reptiles: 0.5 mg/kg i.m. q24h.

Voriconazole see Itraconazole

Xylazine

(Chanazine, Nerfasin, Rompun, Sedaxylan, Virbaxyl, Xylacare, Xylapan) **POM-V**

Formulations: Injectable: 20 mg/ml solution.

Action: Agonist at peripheral and central alpha-2 adrenoreceptors, producing dose-dependent sedation, muscle relaxation and analgesia.

Use: In cats and dogs has been largely superseded by medetomidine or dexmedetomidine and is no longer recommended. Used to provide sedation and premedication when used alone or in combination with opioid analgesics. Xylazine combined with ketamine is used to provide a short duration (20–30 minutes) of surgical anaesthesia. Xylazine is less specific for the alpha-2 adrenoreceptor than are medetomidine and dexmedetomidine and causes significant alpha-1 adrenoreceptor effects. This lack of specificity is likely to be associated with the poorer safety profile of xylazine compared to medetomidine and dexmedetomidine. Xylazine also sensitizes the myocardium to catecholamine arrhythmias, which increases the risk of cardiovascular complications. Xylazine is a potent drug that causes marked changes in the cardiovascular system. It should not be used in animals with cardiovascular or systemic disease affecting cardiovascular performance. Atipamezole is not licensed as a reversal agent for xylazine, but it is effective and can be used to reverse the effects of xylazine if an overdose is given. Spontaneous arousal from deep sedation following stimulation can occur with all alpha-2 agonists; aggressive animals sedated with xylazine must still be managed with caution. Xylazine stimulates growth hormone production and may be used to assess the pituitary's ability to produce this hormone (xylazine stimulation test). Has been used to induce self-limiting emesis in cats where vomiting is desirable (e.g. following the ingestion of toxic, non-caustic foreign material). Emesis generally occurs rapidly and within a maximum of 10 min. Further doses depress the vomiting centre and may not result in any further vomiting.

Safety and handling: Normal precautions should be observed.

Contraindications: Do not use in animals with cardiovascular or other systemic disease. Use of xylazine in geriatric patients is also not advisable. It causes increased uterine motility and should not be used in pregnant animals, nor in animals likely to require or receiving sympathomimetic amines. Due to effects on blood glucose, use in diabetic animals is not recommended. Avoid when vomiting is contraindicated (e.g. foreign body, raised intraocular pressure). Induction of emesis is contraindicated if a strong acid or alkali has been ingested, due to the risk of further damage to the oesophagus. Induction of vomiting is contraindicated if the dog is unconscious, fitting or has a reduced cough reflex, or if the poison has been ingested for >2 hours or if the ingesta contains paraffin, petroleum products or other oily or volatile organic products, due to the risk of inhalation. Do not use for emesis in other species.

Adverse reactions: Xylazine has diverse effects on many organ systems as well as the cardiovascular system. It causes a diuresis by suppressing ADH secretion, a transient increase in blood glucose by decreasing endogenous insulin secretion, mydriasis and decreased intraocular pressure. Vomiting after xylazine is common, especially in cats.

Drug interactions: When used for premedication, xylazine will significantly reduce the dose of all other anaesthetic agents required to maintain anaesthesia.

DOSES
When used for sedation is generally given as part of a combination. See Appendix for sedation protocols in all species.
Dogs: Growth hormone response test: 100 μg (micrograms)/kg i.v.
Cats:
- Emesis: 0.6 mg/kg i.m. or 1 mg/kg s.c. once (effective in >75% of cats).
- Growth hormone suppression test: 100 μg (micrograms)/kg i.v.
Small mammals: See Appendix.
Birds: Do not use.
Reptiles: No information available.

Zidovudine (Azidothymidine, AZT)

(Retrovir*) **POM**

Formulations: Oral: 100 mg, 250 mg capsules; 50 mg/5 ml syrup. Injection: 10 mg/ml solution for use as i.v. infusion.

Action: Competitive inhibition of reverse transcriptase. Requires activation to the 5'-triphosphate form by cellular kinases.

Use: Treatment of FIV-positive cats. In cats not showing clinical signs, it may delay the onset of the clinical phase. In cats showing clinical signs, it may improve recovery in combination with other therapies. In human medicine it is used in combination with other nucleoside reverse transcriptase inhibitors, e.g. abacavir, didanosine, lamivudine, stavudine, tenofovir and zalcitabine. Two of these drugs are usually used with either a non-nucleotide reverse transcriptase inhibitor or a protease inhibitor. Use of drug combinations in HIV-positive people aims to avoid the development of drug resistance. The protease inhibitors currently used in human medicine seem to lack efficacy against FIV, thus hampering this approach for FIV-infected cats in the clinical phase. Haematological monitoring is recommended.

Safety and handling: Normal precautions should be observed.

Contraindications: Animals that are severely anaemic or leucopenic should not be given this drug.

Adverse reactions: Hepatotoxicity and severe anaemia can occur at high doses. Long-term adverse effects of lower doses have not been ascertained.

Drug interactions: No information available.

DOSES
Cats: 5–10 mg/kg daily p.o., s.c. in 2–4 divided doses.
Dogs, Small mammals, Birds, Reptiles: No information available.

Zinc salts

(Numerous trade names) **GSL**

Formulations: Oral: various zinc sulphate, zinc gluconate, zinc acetate and chelated zinc preparations.

Action: Primarily involved in DNA and RNA synthesis, although also involved in essential fatty acid synthesis, WBC function and numerous reactions in intermediary metabolism. When administered orally can reduce GI absorption and hepatic uptake of copper.

Use: Zinc-responsive dermatoses and reduction of copper in dogs with copper-associated liver disease. Proposed benefits also exist in chronic liver disease and hepatic encephalopathy. Bioavailability of elemental zinc varies depending on formulation: zinc acetate and chelated forms: highest; gluconate: intermediate; sulphate: lowest. Higher bioavailability is also associated with improved tolerance.

Safety and handling: Normal precautions should be observed.

Contraindications: Patients with copper deficiency.

Adverse reactions: Nausea, vomiting and occasional diarrhoea. Haemolysis may occur with large doses or serum levels >10 mg/ml particularly if a coexistent copper deficiency exists.

Drug interactions: Significant interactions with other divalent heavy metals such as iron and copper can occur and long-term administration of zinc may lead to decreased hepatic copper or iron stores and functional deficiency. Penicillamine and ursodeoxycholic acid may potentially inhibit zinc absorption; the clinical significance is unclear. Zinc salts may chelate oral tetracycline and reduce its absorption; separate doses by at least 2 hours. Zinc salts may reduce the absorption of fluoroquinolone antibiotics.

DOSES
Dogs, Cats: 1–2 mg elemental zinc p.o. q24h (zinc sulphate: 5 mg/kg p.o. q24h or in divided doses; zinc gluconate: 2 mg/kg p.o. q24h; zinc acetate: 1 mg/kg p.o. q24h). Give on an empty stomach to minimize vomiting.
Small mammals, Birds, Reptiles: No information available.

Zonisamide
(Zonegran) **POM**

Formulations: Oral: 25 mg, 50 mg, 100 mg capsules.

Action: The exact antiepileptic mode of action is unknown, but it is speculated that zonisamide may exert this effect by blocking repetitive firing of voltage-gated sodium channels, inhibition of calcium channels or binding to GABA receptors.

Use: Zonisamide is a sulphonamide anticonvulsant, which is usually used in dogs and cats as an adjunctive therapy in animals refractory to standard anticonvulsant therapy (in dogs, phenobarbital, imepitoin and potassium bromide).

Safety and handling: Normal precautions should be observed.

Contraindications: Avoid use in patients with severe hepatic impairment. Do not use in pregnant animals as toxicity has been demonstrated in experimental studies. Do not discontinue abruptly.

Adverse reactions: Ataxia, sedation, vomiting and anorexia have been reported in a few dogs and, experimentally, in cats. Doses up to 75 mg/kg q24h or divided q12h have been used experimentally for up to 52 weeks in dogs; initially there was weight loss and, in the longer term, minor hepatic and haematological changes.

Drug interactions: No information available.

DOSES
Dogs: Starting dose of 5–10 mg/kg p.o. q12h.
Cats: Starting dose of 5 mg/kg p.o. q12h is suggested.
Small mammals, Birds, Reptiles: No information available.

Appendix I: general information

Abbreviations

In general abbreviations should not be used in prescription writing. However, it is recognized that at present some Latin abbreviations are used when prescribing. These should be limited to those listed here.

Abbreviations used in prescription writing

a.c.	Before meals
ad. lib.	At pleasure
amp.	Ampoule
b.i.d.	Twice a day
cap.	Capsule
g	Gram
h	Hour
i.m.	Intramuscular
i.p.	Intraperitoneal
i.v.	Intravenous
m^2	Square metre
mg	Milligram
ml	Millilitre
o.m.	In the morning
o.n.	At night
p.c.	After meals
prn	As required
q	Every, e.g. q8h = every 8 hours
q.i.d./q.d.s	Four times a day
q.s.	A sufficient quantity
s.c.	Subcutaneous
s.i.d.	Once a day
Sig:	Directions/label
stat	Immediately
susp.	Suspension
tab	Tablet
t.i.d./t.d.s.	Three times a day

Other abbreviations used in this Formulary

ACE	Angiotensin converting enzyme
ACTH	Adrenocorticotrophic hormone
AV	Atrioventricular
CBC	Complete blood count
CHF	Congestive heart failure
CNS	Central nervous system
COX	Cyclo-oxygenase
CRF	Chronic renal failure
CSF	Cerebrospinal fluid
d	Day(s)
DIC	Disseminated intravascular coagulation
ECG	Electrocardiogram
EPI	Exocrine pancreatic insufficiency
GI	Gastrointestinal
h	Hour(s)
Hb	Haemoglobin
min	Minute
p.o.	By mouth, orally
PU/PD	Polyuria/polydipsia
RBC	Red blood cell
SLE	Systemic lupus erythematosus
STC	Special Treatment Certificate
VPC	Ventricular premature contraction
WBC	White blood cell
wk	Week(s)

APPENDIX I: GENERAL INFORMATION

APPENDIX II: PROTOCOLS

INDEX: THERAPEUTIC CLASS

INDEX: GENERIC AND TRADE NAMES

Writing a prescription

A 'veterinary prescription' is defined by EU law as 'any prescription for a veterinary medicinal product issued by a professional person qualified to do so in accordance with applicable national law'. The word 'veterinary' takes its normal meaning 'of or for animals'. In the UK there are two classes of medicines available only on veterinary prescription, POM-V and POM-VPS, described in the Introduction. Only in the case of POM-V medicines does the veterinary prescription have to be issued by a veterinary surgeon. The act of prescribing is taken to mean the decision made by the prescriber as to which product should be supplied, taking account of the circumstances of the animals being treated, the available authorized veterinary medicinal products and the need for responsible use of medicines. Good prescription principles include the following. Only 1, 8, 10 and 12 are legal requirements; the remainder are good practice.

1 Print or write legibly in ink or otherwise so as to be indelible. Sign in ink with your normal signature. Include the date on which the prescription was signed.

2 Use product or approved generic name for drugs **in capital letters – do not abbreviate**. Ensure the full name is stated, to include the pharmaceutical form and strength.

3 State duration of treatment where known and the total quantity to be supplied.

4 Write out microgram/nanogram – **do not abbreviate**.

5 Always put a 0 before an initial decimal point (e.g. 0.5 mg), but avoid the unnecessary use of a decimal point (e.g. 3 mg not 3.0 mg).

6 Give precise instructions concerning route/dose/formulation. Directions should preferably be in English without abbreviation. It is recognized that some Latin abbreviations are used (p.358).

7 Any alterations invalidate the prescription – rewrite.

8 Prescriptions for Schedule 2 and most Schedule 3 Controlled Drugs must be entirely handwritten and include the total quantity in both words and figures, the form and strength of the drug.

9 The prescription should not be repeated more than three times without re-checking the patient.

10 Include both the prescriber's and the client's names and addresses.

11 Include the directions that the prescriber wishes to appear on the labelled product. It is good practice to include the words 'For animal treatment only'.

12 Include a declaration that 'This prescription is for an animal under my care' or words to that effect.

13 If drugs that are not authorized for veterinary use are going to be used when there is an alternative that is 'higher' in the prescribing cascade, there should be a clear clinical justification made on an individual basis and recorded in the clinical notes or on the prescription.

APPENDIX I: GENERAL INFORMATION | APPENDIX II: PROTOCOLS | INDEX: THERAPEUTIC CLASS | INDEX: GENERIC AND TRADE NAMES

The following is a standard form of prescription used:

From: *Address of practice*   *Date*
Telephone No.

Animal's name and identification   *Owner's name*
(species, breed, age and sex)   *Owner's address*

Rx   *Print name, strength and formulation of drug*
      Total quantity to be supplied
      Amount to be administered
      Frequency of administration
      Duration of treatment
      Any warnings
      If not a POM-V and prescribed under the 'Cascade',
      this must be stated

      For animal treatment only
      For an animal under my care

Non-repeat/repeat X *1, 2 or 3*

           Name, qualifications and signature of veterinary surgeon

Topical polypharmaceuticals

The following POM-V preparations contain two or more drugs and are used topically. For further information see relevant monographs. In addition there are a number of AVM-GSL preparations used for ear cleaning etc. that are not listed here.

Name	Antibacterial	Steroid	Antifungal	Antiparasitic	Other
Aurizon	Marbofloxacin	Dexamethasone	Clotrimazole	–	–
Auroto	Neomycin	–	Tiabendazole	Tiabendazole	Amethocaine
Canaural	Fusidic acid Framycetin	Prednisolone	Nystatin	*	–
Easotic	Gentamicin	Hydrocortisone aceponate	Miconazole	–	–
Fuciderm	Fusidic acid	Betamethasone	–	–	–
Otomax	Gentamicin	Betamethasone	Clotrimazole	–	–
Posatex	Orbifloxacin	Mometasone	Posaconazole	–	–
Surolan	Polymixin B	Prednisolone	Miconazole	*	–

* Note that there is some evidence from clinical trials that products that do not contain a specific acaricidal compound may nevertheless be effective at treating infestations of ear mites. The mode of action is unclear but the vehicle for these polypharmaceutical products may be involved.

In addition, there is Dermisol cream which contains a mixture of organic acids to aid removal of embedded debris and dead tissue. None of these products should be used where ear drum perforation is suspected.

Guidelines for responsible antibacterial use

Following these guidelines will help to maximize therapeutic success of antibacterial agents whilst at the same time minimizing the development of antibacterial resistance, thereby safeguarding antimicrobials for future veterinary and human use. These guidelines should be read in conjunction with the updated *BSAVA Guide to the Use of Veterinary Medicines* (available at www.bsava. com/Resources/BSAVAmedicinesGuide.aspx), the PROTECT guidance (www.bsava.com/Resources/PROTECT.aspx) and individual drug monographs. It is important that the veterinary profession uses antibacterials prudently in order to: minimize the selection of resistant veterinary pathogens (and therefore safeguard animal health); minimize possible resistance transfer to human pathogens; and retain the right to prescribe certain antibacterials.

It is important to remember that antibacterials do not make organisms resistant, but they do create selective pressure on populations of organisms. Resistance may be inherent, evolved (by chromosomal DNA changes) or acquired (by plasmid transfer). Resistance is reduced by the following:

1 **Reducing the expectation of antibacterial prescriptions.** Educate clients not to expect antibacterials when they are not appropriate; e.g. viral infections.

2 **Minimizing and ideally avoiding prophylactic use.**
   a. Prophylactic antibacterial use may be appropriate in certain medical situations; for example, when an animal is considered to be at increased risk due to concurrent disease or immunosuppressant therapy and is in contact with other infected animals.
   b. Prophylactic antibacterial use may be appropriate in the perioperative period, although it should not be a substitute for good asepsis. Examples of appropriate criteria for perioperative antibacterial use include:
      • Prolonged surgical procedures (>1.5 hours)
      • Introduction of an implant into the body
      • Procedures where introduction of infection would be catastrophic (e.g. CNS surgery)
      • Where there is an obvious identified break in asepsis
      • Bowel surgery with a risk of leakage
      • Dentistry with associated periodontal disease
      • Contaminated wounds.
   c. In most cases appropriate antibacterials to use would be an intravenous preparation of amoxicillin/clavulanate or a first or second generation cephalosporin administered at induction and repeated at 90-minute intervals during the procedure. In situations where anaerobic involvement is highly likely (e.g. periodontal disease), the addition or substitution of metronidazole would be appropriate. In the case of bowel leakage, a combination of antibacterials may

be most appropriate, e.g. ampicillin combined with an aminoglycoside or a fluoroquinolone.

3 **Culturing appropriate material for sensitivity testing.**
   a. The results from culture and sensitivity tests considerably assist the choice of which antibacterial to use.
   b. Culture is not required in every case, but when prolonged courses of antibacterials are likely to be needed (e.g. pyodermas, otitis externa, deep or surgical wound infections) then culture will improve the animal's treatment.

4 **Knowing the features of antibacterials.** There are three key areas that veterinary surgeons must have a working knowledge of.
   a. <u>Spectrum of activity.</u> Many of the antibacterials in routine veterinary use are broad-spectrum; however, to minimize resistance the narrowest spectrum agent should be chosen. Some specific examples of spectra covered are:
   - Anaerobes – metronidazole, clindamycin, many of the penicillins (especially the narrow spectrum penicillins such as Penicillin G) and cephalosporins
   - Gram-positive bacteria – penicillins, cephalosporins, lincosamides and macrolides
   - Gram-negative bacteria – aminoglycosides and fluoroquinolones.
   b. <u>Distribution.</u> Many of the antibacterial classes are well distributed around the body, and it is important to be aware of some of the specifics of distribution. Key examples include:
   - Aminoglycosides are poorly distributed. They are not absorbed from the GI tract and even if given systemically distribution can be quite restricted. Conversely, it means that they are very appropriate for local delivery
   - Beta lactams attain high concentrations in the urinary tract due to filtration and secretion into the renal tubule. Levels attained may be many times higher than plasma concentrations. Fluoroquinolones also attain extremely high levels in the urinary tract
   - Lipid-soluble basic antibacterials such as the macrolides and lincosamides become ion-trapped (concentrate) in sites such as the prostate gland and the mammary gland.
   c. <u>Adverse effects/toxicity.</u> These must be considered in the context of the individual animal and in relation to concurrent treatment or pre-existing conditions.

5 **Use the antibacterial you have chosen appropriately.**
   a. Consider the practicalities and owner compliance.
   b. Give the appropriate **dose**, for the appropriate **frequency** and the appropriate **duration**. Too little or too much antibacterial will contribute to resistance and inappropriate use will lead to treatment failure.

c. Is the antibacterial **time- or concentration-dependent?** (Refer to the *BSAVA Guide to the Use of Veterinary Medicines* (www.bsava.com/Resources/BSAVAmedicinesGuide.aspx) for an explanation of these terms.)

6 **Assess the response.** Part of this may be carrying out repeated culture and sensitivity testing, where appropriate, and amending treatment if indicated from the results. If you are using an antibacterial which your clinical experience, or the results of culture and sensitivity, suggests should be effective in a particular situation and treatment fails, then this should be reported through the Suspected Adverse Reaction Surveillance Scheme (SARSS) organized by the Veterinary Medicines Directorate (VMD), as this is important in monitoring resistance development.

7 **Certain antibacterials should be used judiciously.** This means that their use as first line agents should be avoided, and they should only be used when other agents are ineffective (ideally determined by culture and sensitivity testing). These include:
- Fluoroquinolones
- Third and fourth generation cephalosporins
- Amikacin.

8 **Certain antibacterials should probably NOT be used in veterinary species.** These are agents of last resort in human patients and include:
- Vancomycin
- Carbapenams such as imipenam.

In addition to written guidelines on which antibacterials should be used and the appropriate dosing regimens, there should be a practice policy in terms of appropriate criteria warranting antibacterials. For example, it is feasible to work out appropriate first option antibacterials for uncomplicated urinary tract infections and surgical prophylaxis, which should then be used by all practice members.

Antibacterials in small mammals

Antibacterial therapy in several small mammal species poses a greater risk when compared with other species due to the suppression of normal bacterial flora, resulting in overgrowth of other species, notably *Clostridium*, resulting in enterotoxaemia and death. Mice, rats, ferrets and usually gerbils are fairly resistant, whereas hamsters, guinea pigs, chinchillas and rabbits are more susceptible. The risk of enterotoxaemia is related to several factors, including the drug selected, the dose, the route of administration and the animal's nutritional status and general health. In general, penicillins, clindamycin and lincomycin are more likely to cause enterotoxaemia, whereas cephalosporins and erythromycin are less likely to do so; aminoglycosides, fluoroquinolones, metronidazole and sulphonamides pose the least risk. Tetracyclines are risky in the guinea pig but appear less so in other species (Prescott *et al.*, 2000). See individual monographs for more details.

Radiographic contrast agents

Barium and iodinated contrast media

See *BSAVA Guide to Procedures in Small Animal Practice.*

MRI contrast media

Several gadolinium chelates are used in magnetic resonance imaging (MRI) studies. None of them is authorized for veterinary use and all are POM.

Action

Gadolinium exerts its paramagnetic effects due to seven unpaired electrons, which cause a shortening of T1 and T2 relaxation times of adjacent tissues. This results in an increased signal on T1-weighted MR images. Gadolinium is toxic so is chelated to reduce toxicity. Gadolinium chelates do not cross the normal blood–brain barrier due to their large molecular size.

Use

During MRI to identify areas of abnormal vascularization or increased interstitial fluid, delineate masses, demonstrate disruption of the blood–brain barrier and areas of inflammation. Gadoteric acid and gadobenic acid are also used for contrast-enhanced magnetic resonance angiography (MRA). Gadobenic acid and gadoxetic acid are also transported across hepatocyte cell membranes (gadoxetic acid via organic anionic-acid transporting peptide 1) and are used in the characterization of liver lesions.

Safety and handling

Contact with skin and eyes may cause mild irritation.

Contraindications

Use with caution in cardiac disease, pre-existing renal disease and neonates. Contraindicated in severe renal impairment.

Adverse reactions

Nephrogenic systemic fibrosis (most commonly with gadodiamide but also gadopentetic acid and gadoversetamide) reported in humans but not in animals. Increase in QT interval and other arrhythmias have also been reported, and cardiac monitoring is recommended in the event of accidental overdosage. Many are hyper-osmolar and irritant if extravasation, therefore should be given through intravenous catheter. Anaphylaxis occurs rarely. May cause transient increase in serum bilirubin if pre-existing hepatic disease. In experimental studies may cause fetal abnormalities in rabbits.

Drug interactions

May have interactions with Class 1a and 3 antiarrhythmics. Gadobenic acid may compete for cannalicular multispecific organic anionic transporter sites. Caution should be used if administering cisplatin, anthracyclines, vinca alkyloids and other drugs using this transporter. Anionic drugs excreted in bile (e.g. rifampicin) may reduce hepatic uptake of gadoxetic acid, reducing contrast enhancement. May affect some laboratory results, e.g. serum iron determination using complexometric methods may be affected, transient increase in liver enzymes, false reduction in calcium.

Generic name	Trade name	Manufacturer	Authorized indications in humans	Excretion	Properties	Protein binding	Dose	Formulations
Gadopentetic acid	Magnevist	Bayer	CNS; whole body (excluding heart); arthrography	Renal	Linear Ionic 1960 mOsm/kg	0	0.1–0.3 mmol/kg	469 mg/ml, 2 mmol/l; 5, 10, 15, 20 ml vials; 10, 15, 20 ml pre-filled syringes; 50, 100 ml pharmacy bulk package
Gadoteric acid	Dotarem	Guerbet Laboratories Ltd	CNS; whole body; MRA	Renal	Cyclic Ionic 1350 mOsm/kg	0	0.1–0.3 mmol/kg	279.3 mg/ml
Gadoteridol	Prohance	Bracco	CNS; whole body	Renal	Cyclic Non-ionic 630 mOsm/kg	0	0.1 mmol/kg	5, 10, 15, 20 ml vials; 15, 20 ml pre-filled syringes
Gadodiamide	Omniscan	Nycomed Amersham	CNS; whole body	Renal	Linear Non-ionic 789 mOsm/kg	0	0.1–0.3 mmol/kg	279.3 mg/ml 5, 10, 15, 20 ml vials; 5, 10, 15, 17 ml pre-filled syringes
Gadobutrol	Gadovist	Bayer	CNS	Renal	Cyclic Non-ionic 1603 mOsm/kg	0	0.1 mmol/kg	287 mg/ml 5, 10, 15, 20, 40, 50 ml vials; 10, 15, 20 ml pre-filled syringes
Gadoxetic acid	Primovist	Bayer	Liver	50% renal, 50% biliary	Linear Ionic 688 mOsm/kg	<15%	0.025 mmol/kg	604.72 mg/ml 7.5, 10, 15 ml vials; 7.5, 10, 15 ml pre-filled syringes; 30, 65 ml bulk packages
Gadobenic acid	MultiHance	Bracco	CNS; liver; MRA; breast	Renal (biliary up to 4%)	Linear Ionic 1970 mOsm/kg	<5%	CNS: 0.1 mmol/kg; liver: 0.05 mmol/kg	181.43 mg/ml 10 ml pre-filled syringes
Gadoversetamide	Optimark	Covidien	CNS; liver	Renal	Linear Non-ionic 1110 mOsm/kg	0	0.1 mmol/kg	334 mg/ml 5, 10, 15, 20 ml vials 330 mg/ml 10, 15, 20, 30 ml pre-filled syringes

Doses and further advice on use

Should be used routinely for MRI examinations of the brain. Use for MRI of other areas if suspect abnormal vascularization, inflammation, neoplasia, for post-surgical evaluation or if MRI study is normal. Post-contrast images should ideally be obtained within 30 minutes of contrast administration. Total doses should not exceed 0.3 mmol/kg (varies with product).

Dogs: 0.1 mmol/kg i.v. (all except gadoxetic acid). Give as bolus if performing MRA or liver studies; 0.025 mmol/kg i.v. bolus of gadoxetic acid for liver studies; 0.05 mmol/kg of gadobenic acid for liver studies. Repeat doses (not gadoxetic acid) of up to 0.3 mmol/kg total dose may be helpful in some cases if poor contrast enhancement with standard dose or for detection of metastases and if using low-field scanner. Enhancement visible up to 45–60 minutes post-administration.

Dosing small and exotic animals

Veterinary surgeons who are unfamiliar with the actions of a particular drug in a given exotic species are advised to consult more complete references (see Further reading).

The size of some animals, particularly 'exotic pets', makes dosing difficult and care must be taken when calculating small doses. Some points to bear in mind when dosing are:

- Where powders are to be dissolved in water, sterile water for injection should be used
- Most **solutions** may be diluted with water for injection or 0.9% saline
- Dilution will be necessary when volumes <0.1 ml are to be administered
- Suspensions cannot be diluted
- Use 1 ml syringes for greatest accuracy
- Specialist laboratories with a Veterinary Specials Authorization should be contacted to reformulate drugs.

Doses provided in this Formulary are for pet birds, small reptiles, etc. They should not be used for commercial poultry, large mammals or reptiles. Established poultry texts should be consulted for treating individual chickens.

Composition of intravenous fluids

Fluid	Na⁺ (mmol/l)	K⁺ (mmol/l)	Ca²⁺ (mmol/l)	Cl⁻ (mmol/l)	HCO₃⁻ (mmol/l)	Dext. (g/l)	Osmol. (mosm/l)
0.45% NaCl	77			77			155
0.9% NaCl	154			154			308
5% NaCl	856			856			1722
Ringer's	147	4	2	155			310
Lactated Ringer's (Hartmann's)	131	5	2	111	29 *		280
Darrow's	121	35		103	53 *		312
0.9% NaCl + 5.5% Dext.	154			154		50	560
0.18% NaCl + 4% Dext.	31			31		40	264
Duphalyte **		2.6	1.0	3.6		454	unknown

Dext. = Dextrose; Osmol. = Osmolality. * Bicarbonate is present as lactate.
** Also contains a mixture of vitamins and small quantities of amino acids and
1.2 mmol/l of MgSO₄

Safety and handling of chemotherapeutic agents

Most drugs used in veterinary practice do not pose a major hazard to the person handling them or handling an animal treated with them (or its waste). Chemotherapeutic agents are the exception. People who are exposed to these drugs during their use in animals risk serious side effects. In addition, chemotherapeutic agents pose a serious risk to patient welfare if not used correctly. They should only be used when absolutely indicated (i.e. histologically confirmed diseases that are known to be responsive to them). Investigational use should be confined to controlled clinical trials.

Personnel

- The preparation and administration of cytotoxic drugs should only be undertaken by trained staff.
- Owners and staff (including cleaners, animal caretakers, veterinary surgeons) involved in the care of animals being treated with cytotoxic drugs must be informed (and proof available that they have been informed) of:
  - The risks of working with cytotoxic agents
  - The potential methods for preventing aerosol formation and the spread of contamination
  - The proper working practices for a safety cabinet
  - The instructions in case of contamination
  - The principles of good personal protection and hygiene practice.

APPENDIX I: GENERAL INFORMATION

APPENDIX II: PROTOCOLS

INDEX: THERAPEUTIC CLASS

INDEX: GENERIC AND TRADE NAMES

- As a general rule, pregnant women and immunocompromised personnel should not be involved in the process of preparing and/or administering cytotoxic agents, caring for animals that have been treated with cytotoxic drugs, or cleaning of the areas these animals have come into contact with. It is the responsibility of the employee to warn their supervisors if they are pregnant, likely to become pregnant or are immunocompromised.

Equipment and facilities

- All areas where cytotoxic agents are prepared and/or administered, or where animals who have received cytotoxic drugs are being cared for, should be identified by a clear warning sign. Access to these areas should be restricted.
- Ideally a negative pressure pharmaceutical isolator with externally ducted exhaust filters, which has been properly serviced and checked, should be used. If such an isolator is not available then a suitably modified Class 2B Biological Safety Cabinet (BSC) may be used.
- There must be adequate materials for cleaning of spilled cytotoxic agents (cytotoxic spill kit).
- Closed or semi-closed systems should be used to prevent aerosol formation and control exposure to carcinogenic compounds. Special spike systems (e.g. Codan and Braun) can be used. Other systems specifically developed for the use of cytotoxic agents are recommended (e.g. Spiros, Tevadaptor, Oncovial and PhaSeal). If such systems are not available, then at the very least infusion sets and syringes with Luer-lock fittings should be used.

Preparation of cytotoxic drugs

- Manipulation of oral or topical medicines containing cytotoxic drugs should be avoided. If a drug concentration is required that is not readily available, then a specialist laboratory with a Veterinary Specials Authorisation should be contacted to reformulate the drug to the desired concentration. This may be useful for drugs such as piroxicam, hydroxycarbamide and lomustine. Tablets should never be crushed or split. If reformulation is not possible then using smaller sized tablets or adjusting the dosage regimen is often sufficient.
- When drug preparation is complete, the final product should be sealed in a plastic bag or other container for transport before it is taken out of the ventilated cabinet. It should be clearly labelled as containing cytotoxic drugs.
- All potentially contaminated materials should be discarded in special waste disposal containers, which can be opened without direct contact with hands/gloves (e.g. a foot pedal). Local regulations as to the disposal of this waste should be followed.
- There should be a clear procedure regarding how to handle cytotoxic drugs following an injection accident.
- During the preparation and administration of cytotoxic drugs, personal protection should be worn, including special disposable

chemoprotective gloves, disposable protective clothing, and eye and face protection.
- After the preparation and/or administration of cytotoxic drugs, or after nursing a treated animal, the area used should be properly cleaned using a specific protocol before other activities commence.

Administration of cytotoxic drugs

- All necessary measures should be taken to ensure that the animal being treated is calm and cooperative. If the temperament of the animal is such that a safe administration is not to be expected, then the veterinary surgeon has the right (and is obliged) not to treat these animals.
- Many cytotoxic drugs are irritant and must be administered via a preplaced i.v. catheter. Administration of bolus injections should be done through a catheter system, which should be flushed with 0.9% NaCl before, during and after the injection.
- Heparinized saline should be avoided as it can interact with some chemotherapeutic drugs (e.g. doxorubicin).
- Drugs should be administered safely using protective medical devices (such as needleless and closed systems) and techniques (such as priming of i.v. tubing by pharmacy personnel inside a ventilated cabinet or priming in line with non-drug solutions).
- The tubing should never be removed from a fluid bag containing a hazardous drug, nor should it be disconnected at other points in the system until the tubing has been thoroughly flushed. The i.v. catheter, tubing and bag should be removed intact when possible.
- Hands should be washed with soap and water before leaving the drug administration area.
- Procedures should be in place for dealing with any spillages that occur and for the safe disposal of waste. In the event of contact with skin or eyes, the affected area should be washed with copious amounts of water or normal saline. Medical advice should be sought if the eyes are affected.

Procedures for nursing patients receiving chemotherapy

- Special wards or designated kennels with clear identification that the patients are being treated with cytotoxic agents are required.
- Excreta (saliva, urine, vomit, faeces) are all potentially hazardous after the animal has been treated with cytotoxic drugs, and should be handled and disposed of accordingly.
- During the period of risk, personal protective equipment (such as disposable gloves and protective clothing) should be worn when carrying out nursing procedures.
- All materials that have come into contact with the animal during the period of risk should be considered as potentially contaminated.
- After the animal has left the ward, the cage should be cleaned according to the cleaning protocol.

APPENDIX I: GENERAL INFORMATION

APPENDIX II: PROTOCOLS

INDEX: THERAPEUTIC CLASS

INDEX: GENERIC AND TRADE NAMES

Guidelines for owners

- All owners should be given written information on the potential hazards of the cytotoxic drugs. Written information on how to deal with the patient's excreta (saliva, urine, vomit, faeces) must also be provided.
- If owners are to administer tablets themselves, then written information on how to do this must also be provided. Drug containers should be clearly labelled with 'cytotoxic contents' warning tape.

Chemotherapy of exotic species

The metabolism of small mammals, birds and reptiles is markedly different from dogs, cats and humans. Therefore, extrapolation of doses is risky to the patient and extrapolation of safety data (such as the length of time that an animal may excrete a cytotoxic drug) is risky to the owners and staff handling the animals. The lack of any proper evidence base for the use of cytotoxic agents in these species means that any attempt to use them cannot be shown to be safe, either to the animal or to the people who come into contact with that animal. For this reason doses of these agents are generally not provided in the *BSAVA Small Animal Formulary*, and the use of these agents in such species is strongly discouraged until such time as better monitoring facilities are available in veterinary practice and there are sufficient cases to undertake effective clinical trials.

Further information

For further information readers are advised to consult specialist texts and the guidelines issued by the European College of Veterinary Medicine – Companion Animals (ECVIM-CA) on 'Preventing occupational and environmental exposure to cytotoxic drugs in veterinary medicine'.

APPENDIX I: GENERAL INFORMATION

APPENDIX II: PROTOCOLS

INDEX: THERAPEUTIC CLASS

INDEX: GENERIC AND TRADE NAMES

Body weight (BW) to body surface area (BSA) conversion tables

Dogs (Formula: BSA (m^2) = 0.101 x (body weight in kg)$^{2/3}$)

BW (kg)	BSA (m^2)	BW (kg)	BSA (m^2)	BW (kg)	BSA (m^2)
0.5	0.06	11	0.50	24	0.84
1	0.1	12	0.53	26	0.89
2	0.16	13	0.56	28	0.93
3	0.21	14	0.59	30	0.98
4	0.25	15	0.61	35	1.08
5	0.30	16	0.64	40	1.18
6	0.33	17	0.67	45	1.28
7	0.37	18	0.69	50	1.37
8	0.4	19	0.72	55	1.46
9	0.44	20	0.74	60	1.55
10	0.47	22	0.79		

Cats (Formula: BSA (m^2) = 0.1 x (body weight in kg)$^{2/3}$)

BW (kg)	BSA (m^2)	BW (kg)	BSA (m^2)	BW (kg)	BSA (m^2)
0.5	0.06	2.5	0.184	4.5	0.273
1	0.1	3	0.208	5	0.292
1.5	0.134	3.5	0.231	5.5	0.316
2	0.163	4	0.252	6	0.33

Percentage solutions

The concentration of a solution may be expressed on the basis of weight per unit volume (w/v) or volume per unit volume (v/v).

% w/v = number of grams of a substance in 100 ml of a liquid
% v/v = number of ml of a substance in 100 ml of liquid

% Solution	g or ml/100 ml	mg/ml	Solution strength
100	100	1000	1:1
10	10	100	1:10
1	1	10	1:100
0.1	0.1	1	1:1000
0.01	0.01	0.1	1:10,000

Drugs usage in renal and hepatic insufficiency

With failure of liver or kidney, the excretion of some drugs may be impaired, leading to increased serum concentrations.

Renal failure

a. Double the dosing interval or halve the dosage in patients with severe renal insufficiency. Use for drugs that are relatively non-toxic.
b. Increase dosing interval 2-fold when creatinine clearance (Ccr) is 0.5–1.0 ml/min/kg, 3-fold when Ccr is 0.3–0.5 ml/min/kg and 4-fold when Ccr is <0.3 ml/min/kg.
c. Precise dose modification is required for some toxic drugs that are excreted solely by glomerular filtration, e.g. aminoglycosides. This is determined by using the dose fraction K_f to amend the drug dose or dosing interval according to the following equations:

Modified dose reduction = normal dose × K_f
Modified dose interval = normal dose interval/K_f
where K_f = patient Ccr/normal Ccr

Where Ccr is unavailable, Ccr may be estimated at 88.4/serum creatinine (μmol/l) (where serum creatinine is <350 μmol/l). Kf may be estimated at 0.33 if urine is isosthenuric or 0.25 if the patient is azotaemic.

Drug	Nephrotoxic	Dose adjustment in renal failure
Amikacin	Yes	c
Amoxicillin	No	a
Amphotericin B	Yes	c
Ampicillin	No	a
Cefalexin	No	b
Chloramphenicol	No	N, A
Digoxin	No	c
Gentamicin	Yes	c
Nitrofurantoin	No	CI
Oxytetracycline	Yes	CI
Penicillin	No	a
Streptomycin	Yes	b
Tobramycin	Yes	c
Trimethoprim/ sulphonamide	Yes	b, A

a, b, c = Refer to section above on dose adjustment; A = Avoid in severe renal failure; CI = Contraindicated; N = normal dose.

Hepatic insufficiency

Drug clearance by the liver is affected by many factors and thus it is not possible to apply a simple formula to drug dosing. The table below is adapted from information in the human literature.

Drug	DI	CI
Aspirin		✓
Azathioprine		✓
Cefotaxime	✓	
Chloramphenicol		✓
Clindamycin		✓
Cyclophosphamide	✓	
Diazepam		✓
Doxorubicin	✓	
Doxycycline	✓	
Fluorouracil		✓
Furosemide	✓	
Hydralazine	✓	
Lidocaine	✓	
Metronidazole	✓	
Morphine	✓	
NSAIDs	✓	
Oxytetracycline		✓
Pentazocine		✓
Pentobarbital	✓	
Phenobarbital	✓	
Propranolol	✓	
Theophylline	✓	
Vincristine	✓	

CI = Contraindicated; avoid use if at all possible. DI = A change in dose or dosing interval may be required.

APPENDIX I: GENERAL INFORMATION

APPENDIX II: PROTOCOLS

INDEX: THERAPEUTIC CLASS

INDEX: GENERIC AND TRADE NAMES

Suspected Adverse Reaction Surveillance Scheme (SARSS)

The Veterinary Medicines Directorate has a website (www.vmd.gov.uk/) to report any and all suspected adverse reactions in an animal or a human to a veterinary medicinal product, or in an animal treated with a human medicine. Anyone can report a suspected adverse reaction in this way. An 'adverse reaction' includes lack of efficacy and known side effects. It is only by completing such forms that the changes in the prevalence of problems can be documented.

The online report form is preferred; however, if you would prefer to use a paper copy you can download and print an Animal Form to report an adverse reaction in an animal to a veterinary medicine or to a human product. Alternatively, download and print a Human Form to report an adverse reaction in a human to a veterinary medicinal product. Post the forms to the address at the top of the reports.

If you have any questions please call the pharmacovigilance team on 01932 338427.

Further reading

British National Formulary No. 66 (2013) British Medical Association and the Royal Pharmaceutical Society of Great Britain

Carpenter JW (2012) *Exotic Animal Formulary, 4th edn*. Saunders Elsevier, St Louis

Compendium of Data Sheets for Animal Medicines (2013) National Office of Animal Health, Enfield, Middlesex

Monthly Index of Medical Specialties (2013) Haymarket Medical Publications, London

Papich MG (2010) *Saunders Handbook of Veterinary Drugs, 3rd edn*. Saunders Elsevier, St Louis

Plumb DC (2011) *Plumb's Veterinary Drug Handbook, 7th edn*. Blackwell Publishing

Giguére S, Prescott JF, Baggot JD and Walker RD (2013) *Antimicrobial Therapy in Veterinary Medicine, 5th edn*. Wiley Blackwell, Iowa

Useful websites

www.bnf.org
British National Formulary – registration required through academic institutions to use BNF online but can order paper copy of BNF from this site.

www.bsava.com
British Small Animal Veterinary Association – useful forums and links to *Journal of Small Animal Practice* and the *BSAVA Guide to the Use of Veterinary Medicines*. Searchable online Formulary available to members.

www.chemopet.co.uk
Chemopet – company that will reformulate a wide range of injectable and oral chemotherapy drugs.

www.emea.europa.eu/ema/
European Medicines Agency.

www.wiley.com
Journal of Small Animal Practice – free for BSAVA members, free abstracts and pay per article for others.

www.ncbi.nlm.nih.gov/pubmed
PubMed is a widely used free service of the U.S. National Library of Medicine and the National Institutes of Health that allows users to search abstracts in the medical literature. All major veterinary publications covered.

www.noahcompendium.co.uk/Compendium/Overview/
NOAH compendium site.

www.novalabs.co.uk/
Site for a company that will reformulate many drugs into conveniently sized tablets.

www.specialslab.co.uk
Site for a company that will reformulate many drugs into conveniently sized tablets.

www.vmd.defra.gov.uk/
Veterinary Medicines Directorate – in particular is useful for repeat applications for special import certificates (SICs) and special treatment certificates (STCs) and the electronic Summary of Product Characteristics (eSPCs).

Appendix II: protocols

Chemotherapy protocols for lymphoma

Various protocols are described in the literature. Three examples are provided below.

Protocol 1: Combination cytotoxic therapy COP (low dose)

Induction:
Cyclophosphamide: 50 mg/m^2 p.o. on alternate days or 50 mg/m^2 p.o. for the first 4 days of each week
Vincristine: 0.5 mg/m^2 i.v. q7d
Prednisolone: 40 mg/m^2 p.o. q24h for first 7 days then 20 mg/m^2 p.o. on alternate days and given with cyclophosphamide

Maintenance after a minimum of 2 months:
Cyclophosphamide: 50 mg/m^2 p.o. on alternate days or 50 mg/m^2 p.o. for the first 4 days of each second week (alternate week therapy)
Vincristine: 0.5 mg/m^2 i.v. q14d
Prednisolone: 20 mg/m^2 p.o. on alternate days of each second week and given with cyclophosphamide

Maintenance after 6 months (if disease in remission):
Cyclophosphamide: 50 mg/m^2 p.o. q48h (one week in three) or 50 mg/m^2 p.o. for the first 4 days of each third week (one week in three)
Vincristine: 0.5 mg/m^2 i.v. q21d
Prednisolone: 20 mg/m^2 p.o. on alternate days of each third week and given with cyclophosphamide

Maintenance after 12 months:
Cyclophosphamide: 50 mg/m^2 p.o. q48h (one week in four) or 50 mg/m^2 p.o. for the first 4 days of each fourth week (one week in four)
Vincristine: 0.5 mg/m^2 i.v. q28d
Prednisolone: 20 mg/m^2 p.o. on alternate days of each fourth week and given with cyclophosphamide

General notes:

- GI protectants: ranitidine 2 mg/kg q12h p.o., sucralfate 500 mg/dog p.o. q8h (dogs up to 20 kg), 1–2 g/dog p.o. q 8h (dogs >20 kg) are recommended for first 14 days. Cimetidine is avoided due to its effect on the hepatic cytochrome P450 enzyme pathway and the potential for altering metabolism of chemotherapeutics.
- Melphalan (5 mg/m^2 p.o.) may be administered as an alternative to cyclophosphamide after 6 months in order to reduce the risk of haemorrhagic cystitis.
- Chlorambucil (5 mg/m^2 p.o. on alternate days) or melphalan may be given as alternatives for cyclophosphamide if haemorrhagic cystitis develops.

APPENDIX I: GENERAL INFORMATION

APPENDIX II: PROTOCOLS

INDEX: THERAPEUTIC CLASS

INDEX: GENERIC AND TRADE NAMES

- Doxorubicin (30 mg/m^2 i.v. q3wk) or crisantaspase (400 IU/kg s.c., i.m. q7d or as necessary) may be used to manage relapsing or recurrent disease. (Refer to specialist texts or advice regarding protocols for treating relapsed lymphoma.)

Recommended monitoring:

- Haematology every 4 weeks
- Urine – dipstick every 1–2 weeks in the first 2 months. Full urinalysis prior to first dose, then as required.

Contraindications and adverse effects

Myelosuppression, haemorrhagic cystitis (cyclophosphamide only) or GI effects may occur. Peripheral neuropathies, although reported, are rare. Discontinue cyclophosphamide therapy if the neutrophil count decreases to <2 x 10^9/l; check count weekly and do not resume treatment until neutrophil count is >3 x 10^9/l. If neutropenia recurs following reinstitution of therapy, decrease dosage by one quarter.

Protocol 2: Combination cytotoxic therapy COP (high dose)

Induction:
Cyclophosphamide: 250 mg/m^2 p.o. q21d
Vincristine: 0.75 mg/m^2 i.v. q7d for 4 weeks then 0.75 mg/m^2 i.v. q21d administered with cyclophosphamide
Prednisolone: 1 mg/kg p.o. q24h for 4 weeks then 1 mg/kg p.o. on alternate days

Maintenance after 6 months:
Cyclophosphamide: 250 mg/m^2 p.o. q28d
Vincristine: 0.75 mg/m^2 i.v. q28d with cyclophosphamide
Prednisolone: 1 mg/kg p.o. on alternate days

Maintenance after 12 months:
Cyclophosphamide: 250 mg/m^2 p.o. q28d
Vincristine: 0.75 mg/m^2 i.v. q5 weeks
Prednisolone: 1 mg/kg p.o. on alternate days

Maintenance after 18 months:
Cyclophosphamide: 250 mg/m^2 p.o. q28d
Vincristine: 0.75 mg/m^2 i.v. q6 weeks
Prednisolone: 1 mg/kg p.o. on alternate days

Maintenance after 24 months:
Stop if in remission

General notes:

- GI protectants: ranitidine 2 mg/kg q12h p.o., sucralfate 500 mg/dog p.o. q8h (dogs up to 20 kg), 1–2 g/dog p.o. q 8h (dogs >20 kg) are recommended for first 14 days. Cimetidine is avoided due to its effect on the hepatic cytochrome P450 enzyme pathway and the potential for altering metabolism of chemotherapeutics.

- Melphalan (5 mg/m^2 p.o.) may be administered as an alternative to cyclophosphamide after 6 months in order to reduce the risk of haemorrhagic cystitis.
- Chlorambucil (5 mg/m^2 p.o. on alternate days) or melphalan may be given as alternatives for cyclophosphamide if haemorrhagic cystitis develops.
- Doxorubicin (30 mg/m^2 i.v. q3wk) or crisantaspase (400 IU/kg i.m. q7d or as necessary) may be used to manage relapsing or recurrent disease. (Refer to specialist texts or advice regarding protocols for treating relapsed lymphoma.)

Recommended monitoring:

- Haematology every 4 weeks
- Urine – dipstick weekly and full urinalysis every 4 weeks.

Contraindications and adverse effects
Myelosuppression, haemorrhagic cystitis (cyclophosphamide only) or GI effects may occur. Peripheral neuropathies, although reported, are rare. Discontinue cyclophosphamide therapy if the neutrophil count decreases to <2 x 10^9/l; check count weekly and do not resume treatment until neutrophil count is >3 x 10^9/l. If neutropenia recurs following reinstitution of therapy, decrease dosage by one quarter.

Protocol 3: Combination cytotoxic therapy Madison–Wisconsin

Week 1
Vincristine: 0.7 mg/m^2 i.v. once
Prednisolone: 2 mg/kg p.o. q24h
Crisantaspase: 400 IU/kg s.c., i.m. once
NB Many oncologists now use the CHOP protocol, which is based on this protocol but with the omission of crisantaspase in weeks 1 and 2

Week 2
Cyclophosphamide: 250 mg/m^2 p.o. once
Prednisolone: 1.5 mg/kg p.o. q24h
Furosemide: 2.0–2.2 mg/kg s.c., i.v.
Crisantaspase: 400 IU/kg s.c., i.m. once *can be administered if remission is not achieved*

Week 3
Vincristine: 0.7 mg/m^2 i.v. once
Prednisolone: 1 mg/kg p.o. q24h

Week 4
Doxorubicin: 30 mg/m^2 i.v. once (in 0.9% NaCl) given over 20 minutes
(Chlorphenamine 2–10 mg/dog i.m. once and maropitant 1 mg/kg s.c. once are given *before* doxorubicin)
Prednisolone: 0.5 mg/kg p.o. q24h for one week

Week 5
No medication (prednisolone is stopped)

APPENDIX I: GENERAL INFORMATION

APPENDIX II: PROTOCOLS

INDEX: THERAPEUTIC CLASS

INDEX: GENERIC AND TRADE NAMES

Week 6
Vincristine: 0.7 mg/m^2 i.v. once

Week 7
Cyclophosphamide: 250 mg/m^2 p.o., i.v.
Furosemide: 2.0–2.2 mg/kg s.c., i.v.

Week 8
Vincristine: 0.7 mg/m^2 i.v. once

Week 9
Doxorubicin: 30 mg/m^2 i.v. once (in 0.9% NaCl) given over 20 minutes.
(Chlorphenamine 2–10 mg/dog i.m. once and maropitant 1 mg/kg s.c.
once are given *before* doxorubicin)

Week 10
No medication

Week 11
Vincristine: 0.7 mg/m^2 i.v. once

Week 12
No medication

Week 13
Cyclophosphamide: 250 mg/m^2 p.o., i.v. once
Furosemide: 2.0–2.2 mg/kg s.c., i.v.

Week 14
No medication

Week 15
Vincristine: 0.7 mg/m^2 i.v. once

Week 16
No medication

Week 17
Doxorubicin: 30 mg/m^2 i.v. (in 0.9% NaCl) given over 20 minutes.
(Chlorphenamine 2–10 mg/dog i.m. once and maropitant 1 mg/kg s.c.
once are given *before* doxorubicin)

Week 18
No medication

Week 19
Vincristine: 0.7 mg/m^2 i.v. once

Week 20
No medication

Week 21
Cyclophosphamide: 250 mg/m^2 p.o., i.v. once
Furosemide: 2.0–2.2 mg/kg s.c., i.v.

Week 22
No medication

Week 23
Vincristine: 0.7 mg/m^2 i.v. once

Week 24
No medication

Week 25
Doxorubicin: 30 mg/m^2 i.v. once (in 0.9% NaCl) given over 20 minutes. (Chlorphenamine 2–10 mg/dog i.m. once and maropitant 1 mg/kg s.c. once are given *before* doxorubicin)

Re-staging (which may include haematology and biochemistry blood tests, thoracic radiography and abdominal ultrasonography) is usually scheduled for 1, 3 and 6 months post cessation of chemotherapy. A post-doxorubicin echocardiogram is usually scheduled for one month post chemotherapy cessation.

General notes:

- In dogs <10 kg, use doxorubicin at a dose of 1 mg/kg i.v. once.
- If reduced cardiac contractility, doxorubicin can be substituted by epirubicin 30 mg/m^2 or mitoxantrone 5.5 mg/m^2 (both i.v. in 0.9% NaCl).
- If sterile haemorrhagic cystitis occurs on cyclophosphamide, discontinue and substitute chlorambucil (1.4 mg/kg p.o.) for subsequently scheduled doses.
- Crisantaspase (400 IU/kg i.m., s.c.) can be given with each vincristine injection until clinical remission is achieved. Chlorphenamine (2–10 mg/dog i.m. once) should be given before the crisantaspase.
- GI protectants: ranitidine 2 mg/kg q12h p.o., sucralfate 500 mg/dog p.o. q8h (dogs up to 20 kg), 1–2 g/dog p.o. q8h (dogs >20 kg) are recommended for first 14 days. Cimetidine is avoided due to its effect on the hepatic cytochrome P450 enzyme pathway and the potential for altering metabolism of chemotherapeutics.
- After initial 6 months all medication is stopped until a relapse occurs.

Suggested monitoring:

- Haematology is done every week with treatment
- Urinalysis is done on weeks 0, 3, 8, 15 and 23
- (Biochemistry may be done on week 8)
- Baseline echocardiography – should be done before giving doxorubicin.

Contraindications and adverse effects
Myelosuppression, haemorrhagic cystitis (cyclophosphamide only), cardiotoxicity (doxorubicin only) or GI effects may occur. Peripheral neuropathies, although reported, are rare. Discontinue chemotherapy

therapy if the neutrophil count decreases to <2 × 10^9/l; check count weekly and do not resume treatment until neutrophil count is >3 × 10^9/l. Patients may require hospitalization or antibiosis if the neutrophil count is <2, or if they have clinical signs of infection/sepsis – consult a specialist text or oncologist for advice as required. If neutropenia recurs following reinstitution of therapy, decrease dosage by 25%.

Immunosuppression protocols

There are many protocols described in the literature for different immune-mediated diseases: three examples are provided here. It is vitally important that the diagnosis of immune-mediated disease is confirmed before undertaking any of these protocols.

Protocol 1: Canine immune-mediated haemolytic anaemia and immune-mediated thrombocytopenia

Induction

Immunosuppression: Prednisolone: 40 mg/m^2 p.o. q24h (<10 kg body weight, 2 mg/kg p.o. q24h) and azathioprine (2 mg/kg p.o. q24h) are preferred to prednisolone on its own. **See Appendix I for safety and handling of chemotherapeutic agents.** Dexamethasone (0.3–0.5 mg/kg i.v. q24h) may be substituted for prednisolone if the patient is unable to tolerate oral medications. Mycophenolate mofetil (MMF) (7–10 mg/kg i.v. q12h) can be substituted for azathioprine if:

- Patient is unable to tolerate oral medications
- Patient has historical evidence of a rapid (>10% in 24 hours) fall in haematocrit prior to presentation
- Patient has gross evidence of spontaneous agglutination (as documented by a haematologist)
- Patient has evidence of intravascular haemolysis (haemoglobinuria, haemoglobinaemia)
- Patient has evidence of pancreatitis on biochemistry or physical examination.

Once patient is able to tolerate oral medications, then substitute prednisolone for dexamethasone and switch to oral dosing of mycophenolate mofetil (10 mg/kg p.o. q12h) or, if preferred, azathioprine at the above doses.

Antithrombotics: Aspirin (0.5 mg/kg p.o. q24h unless thrombocytopenic) may improve survival in dogs. If active GI ulceration, renal disease, or the patient is intolerant of oral medications, then low molecular weight heparin (100 IU s.c. q12h) can be used. There are no studies currently on clopidogrel, but this may be appropriate. Heparin should be administered (concurrently with aspirin unless there are any contraindications) if there is clinical evidence of thromboembolic disease. Discontinue on remission.

Antibiotics: Not required unless there is a documented infection, known risk of infection (e.g. GI barrier compromise, previous endocarditis) or known exposure to ticks.

Gastrointestinal protection: In general not required. Sucralfate is optional, but if given should be given 2 hours before other medications. In cases with known or suspected GI bleeding (particularly cases with immune-mediated thrombocytopenia), effective suppression of gastric acid secretion is required. Current evidence suggests that only famotidine and omeprazole will provide this. The practice of administering ranitidine etc. to every animal receiving high doses of steroids is not necessary and likely ineffective.

Relapse and rescue
If a mild relapse (e.g. a fall in PCV of <5% without any clinical signs of anaemia) occurs following documented remission, this may be treated by re-instigating the drug dosages used at the last visit when the patient was in remission. Severe relapses should be treated by re-instigation of induction doses of all drugs used initially. If this is ineffective (i.e. no response (increase in haemocrit by <5% despite ongoing regenerative response) within 6 days), or if rescue is to be attempted during initial induction phase of treatment (due to progressive deterioration), then ciclosporin (5–7.5 mg/kg p.o. q24h) may be beneficial. If there is no response to the ciclosporin within 5 days and/or the patient continues to deteriorate over that time or if the patient is not tolerant to oral medications, then consider immunoglobulin (0.5–1.0 g/kg i.v. over 6–8 hours). Note that immunoglobulin is best utilized for acute deteriorations. In the non-acute setting, or if long-term control is necessary in a patient that has previously failed all other orally administered drugs, then consider leflunomide (4 mg/kg p.o. q24h).

Decreasing doses
Maintain on induction doses until remission (normal PCV with no evidence of ongoing immune activation) is achieved assuming no suspected/known side effects to the drug(s).

Week	Glucocorticoid	Azathioprine/ MMF	Immunosuppressant 3 (if used)	GI protectants (if used)
Remission	1 mg/kg q24h	UC	UC	UC
2	0.5 mg/kg q24h	UC	UC	STOP
4	0.5 mg/kg every other day	UC	STOP	
6	0.25 mg/kg every other day	UC		
8	STOP	50% dose reduction		
10		UC		
12		UC		
14		STOP		

UC = Dose unchanged.

General notes:
Haematology to be rechecked at each visit (including weeks 14 and 18) and remission confirmed prior to each dose reduction.
Liver parameters should be rechecked at remission and weeks 4 and 8 (if on azathioprine).

Protocol 2: Feline immune-mediated haemolytic anaemia

Induction
Immunosuppression: Prednisolone: 2 mg/kg p.o. q12h and either of the following:

- Chlorambucil: >4 kg body weight, 2 mg p.o. q48h; <4 kg body weight, 2 mg p.o. q72h
- Mycophenolic acid (MPA): 10 mg/kg p.o. q12h
- **See Appendix I for safety and handling of chemotherapeutic agents.**

Mycophenolic acid is preferred if:

- Patient has historical evidence of a rapid (>10% in 24 hours) fall in haematocrit prior to presentation
- Patient has gross evidence of spontaneous agglutination (as documented by a haematologist)
- Patient has evidence of intravascular haemolysis (haemoglobinuria, haemoglobinaemia).

If the patient is unable to tolerate oral medications, then dexamethasone (0.6–1.0 mg/kg i.v. q24h) may be substituted for prednisolone and mycophenolate mofetil (MMF) (7–10 mg/kg i.v. q12h) may be substituted for mycophenolic acid.

Antithrombotics: Avoid in cats as there is no evidence of efficacy and risk of side effects.

Antibiotics: Not required unless there is a documented infection, known risk of infection (e.g. GI barrier compromise, previous endocarditis) or known exposure to ticks.

Gastrointestinal protection: Not required unless GI bleeding has been diagnosed. Effective suppression of gastric acid production is then required. Current evidence suggests that only famotidine and omeprazole will provide this. The practice of administering ranitidine etc. to every animal receiving high doses of steroids is not necessary and likely ineffective.

Relapse and rescue
See Protocol 1: Canine immune-mediated haemolytic anaemia and immune-mediated thrombocytopenia for details.

Decreasing doses
See Protocol 1: Canine immune-mediated haemolytic anaemia and immune-mediated thrombocytopenia for details.
(Note: reports of feline immune-mediated thrombocytopenia are too rare to provide a protocol for treatment, but it is likely that a similar approach should be adopted.)

Protocol 3: Steroid-responsive meningitis

Induction

Immunosuppression: Prednisolone: 2 mg/kg p.o. q12h for 2 days and then reduce to 1 mg/kg p.o. q12h for 12 days. Dexamethasone (0.6 mg/kg i.v. q24h) may be substituted for prednisolone for the first 2 days if the patient is unable to tolerate oral medications at first presentation.

Remission: If remission is achieved, then 0.5 mg/kg p.o. q12h for 6 weeks followed by 0.5 mg/kg p.o. q24h for 6 weeks, followed by 0.5 mg/kg p.o. q48h for 6 weeks, followed by 0.5 mg/kg p.o. q72h for 6 weeks, then stop.

Relapse: In the event of a relapse during or after completion of the protocol (or if remission is not achieved), then 1 mg/kg p.o. q12h can be re-instigated (or continued if remission not achieved) for a further 2 weeks, and then continued as the 24-week remission protocol.

Antibiotics: Not required unless there is a documented infection, known risk of infection (e.g. GI barrier compromise, previous endocarditis) or known exposure to ticks.

Gastrointestinal protection: In general not required. Sucralfate is optional, but if given should be given 2 hours before other medications. The practice of administering ranitidine etc. to every animal receiving high doses of steroids is not necessary and likely ineffective.

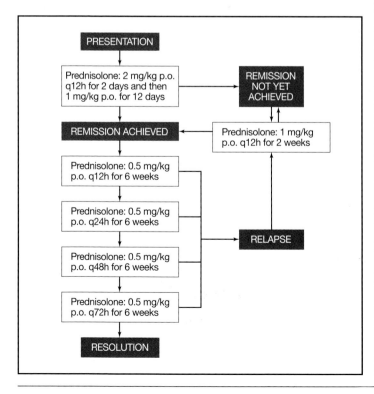

Sedation/immobilization protocols

Sedative combinations for dogs

Acepromazine (ACP) as sole agent: Acepromazine alone is not a particularly effective sedative. For further information see monograph.

ACP/opioid mixtures (neuroleptanalgesia): Acepromazine used in combination with opioid analgesics reduces the dose requirement of both components and also the incidence of adverse effects. Acepromazine (0.01–0.05 mg/kg, except in Boxers 0.005–0.01 mg/kg) can be combined with:

- Pethidine (2–10 mg/kg i.m.)
- Methadone (0.1–0.5 mg/kg i.m., i.v.)
- Papaveretum (0.05–0.4 mg/kg i.v., i.m.)
- Buprenorphine (0.02–0.03 mg/kg i.v., i.m.
- Butorphanol (0.1–0.4 mg/kg i.v., i.m.)

Alpha-2 agonists as sole agents: Although authorized for single-agent use, it is generally preferable to use medetomidine or dexmedetomidine in combination with opioids (see below).

Recommended dose in dogs and cats of medetomidine is 5–20 μg (micrograms)/kg i.m. and of dexmedetomidine is 2.5–10 μg (micrograms)/kg i.m. Repeated dosing is not advised. Although both drugs are authorized for use at up to 4 times these doses, such higher doses are associated with marked effects on cardiopulmonary function. Low doses (2.5–5 μg (micrograms)/kg) of medetomidine or dexmedetomidine may be given intravenously.

Adverse effects may be antagonized with i.m. atipamezole at 5 times the agonist dose rate; the (unauthorized) i.v. route is preferable in critical situations.

For information on xylazine see below.

The use of alpha-2 agonists for sedation is only recommended in healthy animals.

Alpha-2 agonist/opioid mixtures: Including opioids with medetomidine or dexmedetomidine lowers the dose required to achieve a given level of sedation, thereby limiting the marked effects that alpha-2 agonists exert on cardiopulmonary function. If sedation is still inadequate, it is better to proceed to induction of general anaesthesia using an i.v. induction agent, such as alfaxalone or propofol, rather than by giving a repeated or higher dose of alpha-2 agonist.

Medetomidine or dexmedetomidine, at the doses described above, can be combined with:

- Pethidine (2–10 mg/kg i.m.)

- Methadone (0.1–0.4 mg/kg i.m., slow i.v.)
- Buprenorphine (0.02–0.03 mg/kg slow i.v., i.m.)
- Butorphanol (0.1–0.4 mg/kg slow i.v., i.m.).

Although xylazine (1–3 mg/kg) may be used alone or in combinations with opioids, given i.m. or i.v. (unauthorized), its use in dogs and cats has been superseded by use of medetomidine or dexmedetomidine, and it is not recommended. Adverse effects may be antagonized with i.m. or i.v. atipamezole, although this use is unauthorized.

Acepromazine/alpha-2 agonist/opioid mixtures: A mixture of acepromazine (0.05 mg/kg) with any of the combinations given for alpha-2 agonists and alpha-2 agonist/opioid mixtures (higher end of dose ranges) is suitable for the chemical restraint of large, dangerously aggressive dogs. Severe depression can be antagonized using naloxone and atipamezole.

Low doses of acepromazine (0.01 mg/kg) and medetomidine (2.5–5 μg (micrograms)/kg) or dexmedetomidine (2.5–5 μg (micrograms)/kg) combined with opioid agonist drugs provide profound sedation without signs of severe cardiopulmonary depression.

Benzodiazepines and benzodiazepine/opioid mixtures:
Benzodiazepines do not reliably sedate healthy dogs when used alone; indeed, stimulation ranging from increased motor activity to gross excitation may be seen. The risk of excitation is proportional to the health of the recipient: the chances of producing sedation are highest (but not guaranteed) in very sick cases. Diazepam or midazolam (0.2–0.3 mg/kg i.v.) given during anaesthesia can smooth recovery in animals prone to excitability, provided adequate analgesia is present.

Opioid/benzodiazepine mixtures are satisfactory and relatively safe in critically ill animals. These combinations are more effective when given i.v. (with the exception of pethidine). Transient excitation may occur when given by this route. When given i.m., excitation is unlikely although the depth of sedation is also reduced. Midazolam or diazepam at the dose described above can be given with:

- Pethidine (2–10 mg/kg i.m.)
- Methadone (0.2–0.3 mg/kg i.v., i.m.)
- Papaveretum (0.2–0.5 mg/kg i.v., i.m.)
- Buprenorphine (0.02–0.03 mg/kg i.v., i.m.)
- Butorphanol (0.1–0.4 mg/kg i.v., i.m.)
- Fentanyl (0.01 mg/kg slow i.v.).

Alfaxalone: Although not authorized for this use, 2 mg/kg i.m. will provide sedation in dogs lasting 10–15 minutes.

APPENDIX I: GENERAL INFORMATION

APPENDIX II: PROTOCOLS

INDEX: THERAPEUTIC CLASS

INDEX: GENERIC AND TRADE NAMES

General notes:

- A well managed light level of general (inhalational) anaesthesia is frequently safer than heavy sedation in sick animals.
- Neuroleptanalgesic combinations are safer than alpha-2 agonist/opioid mixtures, but are less likely to produce adequate conditions for minor operations or investigations involving abnormal body positions. Furthermore, only the opioid component can be antagonized.
- Most of the aforementioned combinations will have a profound sparing effect on i.v. and inhalational anaesthetics, should a general anaesthetic be required after sedation. This is particularly true of combinations containing alpha-2 agonists.

Sedative combinations for cats

Acepromazine: Acepromazine alone is not a particularly effective sedative and increasing the dose incurs the same problems as in dogs. Doses of 0.01–0.1 mg/kg may be given i.v., i.m. or s.c. Cats often require higher doses of acepromazine than dogs to achieve comparable sedation.

Neuroleptanalgesia: Neuroleptanalgesic combinations confer the same advantages in cats as in dogs. Acepromazine (0.01–0.1 mg/kg) can be combined with:

- Pethidine (2–10 mg/kg i.m.)
- Methadone (0.1–0.5 mg/kg i.v., i.m.)
- Papaveretum (0.05–0.4 mg/kg i.v., i.m.)
- Buprenorphine (0.02–0.03 mg/kg i.v., i.m.)
- Butorphanol (0.1–0.4 mg/kg i.v., i.m.).

Use the lower end of the dose ranges i.v.

Alpha-2 agonists as sole agents and alpha-2 agonist/opioid mixtures: See information given for dogs.

Benzodiazepines:
Diazepam (0.2–0.3 mg/kg) or midazolam (0.2–0.3 mg/kg) i.v. can provide satisfactory sedation in very sick cats. The inclusion of opioids at doses given for alpha-2 agonist/opioid mixtures may improve conditions, but benzodiazepine/opioid combinations do not provide reliable sedation in most cats.

Ketamine and ketamine-based techniques:
Ketamine is relatively safe in ill animals, but high doses cause prolonged recoveries and are associated with muscle rigidity. Acepromazine (0.05–0.1 mg/kg) with midazolam (0.25 mg/kg) or diazepam (0.25 mg/kg) and ketamine at 2.5 or 7.5 mg/kg, mixed and injected i.m., provides good conditions with only modest cardiopulmonary depression. The higher doses of ketamine should

be used in excitable animals undergoing more stimulating interventions. Lower doses of acepromazine and/or ketamine may be used in very ill animals, although acepromazine should be avoided in animals with cardiovascular collapse due to vasodilation.

Alternatives: Ketamine (2.5 mg/kg) combined with diazepam or midazolam (0.2–0.3 mg/kg) i.v. provides profound sedation which lasts for about 15–20 minutes. Higher doses of ketamine (5 mg/kg) may be required if given i.m. This combination is preferred over ketamine/acepromazine combinations in sick cats. Diazepam can cause pain on injection, therefore use of midazolam is preferred.

Ketamine (5 mg/kg) with medetomidine 10–40 μg (micrograms)/kg i.m. produces profound sedation but should only be used in healthy cats. Atipamezole may be given if severe problems are encountered.

Although ketamine elimination depends heavily on renal function in cats, a full recovery still occurs, albeit more slowly, in animals with renal disease or urinary tract obstruction. However, low doses should be used in such cases.

Alfaxalone: Although not authorized for this use, 2 mg/kg i.m. will provide sedation in cats lasting 10–15 minutes.

General notes:

* Careful handling and restraint to achieve injection of sedative is preferred, but a crush cage is useful for restraining violent cats. If injection of sedatives proves impossible, anaesthesia can be induced using a large induction chamber into which volatile anaesthetic agents can be delivered via an anaesthetic machine. Most of the aforementioned combinations will have a profound sparing effect on i.v. and inhalational anaesthetics should a general anaesthetic be required after sedation. This is particularly true of combinations containing alpha-2 agonists.
* The high body surface area to volume ratio of cats results in rapid heat loss compared with dogs. Attention to thermoregulation must be diligent.

Sedative combinations for exotic pets

Ferrets:

* Ketamine (5–8 mg/kg i.m.) plus medetomidine (80–100 μg (micrograms)/kg) i.m.) or dexmedetomidine (40–50 μg (micrograms)/kg i.m.) to which can be added butorphanol (0.1–0.2 mg/kg i.m.) or buprenorphine (0.02 mg/kg i.m.).
* Ketamine (5–20 mg/kg i.m.) plus midazolam (0.25–0.5 mg/kg i.m.) or diazepam (0.25–0.5 mg/kg i.m.) will provide immobilization or, at the higher doses, a short period of anaesthesia.

APPENDIX I: GENERAL INFORMATION

APPENDIX II: PROTOCOLS

INDEX: THERAPEUTIC CLASS

INDEX: GENERIC AND TRADE NAMES

Rabbits:

- Ketamine (3–5 mg/kg i.v. or 5–10 mg/kg i.m., s.c.) in combination with medetomidine (0.05–0.1 mg/kg i.v., 0.1–0.3 mg/kg s.c., i.m.) or dexmedetomidine (0.025–0.05 mg/kg i.v. or 0.05–0.15 mg/kg s.c., i.m.) and butorphanol (0.05–0.1 mg/kg) or buprenorphine (0.02–0.05 mg/kg i.m., i.v., s.c.).
- Fentanyl/fluanisone (0.1–0.3 ml/kg i.m.) plus diazepam (0.5–1 mg/kg i.v., i.m. or 2.5–5.0 mg/kg i.p.) or midazolam (0.25–1.0 mg/kg i.v., i.m., i.p.).

Other small mammals:

- Medetomidine (50 μg (micrograms)/kg i.m.) or dexmedetomidine (25 μg (micrograms)/kg i.m.) plus, if needed, ketamine (2–4 mg/kg i.m.).
- Other combinations as for rabbits.

NB. Reduce doses if animal is debilitated.

Birds:

Injectable anaesthesia is best avoided unless in field situations (i.e. no gaseous anaesthesia available) or for the induction of large (e.g. swans/ratites), diving (e.g. ducks) or high-altitude birds. Even in these species, gaseous induction and maintenance (e.g. with isoflurane/sevoflurane) would still be the normal recommendation wherever possible. Sedation and premedicants are rarely used, as extra handling will add to the general stress of the situation. On occasions, diazepam (0.2–0.5 mg/kg i.m.) or midazolam (0.1–0.5 mg/kg i.m.) may be used; alternatively, either drug may be used at 0.05–0.15 mg/kg i.v. Parasympatholytic agents (such as atropine) are rarely used as their effect is to make respiratory secretions more viscous, thus increasing the risk of tube blockage.

- Propofol (10 mg i.v. by slow infusion to effect: supplemental doses up to 3 mg/kg).
- Alfaxalone (2–4 mg/kg i.v.) is an alternative to propofol for the induction of anaesthesia in large birds or those with a dive response.
- Ketamine/diazepam combinations can be used for induction and muscle relaxation. Ketamine (30–40 mg/kg) plus diazepam (1.0–1.5 mg/kg) are given slowly i.v. to effect.
  May also be given i.m. but this produces different effects in different species and specific literature or specialist advise should be consulted.
- Raptors: ketamine (2–5 mg/kg i.m.) plus medetomidine (25–100 μg (micrograms)/kg) (lower dose rate i.v.; higher rate i.m.). This combination can be reversed with atipamezole at 65 μg (micrograms)/kg i.m. Ketamine should be avoided in vultures.

Reptiles:

- Ketamine (20–60 mg/kg i.m. in chelonians; 25–60 mg/kg i.m. in lizards; 20–80 mg/kg i.m. in snakes). NB. Use lower end of dosage for sedation in all species. Recovery may be prolonged even with low dosages in debilitated, particularly renally compromised, patients. For such patients butorphanol (0.4 mg/kg i.m.) plus midazolam (2 mg/kg i.m.) may be safer.
- Ketamine (5–10 mg/kg i.m.) plus medetomidine (100–200 μg (micrograms)/kg) (deep sedation to light anaesthesia); may reverse medetomidine with atipamezole at 5 times the medetomidine dose (i.e. 0.5–1.0 mg/kg atipamezole).
- Ketamine (10–30 mg/kg i.m.) plus butorphanol (0.5–1 mg/kg i.m.) has also been recommended for deep sedation.
- Chelonians, snakes: sedation to light anaesthesia: ketamine (20–60 mg/kg i.m.) plus midazolam (1–2 mg/kg i.m.) or diazepam (chelonians: 0.2–1 mg/kg i.m.; snakes: 0.2–0.8 mg/kg i.m.).
- Alfaxalone (15 mg/kg i.m. or, preferably, 5–9 mg/kg i.v.) provides deep sedation/anaesthesia in chelonians (preferable to perform intermittent positive pressure ventilation with 100% oxygen after administration to prevent hypoxia). Green iguanas: 10 mg/kg i.m. (light sedation) up to 30 mg/kg i.m. for surgical anaesthesia.
- Midazolam (0.5–2 mg/kg i.m.) provides sedation for imaging and non-noxious procedures.
- Propofol (5–10 mg/kg i.v. or intraosseously) will give 10–15 minutes of sedation/light anaesthesia (preferable to perform intermittent positive pressure ventilation with 100% oxygen after administration to prevent hypoxia). May also be given intracoelomically to small chelonians.

Anti-infectives *continued*

Cardiovascular

Alpha-blockers
Phenoxybenzamine 311
Beta-blockers
Atenolol 31
Carvedilol 60
Propranolol 340
Antiarrhythmics
Amiodarone 17
Digoxin 116
Esmolol 145
Mexiletine 258
Quinidine 348
Sotalol 369
Verapamil 404
Antihypertensives
Amlodipine 20
Antiplatelet aggregators
Aspirin 29
Clopidogrel 88
Diuretics
Amiloride 14

Furosemide 170
Hydrochlorothiazide 188
Spironolactone 371
Torasemide 391
Positive inotropes
Dobutamine 124
Dopamine 128
Pimobendan 319
Vasoconstrictors
Ephedrine 141
Vasodilators
Benazepril 38
Diltiazem 117
Enalapril 137
Glyceryl trinitrate 179
Hydralazine 187
Imidapril 196
Prazosin 331
Ramipril 349
Sildenafil 362
Telmisartan 377

Dermatological

Cleansers and sebolytics
Benzoyl peroxide 39
Chlorhexidine 72
Antifungals
Terbinafine 379
Antihistamines
Cetirizine 67
Chlorphenamine 73
Clemastine 82
Cyproheptadine 95
Diphenhydramine 122
Hydroxyzine 191
Loratadine 228
Promethazine 337
Anti-inflammatory topical steroids
Hydrocortisone aceponate 190
Anti-inflammatory – others
Nicotinamide 280
Oclacitinib 286
Sodium cromoglicate 368

Ecto- and endoparasiticides
Indoxacarb 200
Ivermectin 208
Milbemycin 262
Selamectin 357
Spinosad 370
Ectoparasiticides
Amitraz 19
Deltamethrin 103
Fipronil 159
Imidacloprid 195
Lufenuron 229
Metaflumizone 247
Methoprene 252
Moxidectin 271
Nitenpyram 281
Pyriprole 347
Tiabendazole 385
Hormonal replacements
See Endocrine
Immunosuppressives
Ciclosporin 74
Vasodilator
Pentoxifylline 307

Endocrine

Gastrointestinal and hepatic

Gastrointestinal and hepatic *continued*

Anti-inflammatory drugs
Budesonide 45
Olsalazine 287
Sulfasalazine 375
Chelating agents
Penicillamine 301
Anti-oxidants
S-Adenosylmethionine 355
Silybin 363
Choleretics
Ursodeoxycholic acid 402
Digestive enzymes
Pancreatic enzyme
supplements 295
Emetics
Apomorphine 27

Laxatives
Bisacodyl 42
Bowel cleansing solutions 43
Dantron 100
Docusate sodium 125
Lactulose 215
Paraffin 299
Phosphate enema 317
Sodium citrate 367
Ulcer-healing drugs
Aluminium antacids 12
Cimetidine 76
Famotidine 150
Misoprostol 265
Nizatidine 284
Omeprazole 288
Ranitidine 350
Sucralfate 373

Genito-urinary tract

Antifibrotic
Colchicine 92
Urinary acidifiers
Methionine 251
Urinary alkalinizers
Potassium citrate 326
Urinary antiseptics
Methenamine 249
Urethral relaxants
Diazepam 109
Phenoxybenzamine 311
Urinary incontinence
Ephedrine 141
Estriol 146

Phenylpropanolamine 314
Propantheline 337
Urinary retention
Bethanecol 41
Urolithiasis
Allopurinol 10
Penicillamine 301
Potassium citrate 326
Walpole's solution 364
Phosphate binders
Calcium acetate 53
Chitosan 68
Lanthanum carbonate
octahydrate 216
Sevelamer hydrochloride 360

Metabolic

Antidotes
Acetylcysteine 3
Antivenom (European Adder)
26
Charcoal 68
Colestyramine 92
Deferoxamine 102
Dimercaprol 119
Edetate calcium disodium 135

Ethanol 147
Fomepizole 169
Methylthioninium chloride 255
Penicillamine 301
Pralidoxime 329
Protamine sulphate 342
Anti-hypercalcaemics
Clodronate 84
Pamidronate 295

Ophthalmic *continued*

Respiratory system

APPENDIX I: GENERAL INFORMATION

APPENDIX II: PROTOCOLS

INDEX: THERAPEUTIC CLASS

INDEX: GENERIC AND TRADE NAMES

Generic names are in plain type. Trade names are in italics; asterisks denote products not authorized for use in veterinary species.

CIL Client Information Leaflets available for BSAVA members to download from the BSAVA website (**www.bsava.com**)